Infection Control

Editors

JASON W. STULL
J. SCOTT WEESE

VETERINARY CLINICS
OF NORTH AMERICA:
SMALL ANIMAL PRACTICE

www.vetsmall.theclinics.com

March 2015 • Volume 45 • Number 2

ELSEVIER
1600 John F. Kennedy Boulevard • Suite 1800 • Philadelphia, Pennsylvania, 19103-2899
http://www.vetsmall.theclinics.com

VETERINARY CLINICS OF NORTH AMERICA: SMALL ANIMAL PRACTICE Volume 45, Number 2 March 2015 ISSN 0195-5616, ISBN-13: 978-0-323-35669-5

Editor: Patrick Manley
Developmental Editor: Meredith Clinton

Veterinary Clinics of North America: Small Animal Practice (ISSN 0195-5616) is published bimonthly by Elsevier Inc., 360 Park Avenue South, New York, NY 10010-1710. Months of issue are January, March, May, July, September, and November. Business and Editorial Offices: 1600 John F. Kennedy Blvd., Ste. 1800, Philadelphia, PA 19103-2899. Customer Service Office: 3251 Riverport Lane, Maryland Heights, MO 63043. Periodicals postage paid at New York, NY and additional mailing offices. Subscription prices are $310.00 per year (domestic individuals), $500.00 per year (domestic institutions), $150.00 per year (domestic students/residents), $410.00 per year (Canadian individuals), $621.00 per year (Canadian institutions), $455.00 per year (international individuals), $621.00 per year (international institutions), and $220.00 per year (international and Canadian students/residents). To receive student/resident rate, orders must be accompanied by name of affiliated institution, date of term, and the *signature* of program/residency coordinator on institution letterhead. Orders will be billed at individual rate until proof of status is received. Foreign air speed delivery is included in all *Clinics* subscription prices. All prices are subject to change without notice. **POSTMASTER:** Send address changes to *Veterinary Clinics of North America: Small Animal Practice*, Elsevier Health Sciences Division, Subscription Customer Service, 3251 Riverport Lane, Maryland Heights, MO 63043. Customer Service (orders, claims, online, change of address): Elsevier Periodicals Customer Service, Elsevier Health Sciences Division Subscription Customer Service 3251 Riverport Lane Maryland Heights, MO 63043. Tel: 1-800-654-2452 (U.S. and Canada); 314-447-8871 (outside U.S. and Canada). Fax: 314-447-8029. E-mail: journalscustomerservice-usa@elsevier.com (for print support); journalsonlinesupport-usa@elsevier.com (for online support).

Reprints. For copies of 100 or more of articles in this publication, please contact the Commercial Reprints Department, Elsevier Inc., 360 Park Avenue South, New York, NY 10010-1710. Tel.: 212-633-3874; Fax: 212-633-3820; E-mail: reprints@elsevier.com.

Veterinary Clinics of North America: Small Animal Practice is also published in Japanese by Inter Zoo Publishing Co., Ltd., Aoyama Crystal-Bldg 5F, 3-5-12 Kitaaoyama, Minato-ku, Tokyo 107-0061, Japan.

Veterinary Clinics of North America: Small Animal Practice is covered in *Current Contents/Agriculture, Biology and Environmental Sciences, Science Citation Index, ASCA, MEDLINE/PubMed (Index Medicus), Excerpta Medica, and BIOSIS.*

Contributors

EDITORS

JASON W. STULL, VMD, MPVM, PhD
Diplomate, American College of Veterinary Preventive Medicine; Assistant Professor, Department of Veterinary Preventive Medicine, College of Veterinary Medicine, The Ohio State University, Columbus, Ohio

J. SCOTT WEESE, DVM, DVSc
Diplomate, American College of Veterinary Internal Medicine; Professor, Department of Pathobiology, Ontario Veterinary College, University of Guelph, Guelph, Ontario, Canada

AUTHORS

HELEN ACETO, PhD, VMD
Associate Professor of Epidemiology; Director of Biosecurity; Department of Clinical Studies, New Bolton Center, University of Pennsylvania, Kennett Square, Pennsylvania

MAUREEN E.C. ANDERSON, DVM, DVSc, PhD
Diplomate, American College of Veterinary Internal Medicine; Lead Veterinarian - Animal Health and Welfare Branch, Ontario Ministry of Agriculture, Food and Rural Affairs (OMAFRA), Guelph, Ontario, Canada

SARAH BABCOCK, DVM, JD
Animal and Veterinary Legal Services, PLLC, Harrison Township, Michigan

BRANDY A. BURGESS, DVM, MSc, PhD
Diplomate, American College of Veterinary Internal Medicine; Diplomate, American College of Veterinary Preventive Medicine; Assistant Professor, Department of Population Health Sciences, Virginia Maryland Regional College of Veterinary Medicine, Virginia Tech, Blacksburg, Virginia

JOHN D. GIBBINS, DVM, MPH
Diplomate, American College of Veterinary Preventive Medicine; Veterinary Epidemiologist; Division of Surveillance, Hazard Evaluations, and Field Studies, National Institute for Occupational Safety and Health, Centers for Disease Control and Prevention, Cincinnati, Ohio

LUCA GUARDABASSI, DVM, PhD
Professor (PMSO), Diplomate, European College of Veterinary Public Health; Department of Veterinary Disease Biology, Faculty of Health and Medical Sciences, University of Copenhagen, Copenhagen, Denmark

LYNN GUPTILL, DVM, PhD
Diplomate, American College of Veterinary Internal Medicine (Small Animal Internal Medicine); Associate Professor, Small Animal Internal Medicine, Department of Veterinary Clinical Sciences, Purdue University, West Lafayette, Indiana

KATHLEEN MACMAHON, DVM, MS
Senior Health Scientist, Education and Information Division, National Institute for Occupational Safety and Health, Centers for Disease Control and Prevention, Cincinnati, Ohio

ANTOINETTE E. MARSH, MS, PhD, JD
Veterinary Preventive Medicine, College of Veterinary Medicine, The Ohio State University, Columbus, Ohio

PAUL S. MORLEY, DVM, PhD
Diplomate, American College of Veterinary Internal Medicine; Professor, Department of Clinical Sciences, James L. Voss Veterinary Teaching Hospital, Colorado State University, Fort Collins, Colorado

JOHN F. PRESCOTT, VetMB, DVM, PhD
Professor, Department of Pathobiology, Ontario Veterinary College, University of Guelph, Guelph, Ontario, Canada

AMEET SINGH, DVM, DVSc
Diplomate, American College of Veterinary Surgeons; Assistant Professor of Small Animal Surgery; Department of Clinical Studies, Ontario Veterinary College, University of Guelph, Guelph, Ontario, Canada

KURT B. STEVENSON, MD, MPH
Professor of Medicine and Epidemiology; Department of Internal Medicine, Wexner Medical Center, Colleges of Medicine and Public Health, The Ohio State University, Columbus, Ohio

JASON W. STULL, VMD, MPVM, PhD
Diplomate, American College of Veterinary Preventive Medicine; Assistant Professor, Department of Veterinary Preventive Medicine, College of Veterinary Medicine, The Ohio State University, Columbus, Ohio

MICHELLE TRAVERSE, BS, CVT
Infection Control Coordinator, Department of Clinical Studies, Matthew J. Ryan Veterinary Hospital, University of Pennsylvania, Philadelphia, Pennsylvania

DENIS VERWILGHEN, DVM, MSc, PhD, DES
Diplomate, European College of Veterinary Surgeons; Associate Professor in Large Animal Surgery, Department of Large Animal Sciences, University of Copenhagen, Taatsrup, Denmark

J. SCOTT WEESE, DVM, DVSc
Diplomate, American College of Veterinary Internal Medicine; Professor, Department of Pathobiology, Ontario Veterinary College, University of Guelph, Guelph, Ontario, Canada

Contents

VETERINARY CLINICS OF NORTH AMERICA: SMALL ANIMAL PRACTICE

FORTHCOMING ISSUES

May 2015
Soft Tissue Surgery
Lisa M. Howe and Harry W. Boothe Jr, *Editors*

July 2015
Urology
Joseph W. Bartges, *Editor*

September 2015
Perioperative Care
Lori Waddell, *Editor*

RECENT ISSUES

January 2015
Rehabilitation and Physical Therapy
David Levine, Darryl L. Millis, and Denis Marcellin-Little, *Editors*

November 2014
Advances in Veterinary Neurology
Natasha J. Olby and Nicholas Jeffery, *Editors*

September 2014
Advances in Veterinary Oncology
Annette N. Smith, *Editor*

RELATED INTEREST

Veterinary Clinics of North America: Equine Practice
December 2014, Volume 30, Issue 3
New Perspectives in Infectious Diseases
Robert H. Mealey, *Editor*

Preface

Infection Control in Veterinary Small Animal Practice

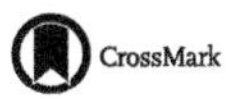

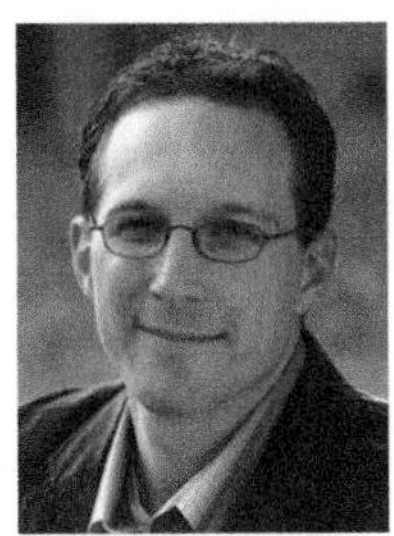

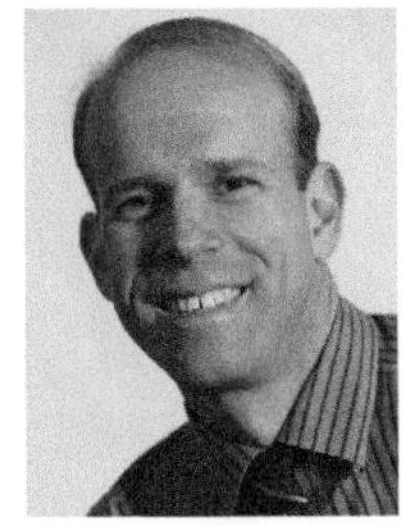

Jason W. Stull, VMD, MPVM, PhD, DACVPM J. Scott Weese, DVM, DVSc, DACVIM
Editors

This issue of *Veterinary Clinics of North America: Small Animal Practice* addresses the topic of "Infection Control in Veterinary Small Animal Practice." Infection control has been acknowledged as a cornerstone of human medicine for decades. Attention to, and progress in, this area is regarded as one of the most important advances in human health care. Despite this recognized prominence, veterinary medicine has been slow to adopt infection control principles. This is particularly evident in small animal practice. Although there are likely a number of reasons for this deficiency (eg, lack of perceived importance, minimal local or national regulations), perhaps one of the greatest obstacles has been limited published practical guidance and recommendations for all scopes of practice, from the smaller single veterinarian private practice to larger referral or teaching hospitals. In this issue, we have carefully selected topics and authors to address these information gaps, ensuring practical guidance is finally available for all small animal veterinary clinic types and sizes.

The topics were carefully selected to cover (in our minds) all key areas of infection control pertinent to small animal practice. The first articles in this issue introduce the topic, providing evidence for the utility of infection control in our practices and directing practitioners and staff toward key areas to address identifying and preventing the major types of hospital-associated infections in veterinary patients: urinary tract infections, pneumonia, bloodstream infections, surgical site infections, and infectious diarrhea. The next articles target crucial strategies aimed at reducing hospital environmental, equipment, and staff contamination by pathogens and antimicrobial stewardship approaches to reduce the occurrence of multi-drug-resistant organisms. The final articles address veterinary workplace safety, including zoonotic disease risk for immunocompromised clients and staff, as well as legal implications for such hazards. Together, these eleven articles provide the key elements and practical examples for the development of a clinic-specific infection control plan, allowing for a safer environment for patients, staff, and clients.

Vet Clin Small Anim 45 (2015) xi–xii
http://dx.doi.org/10.1016/j.cvsm.2014.12.001 vetsmall.theclinics.com
0195-5616/15/$ – see front matter

We would like to thank the staff at *Veterinary Clinics of North America: Small Animal Practice* for inviting us to edit this issue, ensuring this critical information is available to all. Many thanks to the authors, who generously took time out of their busy lives to provide the material and insight to make this an important and long-lasting contribution to the field. Finally, we are grateful to our families, colleagues, and students, who offer us support, inspire us to continuously improve, and help us to remember to enjoy the journey.

Jason W. Stull, VMD, MPVM, PhD, DACVPM
Department of Veterinary Preventive Medicine
College of Veterinary Medicine
The Ohio State University
Columbus, OH 43210, USA

J. Scott Weese, DVM, DVSc, DACVIM
Department of Pathobiology
Ontario Veterinary College
University of Guelph
Guelph, Ontario N1G 2W1, Canada

E-mail addresses:
Stull.82@osu.edu (J.W. Stull)
jsweese@uoguelph.ca (J.S. Weese)

Hospital-Associated Infections in Small Animal Practice

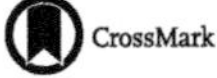

Jason W. Stull, VMD, MPVM, PhD[a,*], J. Scott Weese, DVM, DVSc[b]

KEYWORDS

• Nosocomial • Infection • Hospital • Veterinary • Control • Hospital-associated

KEY POINTS

- Hospital-associated infections (HAIs) occur in veterinary medicine, and their frequency is likely to increase.
- Urinary tract infections, pneumonia, bloodstream infections, surgical site infections, and infectious diarrhea are the HAIs most frequently identified in veterinary medicine.
- All staff members should be educated on the risks and signs associated with HAIs so that cases can be detected early and managed appropriately.
- A hospital infection-control program, consisting of an infectious disease control officer, a written protocol, and staff training, is critical to reducing HAIs and promoting patient, staff, and client health.

INTRODUCTION: NATURE OF THE PROBLEM

Hospital-associated infections (HAIs), sometimes referred to as nosocomial infections, are infections acquired by patients during hospitalization and are an inherent risk in human and veterinary medicine. In human hospitals, HAIs are a well-recognized contributor to illness and death, with an estimated 5% of patients developing an HAI and tens of thousands dying each year from HAIs.[1] It is estimated that, in the United States, human HAIs account for \$28 to \$45 billion in direct costs annually, not including the substantial indirect costs (eg, community care costs, lost wages, and productivity by the patient and caregivers).[2]

Veterinary data for this field are limited. In some aspects, risks may be lower because of the generally lower proportion of veterinary patients that have long hospital stays, are profoundly immunocompromised, and undergo highly invasive procedures

The authors have nothing to disclose.

[a] Department of Veterinary Preventive Medicine, The Ohio State University, College of Veterinary Medicine, 1920 Coffey Road, Columbus, OH 43210, USA; [b] Department of Pathobiology, Ontario Veterinary College, University of Guelph, 50 Stone Road East, Guelph, Ontario N1G2W1, Canada

* Corresponding author.

E-mail address: Stull.82@osu.edu

http://dx.doi.org/10.1016/j.cvsm.2014.11.009 **vetsmall.theclinics.com** compared with people. However, this may be countered with greater patient hygiene challenges, greater difficulty with patient compliance (eg, licking wounds), and a lesser "culture" of infection control. Although current data are limited for the veterinary field, similar (or even higher) HAI rates have been reported compared with human studies, such as HAIs in 16% of intensive care unit patients in one study.[3] During a 5-year period, 82% of veterinary teaching hospitals in North America and Europe reported at least one HAI outbreak and 45% reported multiple outbreaks. Many of these outbreaks required restricted patient admissions (58%) or closure of the hospital or section (32%).[4] Therefore, although HAIs are poorly quantified in veterinary medicine, they are undeniably a concern.

There are many potential adverse events from HAIs in veterinary patients. Animals suffering from HAIs may have an increased hospital stay (with accompanying increased cost to the client or clinic). These patients may also suffer permanent health consequences, or HAIs may result in death of the pet. Multidrug-resistant organisms (MDROs) are often involved in HAIs, complicating treatment and resulting in poor patient outcomes and extensive outbreaks. Furthermore, some veterinary hospital-associated (HA) pathogens (eg, methicillin-resistant *Staphylococcus aureus* [MRSA], *Salmonella*) can be transmitted to staff or pet owners, resulting in human illness. Additionally, as veterinary medicine advances, there may be parallel *increases* in HAI risk through the use of more invasive procedures, more use of invasive devices (eg, urinary catheters, intravenous catheters), more immunosuppressant therapies, and a greater intensity of critical care management. Patients that might not have survived their underlying disease in the past may now be alive, but highly susceptible to infection.

Perhaps most important to this topic is the assumption in human medicine that 10% to 70% of all HAIs are preventable through the use of practical infection-control measures.[5] Large economic benefits are estimated to occur with the implementation of infection-control interventions ($6-$32 billion cost savings in the United States alone).[2] The proportion of HAIs that are preventable in veterinary medicine is unknown, but is likely to be similar, and even a 10% reduction in infections could constitute a major impact on patient health, owner cost, and owner and clinician satisfaction. The routine use of simple infection prevention practices can likely dramatically reduce HAIs.

APPROACH/GOALS

Infection control is the term best suited to the goal in small animal veterinary medicine of preventing (or, more practically speaking, limiting) the introduction and/or spread of pathogens with a group of patients and caregivers. Central to this goal is the establishment and refinement of an infection-control program at each animal hospital. Every hospital's infection-control program will be different, reflecting the unique pathogen risks, facility and personnel characteristics, animal populations served, and level of risk tolerance of the practice. However, at a minimum, each practice's program should include the following:

- An infectious disease control officer (otherwise known as an infection-control practitioner);
- A written infection-control protocol (plan);
- Regular training of staff about hospital infection-control protocols (and documentation of this training and assessment of comprehension);
- Monitoring of both disease rates and infection-control protocol compliance.

Together, the components of the program should address the HAI risks for patients and staff and recommended or required protocols to reduce these risks. The end result will be a safer working environment for staff, optimal care for all patients, and protection of public health. Although good infection-control practices are not the only feature defining excellence in patient care, it is impossible to achieve excellent patient care without them. The standard of what is "acceptable" from an infection-control standpoint is changing in veterinary medicine, and it is clear that the "bar" is being raised in terms of the expected standard of care.

EPIDEMIOLOGY

In human medicine, urinary tract infections (UTIs), pneumonia, surgical site infections (SSIs), and bloodstream infections (BSIs) account for approximately 80% of all HAIs.[6] In veterinary medicine, these sites along with gastrointestinal disease (infectious diarrhea) are likely to be the most common HAIs, although other conditions, such as upper respiratory tract infection, dermatophyte infection, iatrogenic blood-borne pathogen infection, and infections of a wide range of invasive devices can also occur. Each of these main areas is discussed later, highlighting (where available) incidence, risk factors for disease, and commonly identified pathogens. Because SSIs are being exclusively covered in a separate article in this issue, they are not discussed here.

Sites of Infections

Urinary tract infections

Catheter-associated UTIs are one of the more common HAIs in small animal veterinary medicine, although veterinary data are often limited by the failure to differentiate bacteriuria (a potentially benign condition) from UTI (disease). Studies have reported catheter-associated bacteriuria occurring in 10% to 32% of hospitalized dogs, with a subset of these exhibiting clinical signs or other evidence of infection.[7–10] The interference of normal defense mechanisms by urinary catheters, such as mucosal-secreted adhesion inhibitors, along with patient comorbid factors and some catheter handling factors, facilitate bacterial colonization of the catheter and ascension of the organism or organisms into the bladder. These pathogens may be endogenous to the patient, arising from the rectum or perineum, or directly from the hospital environment or people through contamination of the drainage system or bag. If the collection system has been contaminated, bacteria can ascend into the bladder through the catheter if there is retrograde flow of urine. Retrograde urine flow can occur if the collection system is elevated above the level of the patient; if collection lines are flushed, or if there is obstruction to flow in the collection system. In addition, biofilms (a complex structure of microorganisms and extracellular matrix) can be produced by bacteria on surfaces of urinary catheters. Biofilm formation can be associated with poor antimicrobial penetration, antimicrobial resistance, and treatment failure.[11]

Pneumonia

In human medicine, several factors, such as recumbent position, mechanical ventilation, and use of endotracheal or nasogastric tubes, are likely to increase the risk for HA pneumonia.[12,13] This topic has been minimally investigated in the veterinary field, in large part because of the limited use of mechanical ventilation. In one study, *Escherichia coli* and *Acinetobacter* spp were commonly identified in feline HA ventilator-associated pneumonia cases.[14] Although not included in the human surveillance definition, aspiration pneumonia is not uncommon in small animal medicine and can occur in patients hospitalized for a wide range of disorders as well as otherwise healthy patients undergoing sedation or anesthesia. In addition to those factors listed for human HA pneumonia, factors that increase aspiration pneumonia, such as laryngeal or esophageal disorders and decreased mentation or recumbency, likely increase HAI risk.[15–17] If these patients have been hospitalized for multiple days before aspiration, it is more likely that the oropharynx is colonized with organisms from the hospital environment or hands of staff, and the pneumonia may be more likely to involve MDROs, particularly if patients have been treated with antimicrobials.

Bloodstream infections

In the human literature, most HA BSIs are associated with intravascular devices. Duration of catheterization has been recognized as the most important risk factor for the development of catheter-related (CR) BSIs (most developing 4–5 days after placement).[18] Despite this increased risk, studies have not documented a benefit with prophylactic catheter changes (eg, every 3 days). In human medicine, the current recommendation is for catheters to be removed as soon as medically indicated, but for routine changes to be avoided. A similar approach is appropriate in veterinary medicine.

Veterinary studies have revealed that jugular and intravenous catheters are frequently contaminated with enteric or environmental pathogens.[9,19] Several factors have been positively associated with intravenous catheter contamination/colonization in dogs and cats, including receipt of dextrose infusion, longer duration of catheter placement, and patient immunosuppression (presence of immunosuppressive diseases or receipt of immunosuppressive drugs).[20] Commonly isolated organisms include staphylococci, *E coli*, *Enterobacter* spp, *Proteus* spp, and *Klebsiella* spp.[19–21] Contamination may occur from the hands of people placing or handling the catheter, the patient's own flora, or the hospital environment. However, there is little evidence indicating that contaminated but not infected catheters (ie, catheters from which bacteria can be isolated but where the catheter insertion site and vein are clinically normal) pose a risk for subsequent BSI. As a result, routine culture of catheters at time of removal or culture of catheter insertion sites is not recommended because skin bacteria are expected to be present. Veterinary outbreaks involving CR BSIs have been associated with inadequate skin preparation or contaminated materials used in skin preparation,[21,22] something that is of most concern when antiseptic solutions or wipes are prepared by refilling bottles or containers, which can become contaminated with biocide-resistant bacteria over time.

Infectious diarrhea

HA gastrointestinal infections are usually recognized when there is a noted increase (outbreak) of infectious diarrhea in hospital patients. Although identification of diarrhea is simple, determination of the cause is often difficult, even for known pathogens. In small animal veterinary facilities, salmonellosis is the most frequently reported gastrointestinal HAI[4,23]; however, it is unclear whether that is because it poses the greatest risk or (more likely) it is more readily identified and reported compared with other potential causes. In nonhospitalized small animal populations, several risk factors for *Salmonella* colonization or infection have been identified, including animal species (eg, reptiles, amphibians, young poultry, exotics), consuming a raw animal–based diet or treats (eg, raw meat/eggs, rawhides), exposure to livestock, and recently receiving a probiotic.[24,25] These factors may substantially increase the risk of shedding *Salmonella*, 14% to 69% shedding in dogs with one or more of these risk factors as compared with less than 5% typically noted in dogs without these risk factors.[25,26] However, the true scope of this issue is unclear because most outbreaks go unnoticed or testing is not performed, but, conversely, clusters of diarrhea seem to be uncommon in most facilities.

Pathogens of Concern

Pathogens involved in small animal HAIs often have one or more of the following characteristics: opportunistic pathogen in companion animals and/or humans, environmentally stable, or multidrug-resistant. Many pathogens involved in HAIs are opportunistic pathogens that can be found in healthy animals, highlighting the inability to prevent entrance of all potential pathogens into a veterinary facility. The frequency of each pathogen varies for each veterinary practice (in part influenced by antimicrobial use/pressure, geography, animal species, vaccine coverage of animals in "catchment" area, level of care provided). In addition, environmentally stable pathogens (eg, parvovirus, clostridial spores, dermatophytes) have a demonstrated clear "advantage," increasing the chance of transmission. Given the close interaction between veterinary staff and patients as well as the often poor hand hygiene practices documented in veterinary practices, human commensals with zoonotic potential are represented by HAIs in veterinary medicine. Finally, increased resistance to antimicrobials is a common feature of most nosocomial bacteria.

Several pathogens are a concern from a small animal infection-control standpoint (**Box 1**). Although a wide range of pathogens may be involved in HAIs, currently there is a strong focus on the emerging epidemic of multidrug-resistant bacteria because of dramatic increases in infections, limited antimicrobial options, and potential public health consequences. These MDROs are not inherently more virulent than antimicrobial susceptible organisms, but treatment options are limited, something that ultimately can worsen the prognosis. The US Centers for Disease Control and Prevention has recently assessed domestic antibiotic resistance threats for people based on

Box 1
Pathogens of concern in a small animal clinic

- Adenovirus (canine)
- *Bordetella bronchiseptica*
- Calicivirus (feline)
- *Chlamydophila* (feline)
- Distemper virus (canine)
- Herpes virus (feline)
- Influenza viruses (canine, novel)
- *Microsporum canis*
- Parainfluenza virus (canine)
- Parvoviruses (canine, feline)
- Respiratory coronavirus (canine)
- Multidrug-resistant organisms
  - *Acinetobacter* spp
  - *Escherichia coli*
  - *Enterococcus* spp
  - *Salmonella* spp
  - *Staphylococcus* spp
  - *Pseudomonas* spp

clinical and economic impact, incidence, transmissibility, availability of effective antimicrobials, and barriers to prevention. Several pathogens of importance relative to veterinary HAIs were included as "serious antibiotic resistance threats," namely, *Acinetobacter* spp, extended spectrum β-lactamase-producing Enterobacteriaceae (ESBLs), *Pseudomonas aeruginosa*, *Salmonella* spp, and MRSA.[27] As animals and people may share common infection sources or transmit these pathogens to each other, this concern is equally important in the veterinary field, and all of the above-named pathogens can be found in veterinary patients. Given these relatively novel threats and the often limited knowledge by veterinary personnel on this group of pathogens, the attention here is focused on MDROs as HAIs.

In human medicine, HAIs are often captured through voluntary or mandatory hospital reporting. As such, the occurrence (and trends) of HAIs are fairly well-established. In the United States, recent data indicate bacteria are responsible for 90% of HAIs, with commonly identified groups including *Staphylococcus aureus*, *Enterococcus* spp, *E coli*, coagulase-negative staphylococci (CoNS), *Klebsiella* spp, *P aeruginosa*, *Enterobacter* spp, and *Acinetobacter baumannii*.[28]

Despite the importance of this field, current knowledge of many aspects of the epidemiology of important MDROs and pathogens responsible for HAIs in veterinary medicine is unclear (eg, prevalence, risk factors, and transmission dynamics). Unfortunately, companion animal veterinary medicine has been slow to implement surveillance systems; however, this is changing. Currently, most data come from limited retrospective studies of clinical isolates, likely resulting in geographic and culture-based bias, potentially misrepresenting the frequency of these pathogens and potentially overestimating the prevalence of antimicrobial resistance if culture submissions are biased toward infections that failed to respond to empirical therapy. Regardless, based on the reported veterinary HA outbreaks or supposition from the human literature, several important MDROs responsible for HAIs are identifiable: *S aureus*, *Staphylococcus pseudintermedius*, Enterococci, *Salmonella* spp, *Acinetobacter* spp, *E coli*, and other Enterobacteriaceae, and *Pseudomonas* spp. The specific resistance profiles and treatment options for common multidrug-resistant (MDR) pathogens have recently been summarized.[29] The reader is directed to the article elsewhere in this issue of *Veterinary Clinics of North America: Small Animal Practice* by Guardabassi and Prescott entitled, "Antimicrobial stewardship in small animal veterinary practice: from theory to practice," which expands on the topic of MDROs in HAIs and antimicrobial stewardship.

Current Examples of Multidrug-Resistant Organisms Involved in Hospital-Associated Infections

Staphylococcus

S pseudintermedius and to a lesser extent *S aureus* are common causes of veterinary HAIs.[30] Both are frequently carried on the skin and mucosal surfaces of dogs and people (respectively), creating the potential for both endogenous infection (infection caused by bacteria the animal was harboring at the time of hospital admission) and acquisition of the pathogen during hospitalization directly or indirectly from other patients, the environment, or human caregivers. The emergence of methicillin resistance in these species (methicillin-resistant *S pseudintermedius* [MRSP] and MRSA) has had important implications for HAI prevention and control. Methicillin resistance is mediated by the *mecA* gene, which results in resistance to β-lactam antimicrobials (penicillins, cephalosporins, and carbapenems). In addition, resistance to other classes of antimicrobials is frequently observed: lincosamides (clindamycin), fluoroquinolones, macrolides (erythromycin), tetracyclines, trimethoprim-sulfonamides.[29,31,32]

MRSA is an important pathogen in human HAIs, being a common cause of SSIs and various other types of infections.[33] To a lesser extent, MRSA has also been noted in veterinary HAIs.[34] Risk factors for veterinary MRSA HAIs have not been well studied, but prior antimicrobial use, prior hospitalization, ownership by veterinary or human health care workers/students, and longer hospitalization (>3 days) have been associated with MRSA colonization or infection in dogs.[35–38] Furthermore, the use of fluoroquinolones and cephalosporins has been linked to the emergence of MRSA in people and may play a role in veterinary species.[39] It is important to note that an abnormally high proportion of veterinarians are colonized with MRSA as compared with the general public.[40] As such, they may serve as a source for HAIs in their patients if infection-control practices (notably hand hygiene) are substandard. This also likely indicates deficiencies in standard infection control and hygiene practices that allow for transmission of MRSA between veterinary personnel and animals.

MRSP has rapidly spread in canine populations, often with high levels of antimicrobial resistance,[41] something that is of tremendous concern because *S pseudintermedius* is the leading opportunistic pathogen in dogs (and, to a lesser degree, cats). It is the most common cause of SSIs in some regions,[42] and treatment may be complicated because of the high level of resistance. In one study, more than 90% of MRSP isolates were also resistant to 4 additional antimicrobial classes.[43] Recent prior hospitalization and β-lactam antimicrobial administration have been associated with MRSP infections,[44] suggesting hospital-associated transmission may be a factor in MRSP disease.

The topic of CoNS deserves mention. Veterinary diagnostic laboratories often consider these species as a group and speciation is rarely performed. CoNS are frequently identified as commensals in small animal species, with high methicillin resistance in healthy animals. With the exception of highlycompromised individuals, it has been generally assumed that CoNS, even those that are multidrug resistant, are of limited clinical concern. That assumption has been challenged to some degree and some CoNS species may be more clinically relevant than others; however, this group remains a less common cause for concern compared with *S pseudintermedius* and *S aureus*. However, their commonness as skin or mucous membrane commensals can complicate interpretation of culture results because differentiating infection from contamination may be challenging.

Escherichia coli

E coli is a frequent component of the commensal gastrointestinal microbiota and is an important pathogen, particularly in UTIs. MDR*E coli* is frequently shed in the feces of both community and hospitalized small animals.[45–47] Multiple factors have been associated with dogs shedding or acquiring MDR *E coli* during hospitalization, including duration of hospitalization (>3 days) and treatment with antimicrobials shortly before or while hospitalized (cephalosporins, metronidazole).[38,48]

Antimicrobial resistance is an important problem with *E coli* and other Enterobacteriaceae (eg, *Enterobacter*). Although β-lactamase-producing isolates have been common for some time, there has been a recent emergence of ESBLs producers, which provide resistance to a broad range of β-lactam antimicrobials, including third-generation cephalosporins. In addition, ESBLs are conferred resistance to other antimicrobial classes through genetic linkage with resistance mechanisms.[49] Extended spectrum β-lactamase-producing *E coli* has been identified as the source of veterinary HAIs, occurring as SSIs and catheter-associated UTIs, with observed hospital contamination.[50,51] Other genera in the Enterobacteriaceae family (ie, *Klebsiella*,

Enterobacter) are considered to be important in human HAIs; however, less is known of their involvement in veterinary infections.

One of the most important drug classes for treatment of ESBL-producing bacteria is carbapenems (eg, meropenem). Unfortunately, carbapenemase-producing Enterobacteriaceae (or carbapenem-resistant Enterobacteriaceae; CRE) (including *E coli*) have emerged as a significant problem in human health care. Additional resistance mechanisms are often present, rendering isolates virtually pan-resistant, and ability for CREs to spread rapidly in health care settings with extension into the community.[52] High mortality (>40%) has been documented for invasive human CRE infections.[53] Carbapenemase-producing *E coli* have recently been identified in small animals, with suggested nosocomial transmission.[54] Nosocomial transmission currently seems to be a rare, albeit concerning, occurrence, and one that is likely to increase as CREs increase in prevalence in the human population, with subsequent exposure of pets.

Enterococci

Enterococci are often found in the gastrointestinal tract of animals and humans. Two species, *Enterococcus faecium* and *Enterococcus faecalis*, are most often involved in disease, including HAIs, although enterococci tend to be of limited virulence and typically cause infections in compromised hosts. Enterococci are inherently resistant to several antimicrobial classes, including cephalosporins, some penicillins, fluoroquinolones, clindamycin, and trimethoprim.[55] They may also acquire resistance to various other antimicrobial classes and, although they are typically of limited virulence, they may be difficult to eliminate in cases when disease develops.

Vancomycin-resistant enterococci (VRE) are an increasing concern in human medicine, with vancomycin resistance noted in up to 83% of *E faecium* involved in HAIs.[28] To date, VRE appears to be rare in companion animals.[56] However, other MDR enterococci are regularly recognized in small animals and have been identified in HAIs.[30,57,58] Enterococci are often identified as UTIs (including catheter-associated); however, infections at other anatomic sites occur (eg, SSIs, BSIs, pneumonia). The high degree of antimicrobial resistance, ability to propagate for extended periods in small animal hosts as a commensal, and environmental persistence make enterococci particularly challenging when involved in HAIs.

It is important to note that isolation of *Enterococcus* species (regardless of antimicrobial resistance) does not always indicate treatment is indicated. Without clinical signs in an otherwise immune-competent animal, it may be warranted to withhold treatment and monitor the patient. When isolated in a patient with clinical signs (notably infections of the urinary tract, wound, or body cavity), treatment should often be directed at the organism or organisms also isolated that are thought to be primarily responsible for clinical disease.[29] Often, that involves ignoring the *Enterococcus* and targeting therapy toward another, more convincing, pathogen, such as *E coli*.

Salmonella spp

Salmonella is most frequently a concern in equine facilities, but has been identified as a source of sporadic illness and hospital-associated outbreaks in small animal hospitals.[23,59] An important concern with *Salmonella* HAIs is the occurrence of zoonotic transmission with accompanying human infections.[23,59] Because most infections in dogs and cats are subclinical, there is a high risk for inadvertent hospital-wide environmental contamination and nosocomial transmission. Reported factors leading to an increased risk of *Salmonella* shedding in small animals include consumption of raw meat diets, exposure to livestock, and receiving a probiotic in the previous 30 days.[25,60] As with *E coli*, ESBL-producing strains are a concern for antimicrobial resistance and have been identified in small animals.[61] Given its environmental stability, potential shedding by healthy animals, and significant zoonotic health hazard to clinic staff and clients, *Salmonella* needs to be considered an important companion animal nosocomial pathogen.

Acinetobacter spp

Acinetobacter is well-recognized as an important HA pathogen in human medicine, in part because of recently recognized high levels of antimicrobial resistance in *A baumannii*. More than 60% of *A baumannii* human isolates involved in HAIs were MDR in one study.[28] Given its role as an opportunistic pathogen in small animals, ability to persist in the environment for extended periods, and documented outbreaks in veterinary facilities, it is also a concern for veterinary medicine.[30,62,63] Documented HAIs involving *A baumannii* include intravenous and urinary catheters, surgical drain infections, SSIs, pneumonia, and BSIs.[62]

Pseudomonas spp

Multidrug resistance is frequently encountered with *Pseudomonas* spp. This along with their noted persistence in the hospital environment makes *Pseudomonas* spp a concern for HAIs. In humans, most infections are HA and occur in immunocompromised hosts.[64] In companion animal species, *Pseudomonas* spp infections often involve the skin, urinary system, and ears,[65–67] along with SSIs and invasive device infections.[68,69] Biofilm formation by *Pseudomonas* spp can further complicate treatment. Identification of within hospital clusters of *Pseudomonas* infections should prompt investigation of potentially contaminated environmental, equipment (eg, endoscope), or consumable (eg, catheter preparation supplies) sources.

CHALLENGES/RISKS

The admission of sick animals occurs daily in most if not all small animal veterinary facilities. Furthermore, every animal admitted to the veterinary clinic, healthy or not, can reasonably be assumed to be shedding multiple microorganisms that could cause infection in humans or animals, given the opportunity. As such, there is always a risk for the introduction and spread of HAIs and for exposure to zoonotic pathogens. The level of risk will be determined, in part, by the population of animals served (eg, young, elderly, immunocompromised), pathogens circulating in the community animals, proportion of patients for which protective or increased-risk practices are taken by their owners (eg, vaccination, husbandry practices to reduce pathogen acquisition), intensity of care typically provided for patients, and clinic infection-control practices and adherence to these practices by staff and clients. Veterinary clinic staff will not be able to alter many of these risks; however, infection-control practices is an area that with some planning and dedicated time, can be relatively easy to address.

PREVENTION

Although complete prevention of HAIs is the goal, given the nature of patient care, bacterial adaptation, and complexity of many pathogens (subclinical shedding, insensitive diagnostic tests), it is inevitable they will continue to occur. Methods to reduce the risk of HAIs are paramount. In general, methods to reduce HAIs can be divided into the following main categories:

- Hand hygiene and use of personal protective equipment (PPE; ie, clothing and/or gloves to reduce contamination of staff, patients, and the environment);
- Cleaning and disinfection (environmental surfaces and patient equipment);

- Patient management (eg, cohorting patients based on risk, isolating high-risk patients, discontinuing the use of higher risk devices when indicated);
- Surveillance (identification of infected or colonized patients, HAIs, and source/risk factors);
- Antimicrobial stewardship (prudent antimicrobial use);
- Education and training (clients, staff).

These methods will not only reduce overt problems such as hospital-associated outbreaks but also reduce the likelihood of patient colonization with a HA pathogen, which can become part of the patient's resident microbiota, potentially increasing disease risk at a later date and posing a risk to other animals and humans. Each of these areas should be addressed in a hospital's infection-control manual. Several "model" plans are widely available to use as a starting point for developing an individualized hospital plan; infection-control officers are encouraged to review these resources.[70,71] Individual articles in this issue of *Veterinary Clinics of North America: Small Animal Practice* are devoted to each of these areas, so they are only briefly discussed here. Unfortunately, studies on the area indicate only a minority of small animal veterinary hospitals have written infection-control plans (0%–31%).[72,73] Given the relative ease of putting together an infection-control plan and potential health, legal, and financial benefits of doing so, every clinic should invest the time and effort to make this a priority.

Hand Hygiene and Personal Protective Equipment

Hand hygiene (washing hands with soap and water or using an alcohol-based hand rub) and use of PPE, such as nonsterile gloves and gowns, are simple techniques that can reduce the risk of HAIs. Effective use of hand hygiene and appropriate PPE use reduces the risk of contamination of personal clothing, reduces exposure of skin and mucous membranes of veterinary staff to pathogens, and reduces transmission of pathogens between patients by veterinary personnel. Unfortunately, several studies indicate that veterinarians and staff do a poor job at performing hand hygiene between patients (~20%) or using PPE when indicated (6%–37% depending on the situation).[72,74]

Cleaning and Disinfection

Recent evidence suggests environmental contamination in human hospitals increases the risk for HAIs,[75] whereas interventions that reduce environmental contamination have assisted with cessation of HA outbreaks or reduction of HAIs.[76,77] The same connection is assumed to occur in veterinary medicine. Effective cleaning and disinfection of hospital equipment and environmental surfaces play an important role in reducing HAIs. In order for a disinfectant to work properly, the surface or item must first be clean (free of visible organic material) and the product must be applied at the manufacturer's suggested dilution and contact time (amount of time the disinfectant is in contact with the item before being removed). Disinfectants should be selected based on several criteria, including the product's spectrum of activity, susceptibility to inactivation by organic matter, and potential pathogens in the environment.

Patient Management

Given the close contact between veterinary patients and their hospital housing, environmental contamination is inevitable. Furthermore, staff caring for these patients is at increased risk for spreading the pathogen through contact with the patient or its environment. To protect other patients and clinic staff, special attention to patient housing is important in managing infectious patients. Isolation procedures, use of dedicated medical equipment, and patient cohorting are important stopgaps in the transmission of HAIs for animals suspected to be infectious. In addition, specific patient care procedures may be helpful in reducing HAIs associated with catheters, aspiration pneumonia, BSIs, infectious diarrhea, and SSIs.

Resident small animals are sometimes kept at veterinary facilities as blood donors, companionship for staff, or other reasons. Because these animals may harbor MDR pathogens and be sources or propagation of hospital contamination or outbreaks, special attention should be devoted to hospital policies for these animals regarding staff-animal contact and restricted movement (not permitting direct contact with patients or patient areas, including areas for exercise and elimination).[78,79]

Surveillance

The early identification of HAIs is critical for effective infection control. Identification of "abnormal" (increases in disease incidence or patterns) depends on a reasonable understanding of "normal." Understanding of endemic rates can be useful to allow for comparison with other facilities, to establish benchmarks for ongoing surveillance, to serve as a baseline for interventions, to allow for more accurate counseling of clients about risks (eg, SSI rates), and to provide a greater overall awareness of the importance of HAIs and corresponding control measures. It is not unusual for HAI outbreaks to "smolder" below the radar of veterinary staff for extended periods because of the lack of centralized data reporting or communication, resulting in substantial environmental contamination, patient morbidity (and potentially mortality), and even increased zoonotic disease risk for staff and clients. Key elements of early HAI identification include (1) a surveillance program tailored to the risks and needs of the veterinary practice and (2) routine use of diagnostic culture and susceptibility data to establish practice-specific baseline levels of pathogen prevalence and antimicrobial resistance and detect changes from this baseline.

Antimicrobial Stewardship

Careful selection and appropriate use of antimicrobials are important steps in combating patient MDRO development and subsequent contamination and transmission in the hospital environment. Antimicrobials should be avoided when a bacterial infection has not been confirmed. Antimicrobials used in the initial treatment of an infection should be selected based on the effectiveness against the most likely organisms causing the infection (something that can be facilitated by having good passive surveillance data) as well as patient (eg, renal function, comorbidities) or drug (eg, penetration, route of administration, frequency of administration) factors. Whenever possible, a culture should be submitted to determine the true susceptibility pattern of the bacteria involved. Local therapy can be an important option that is often overlooked.

Education and Training

During their careers, approximately two-thirds of veterinarians report a major animal-related injury resulting in lost work or hospitalization.[71,80] Animal bite injuries and infections are a large contributor to this hazard, but zoonotic infections (eg, MRSA, dermatophytosis [ringworm], salmonellosis) are also frequently reported.[23,81] Educating staff and clients on zoonotic disease risks and enforcing in-hospital infection-control protocols to reduce these risks will be beneficial to the health of people and patients.

All veterinary personnel and visitors should be familiar with the hospital's infection-control plan and policies.

The Infection-Control Officer/Infection-Control Practitioner

The infection-control officer is integral to the successful development, maintenance, and enforcement of an infection-control plan. In the human health care field, infection-control practitioners are formally trained and certified, with the infection-control program typically overseen by a physician with specialized training in infectious diseases, infection control, and/or microbiology. In veterinary medicine, this type of approach is only practiced in large facilities (mainly teaching hospitals), yet the basic concepts remain the same for veterinary facilities of any type and size. A functional infection-control program can be directed by a single infection-control practitioner in a veterinary hospital, with minimal time requirements. This individual can be a technician or veterinarian who has an interest in infection control. The skills required (eg, general understanding of infection-control concepts) can be obtained on the job and need not be a prerequisite for the position, and the limited time requirement under normal circumstances means that a new position does not need to be added. Rather, direction of the infection control can usually be undertaken by an existing staff member. Of greatest importance for the individual filling this position is an interest in the topic, motivation to make improvements in the clinic's infection-control policies, and the support of clinic leaders (eg, practice owners, veterinarians). Without full support by clinic leaders (eg, time to perform the required duties, financial investments, serving as a role model by following clinic infection-control policies), the infection-control officer, and resulting program, is unlikely to be successful.

SUMMARY

HAIs have been reported in veterinary medicine and their frequency is likely to increase with the increase in intensive care practices in many veterinary hospitals. Prolonged hospitalization and the use of invasive devices and procedures increase the risk of HAIs. All staff members should be educated on the risks and signs associated with HAIs so that cases can be detected early and managed appropriately. Ultimately, a multifaceted approach is necessary to address HAIs in small animal veterinary medicine, including prudent antimicrobial use, strengthening surveillance of HAIs in companion animals, improving infection-control practices (eg, hand hygiene, PPE, cleaning and disinfection, patient management), instilling an infection-control culture among veterinary staff, and improving health care and public education of antimicrobials. A hospital infection-control program, consisting of an infectious disease control officer, a written protocol, and staff training, is a key component to unifying these elements and successful reduction of HAIs in small animal veterinary practice.

REFERENCES

1. Klevens RM, Edwards JR, Richards CL Jr, et al. Estimating health care-associated infections and deaths in U.S. hospitals, 2002. Public Health Rep 2007;122(2):160–6.
2. Scott RD. The direct medical costs of healthcare-associated infections in U.S. hospitals and the benefits of prevention. Atlanta (GA): Centers for Disease Control and Prevention; Division of Healthcare Quality Promotion; 2009.

3. Ruple-Czerniak A, Aceto HW, Bender JB, et al. Using syndromic surveillance to estimate baseline rates for healthcare-associated infections in critical care units of small animal referral hospitals. J Vet Intern Med 2013;27(6):1392–9.
4. Benedict KM, Morley PS, Van Metre DC. Characteristics of biosecurity and infection control programs at veterinary teaching hospitals. J Am Vet Med Assoc 2008; 233(5):767–73.
5. Harbarth S, Sax H, Gastmeier P. The preventable proportion of nosocomial infections: an overview of published reports. J Hosp Infect 2003;54(4): 258–66.
6. Horan TC, Andrus M, Dudeck MA. CDC/NHSN surveillance definition of health care–associated infection and criteria for specific types of infections in the acute care setting. Am J Infect Control 2008;36(5):309–32.
7. Ogeer-Gyles J, Mathews K, Weese JS, et al. Evaluation of catheter-associated urinary tract infections and multi-drug-resistant *Escherichia coli* isolates from the urine of dogs with indwelling urinary catheters. J Am Vet Med Assoc 2006; 229(10):1584–90.
8. Smarick SD, Haskins SC, Aldrich J, et al. Incidence of catheter-associated urinary tract infection among dogs in a small animal intensive care unit. J Am Vet Med Assoc 2004;224(12):1936–40.
9. Lippert A, Fulton R Jr, Parr A. Nosocomial infection surveillance in a small animal intensive care unit. J Am Anim Hosp Assoc 1988;24(6):627–36.
10. Biertuempfel PH, Ling GV, Ling GA. Urinary tract infection resulting from catheterization in healthy adult dogs. J Am Vet Med Assoc 1981;178(9):989–91.
11. Saint S, Chenoweth CE. Biofilms and catheter-associated urinary tract infections. Infect Dis Clin North Am 2003;17(2):411–32.
12. von Dossow V, Rotard K, Redlich U, et al. Circulating immune parameters predicting the progression from hospital-acquired pneumonia to septic shock in surgical patients. Crit Care 2005;9(6):R662–9.
13. Drakulovic MB, Torres A, Bauer TT, et al. Supine body position as a risk factor for nosocomial pneumonia in mechanically ventilated patients: a randomised trial. Lancet 1999;354(9193):1851–8.
14. Lee JA, Drobatz KJ, Koch MW, et al. Indications for and outcome of positive-pressure ventilation in cats: 53 cases (1993-2002). J Am Vet Med Assoc 2005; 226(6):924–31.
15. MacPhail CM, Monnet E. Outcome of and postoperative complications in dogs undergoing surgical treatment of laryngeal paralysis: 140 cases (1985-1998). J Am Vet Med Assoc 2001;218(12):1949–56.
16. Brainard BM, Alwood AJ, Kushner LI, et al. Postoperative pulmonary complications in dogs undergoing laparotomy: anesthetic and perioperative factors. J Vet Emerg Crit Care 2006;16(3):184–91.
17. Java MA, Drobatz KJ, Gilley RS, et al. Incidence of and risk factors for postoperative pneumonia in dogs anesthetized for diagnosis or treatment of intervertebral disk disease. J Am Vet Med Assoc 2009;235(3):281–7.
18. Collins RN, Braun PA, Zinner SH, et al. Risk of local and systemic infection with polyethylene intravenous catheters. A prospective study of 213 catheterizations. N Engl J Med 1968;279(7):340–3.
19. Marsh-Ng ML, Burney DP, Garcia J. Surveillance of infections associated with intravenous catheters in dogs and cats in an intensive care unit. J Am Anim Hosp Assoc 2007;43(1):13–20.
20. Seguela J, Pages JP. Bacterial and fungal colonisation of peripheral intravenous catheters in dogs and cats. J Small Anim Pract 2011;52(10):531–5.

21. Burrows CF. Inadequate skin preparation as a cause of intravenous catheter-related infection in the dog. J Am Vet Med Assoc 1982;180(7):747–9.
22. Mathews KA, Brooks MJ, Valliant AE. A prospective study of intravenous catheter contamination. J Vet Emerg Crit Care 1996;6(1):33–43.
23. Cherry B, Burns A, Johnson GS, et al. *Salmonella* Typhimurium outbreak associated with veterinary clinic. Emerg Infect Dis 2004;10(12):2249–51.
24. Leonard EK, Pearl DL, Finley RL, et al. Evaluation of pet-related management factors and the risk of *Salmonella* spp. carriage in pet dogs from volunteer households in Ontario (2005-2006). Zoonoses Public Health 2011;58(2):140–9.
25. Lenz J, Joffe D, Kauffman M, et al. Perceptions, practices, and consequences associated with foodborne pathogens and the feeding of raw meat to dogs. Can Vet J 2009;50(6):637–43.
26. Cantor GH, Nelson S Jr, Vanek JA, et al. *Salmonella* shedding in racing sled dogs. J Vet Diagn Invest 1997;9(4):447–8.
27. Centers for Disease Control and Prevention. Antibiotic resistance threats in the United States, 2013. Atlanta (GA): Centers for Disease Control and Prevention; 2013.
28. Sievert DM, Ricks P, Edwards JR, et al. Antimicrobial-resistant pathogens associated with healthcare-associated infections: summary of data reported to the National Healthcare Safety Network at the Centers for Disease Control and Prevention, 2009-2010. Infect Control Hosp Epidemiol 2013;34(1):1–14.
29. Papich MG. Antibiotic treatment of resistant infections in small animals. Vet Clin North Am Small Anim Pract 2013;43(5):1091–107.
30. Boerlin P, Eugster S, Gaschen F, et al. Transmission of opportunistic pathogens in a veterinary teaching hospital. Vet Microbiol 2001;82(4):347–59.
31. Faires MC, Gard S, Aucoin D, et al. Inducible clindamycin-resistance in methicillin-resistant *Staphylococcus aureus* and methicillin-resistant *Staphylococcus pseudintermedius* isolates from dogs and cats. Vet Microbiol 2009; 139(3–4):419–20.
32. Sasaki T, Kikuchi K, Tanaka Y, et al. Methicillin-resistant *Staphylococcus pseudintermedius* in a veterinary teaching hospital. J Clin Microbiol 2007;45(4):1118–25.
33. Anderson DJ, Sexton DJ, Kanafani ZA, et al. Severe surgical site infection in community hospitals: epidemiology, key procedures, and the changing prevalence of methicillin-resistant *Staphylococcus aureus.* Infect Control Hosp Epidemiol 2007; 28(9):1047–53.
34. Weese JS, Dick H, Willey BM, et al. Suspected transmission of methicillin-resistant *Staphylococcus aureus* between domestic pets and humans in veterinary clinics and in the household. Vet Microbiol 2006;115(1–3):148–55.
35. Hoet AE, van Balen J, Nava-Hoet RC, et al. Epidemiological profiling of methicillin-resistant *Staphylococcus aureus*-positive dogs arriving at a veterinary teaching hospital. Vector Borne Zoonotic Dis 2013;13(6):385–93.
36. Faires MC, Traverse M, Tater KC, et al. Methicillin-resistant and -susceptible *Staphylococcus aureus* infections in dogs. Emerg Infect Dis 2010;16(1):69–75.
37. Soares Magalhaes RJ, Loeffler A, Lindsay J, et al. Risk factors for methicillin-resistant *Staphylococcus aureus* (MRSA) infection in dogs and cats: a case-control study. Vet Res 2010;41(5):55.
38. Hamilton E, Kruger JM, Schall W, et al. Acquisition and persistence of antimicrobial-resistant bacteria isolated from dogs and cats admitted to a veterinary teaching hospital. J Am Vet Med Assoc 2013;243(7):990–1000.
39. Dancer SJ. The effect of antibiotics on methicillin-resistant *Staphylococcus aureus.* J Antimicrob Chemother 2008;61(2):246–53.

40. Hanselman BA, Kruth SA, Rousseau J, et al. Methicillin-resistant *Staphylococcus aureus* colonization in veterinary personnel. Emerg Infect Dis 2006;12(12):1933–8.
41. Perreten V, Kadlec K, Schwarz S, et al. Clonal spread of methicillin-resistant *Staphylococcus pseudintermedius* in Europe and North America: an international multicentre study. J Antimicrob Chemother 2010;65(6):1145–54.
42. Nicoll C, Singh A, Weese JS. Economic impact of tibial plateau leveling osteotomy surgical site infection in dogs. Vet Surg 2014;43:899–902.
43. Bemis DA, Jones RD, Frank LA, et al. Evaluation of susceptibility test breakpoints used to predict *mec*A-mediated resistance in *Staphylococcus pseudintermedius* isolated from dogs. J Vet Diagn Invest 2009;21(1):53–8.
44. Weese JS, Faires MC, Frank LA, et al. Factors associated with methicillin-resistant versus methicillin-susceptible *Staphylococcus pseudintermedius* infection in dogs. J Am Vet Med Assoc 2012;240(12):1450–5.
45. Wedley AL, Maddox TW, Westgarth C, et al. Prevalence of antimicrobial-resistant *Escherichia coli* in dogs in a cross-sectional, community-based study. Vet Rec 2011;168(13):354.
46. Murphy C, Reid-Smith RJ, Prescott JF, et al. Occurrence of antimicrobial resistant bacteria in healthy dogs and cats presented to private veterinary hospitals in southern Ontario: a preliminary study. Can Vet J 2009;50(10):1047–53.
47. Gibson JS, Morton JM, Cobbold RN, et al. Risk factors for multidrug-resistant *Escherichia coli* rectal colonization of dogs on admission to a veterinary hospital. Epidemiol Infect 2011;139(2):197–205.
48. Gibson JS, Morton JM, Cobbold RN, et al. Risk factors for dogs becoming rectal carriers of multidrug-resistant *Escherichia coli* during hospitalization. Epidemiol Infect 2011;139(10):1511–21.
49. Pitout JD. Infections with extended-spectrum beta-lactamase-producing *enterobacteriaceae*: changing epidemiology and drug treatment choices. Drugs 2010;70(3):313–33.
50. Sanchez S, McCrackin Stevenson MA, Hudson CR, et al. Characterization of multidrug-resistant *Escherichia coli* isolates associated with nosocomial infections in dogs. J Clin Microbiol 2002;40(10):3586–95.
51. Sidjabat HE, Townsend KM, Lorentzen M, et al. Emergence and spread of two distinct clonal groups of multidrug-resistant *Escherichia coli* in a veterinary teaching hospital in Australia. J Med Microbiol 2006;55(Pt 8):1125–34.
52. Centers for Disease Control and Prevention (CDC). Vital signs: carbapenem-resistant Enterobacteriaceae. Morb Mortal Wkly Rep 2013;62(9):165–70.
53. Patel G, Huprikar S, Factor SH, et al. Outcomes of carbapenem-resistant *Klebsiella pneumoniae* infection and the impact of antimicrobial and adjunctive therapies. Infect Control Hosp Epidemiol 2008;29(12):1099–106.
54. Stolle I, Prenger-Berninghoff E, Stamm I, et al. Emergence of OXA-48 carbapenemase-producing *Escherichia coli* and *Klebsiella pneumoniae* in dogs. J Antimicrob Chemother 2013;68:2802–8.
55. Mascini EM, Bonten MJ. Vancomycin-resistant enterococci: consequences for therapy and infection control. Clin Microbiol Infect 2005;11(Suppl 4):43–56.
56. Damborg P, Sorensen AH, Guardabassi L. Monitoring of antimicrobial resistance in healthy dogs: first report of canine ampicillin-resistant *Enterococcus faecium* clonal complex 17. Vet Microbiol 2008;132(1–2):190–6.
57. Ossiprandi MC, Bottarelli E, Cattabiani F, et al. Susceptibility to vancomycin and other antibiotics of 165 *Enterococcus* strains isolated from dogs in Italy. Comp Immunol Microbiol Infect Dis 2008;31(1):1–9.

58. Ghosh A, Dowd SE, Zurek L. Dogs leaving the ICU carry a very large multi-drug resistant enterococcal population with capacity for biofilm formation and horizontal gene transfer. PLoS One 2011;6(7):e22451.
59. Wright JG, Tengelsen LA, Smith KE, et al. Multidrug-resistant *Salmonella* Typhimurium in four animal facilities. Emerg Infect Dis 2005;11(8):1235–41.
60. Leonard EK, Pearl DL, Finley RL, et al. Comparison of antimicrobial resistance patterns of *Salmonella* spp. and *Escherichia coli* recovered from pet dogs from volunteer households in Ontario (2005-06). J Antimicrob Chemother 2012;67:174–81.
61. Frye JG, Fedorka-Cray PJ. Prevalence, distribution and characterisation of ceftiofur resistance in *Salmonella enterica* isolated from animals in the USA from 1999 to 2003. Int J Antimicrob Agents 2007;30(2):134–42.
62. Francey T, Gaschen F, Nicolet J, et al. The role of *Acinetobacter baumannii* as a nosocomial pathogen for dogs and cats in an intensive care unit. J Vet Intern Med 2000;14(2):177–83.
63. Zordan S, Prenger-Berninghoff E, Weiss R, et al. Multidrug-resistant *Acinetobacter baumannii* in veterinary clinics, Germany. Emerg Infect Dis 2011;17(9):1751–4.
64. Agodi A, Barchitta M, Cipresso R, et al. *Pseudomonas aeruginosa* carriage, colonization, and infection in ICU patients. Intensive Care Med 2007;33(7):1155–61.
65. Lin D, Foley SL, Qi Y, et al. Characterization of antimicrobial resistance of *Pseudomonas aeruginosa* isolated from canine infections. J Appl Microbiol 2012;113(1):16–23.
66. Nuttall T, Cole LK. Evidence-based veterinary dermatology: a systematic review of interventions for treatment of *Pseudomonas* otitis in dogs. Vet Dermatol 2007;18(2):69–77.
67. Gatoria IS, Saini NS, Rai TS, et al. Comparison of three techniques for the diagnosis of urinary tract infections in dogs with urolithiasis. J Small Anim Pract 2006;47(12):727–32.
68. Fine DM, Tobias AH. Cardiovascular device infections in dogs: report of 8 cases and review of the literature. J Vet Intern Med 2007;21(6):1265–71.
69. Peremans K, De Winter F, Janssens L, et al. An infected hip prosthesis in a dog diagnosed with a 99mTc-ciprofloxacin (infecton) scan. Vet Radiol Ultrasound 2002;43(2):178–82.
70. Canadian Committee on Antibiotic Resistance. Infection prevention and control best practices for small animal veterinary clinics. 2008. Available at: http://www.wormsandgermsblog.com/uploads/file/CCAR%20Guidelines%20Final(2).pdf. Accessed December 6, 2014.
71. Scheftel JM, Elchos BL, Cherry B, et al. Compendium of veterinary standard precautions for zoonotic disease prevention in veterinary personnel: National Association of State Public Health Veterinarians Veterinary Infection Control Committee 2010. J Am Vet Med Assoc 2010;237(12):1403–22. Available at: http://www.nasphv.org/Documents/VeterinaryPrecautions.pdf.
72. Wright JG, Jung S, Holman RC, et al. Infection control practices and zoonotic disease risks among veterinarians in the United States. J Am Vet Med Assoc 2008;232(12):1863–72.
73. Murphy CP, Reid-Smith RJ, Weese JS, et al. Evaluation of specific infection control practices used by companion animal veterinarians in community veterinary practices in southern Ontario. Zoonoses Public Health 2010;57(6):429–38.
74. Shea A, Shaw S. Evaluation of an educational campaign to increase hand hygiene at a small animal veterinary teaching hospital. J Am Vet Med Assoc 2012;240(1):61–4.

75. Donskey CJ. Does improving surface cleaning and disinfection reduce health care-associated infections? Am J Infect Control 2013;41(Suppl 5):S12–9.
76. Orenstein R, Aronhalt KC, McManus JE Jr, et al. A targeted strategy to wipe out *Clostridium difficile.* Infect Control Hosp Epidemiol 2011;32(11):1137–9.
77. Denton M, Wilcox MH, Parnell P, et al. Role of environmental cleaning in controlling an outbreak of *Acinetobacter baumannii* on a neurosurgical intensive care unit. J Hosp Infect 2004;56(2):106–10.
78. Weese JS, Armstrong J. Outbreak of *Clostridium difficile*-associated disease in a small animal veterinary teaching hospital. J Vet Intern Med 2003;17(6):813–6.
79. Ghosh A, Kukanich K, Brown CE, et al. Resident cats in small animal veterinary hospitals carry multi-drug resistant enterococci and are likely involved in cross-contamination of the hospital environment. Front Microbiol 2012;3:62.
80. Baker WS, Gray GC. A review of published reports regarding zoonotic pathogen infection in veterinarians. J Am Vet Med Assoc 2009;234(10):1271–8.
81. Lipton BA, Hopkins SG, Koehler JE, et al. A survey of veterinarian involvement in zoonotic disease prevention practices. J Am Vet Med Assoc 2008;233(8):1242–9.

Veterinary Hospital Surveillance Systems

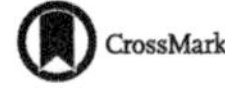

Brandy A. Burgess, DVM, MSc, PhD[a,*], Paul S. Morley, DVM, PhD[b]

KEYWORDS

• Infection control • Surveillance systems • Veterinary medicine

KEY POINTS

- There is a recognized and evolving standard of practice with respect to veterinary infection control; one can do too little.
- Organized surveillance efforts should inform infection control and prevention program development and maintenance.
- Endemic rates of infection account for the majority of health care-associated infections and should be the emphasis of ongoing surveillance efforts.
- There is no "one size fits all" infection control and prevention program. Each program should be tailored to a facility's unique operational limits.

"Good surveillance does not necessarily ensure the making of the right decisions, but it reduces the chances of wrong ones."

—Alexander D. Langmuir (1963)[1]

IMPORTANCE OF VETERINARY INFECTION CONTROL AND SURVEILLANCE SYSTEMS

One cannot manage what one does not measure. In veterinary infection control, one tends to respond to theoretic threats based on first principles rather than establishing prevention practices based upon the evidence.[2,3] Quite simply, this is because, as a discipline, veterinary infection control is relatively new; thus there are very limited data upon which to base strategies for the prevention of infectious disease transmission within veterinary facilities (ie, health care-associated infections [HAIs]). Further, limited data from a survey of veterinary teaching hospitals suggests that even when monitoring of specific pathogens or diseases occurs in veterinary facilities, it is not

The authors have nothing to disclose.

[a] Department of Population Health Sciences, Virginia Maryland Regional College of Veterinary Medicine, Virginia Tech, 100 Sandy Hall (MC0395), Blacksburg, VA 24061, USA; [b] Department of Clinical Sciences, James L. Voss Veterinary Teaching Hospital, Colorado State University, 1678 Campus Delivery, Fort Collins, CO 80526, USA

* Corresponding author.

E-mail address: burgessb@vt.edu

Vet Clin Small Anim 45 (2015) 235–242

http://dx.doi.org/10.1016/j.cvsm.2014.11.002 **vetsmall.theclinics.com**

0195-5616/15/$ – see front matter

conducted at predetermined intervals, suggesting that there is very little systematic effort used to identify latent issues regarding HAI.[3]

If one looks to human health care for guidance, one finds the initial comprehensive studies conducted in the United States from 1970 to 1976, collectively called the Study on the Efficacy of Nosocomial Infection Control (SENIC). This pivotal work found that the occurrence of nosocomial (or health care-associated) infections could be reduced by an estimated 32% following implementation of a "comprehensive" infection control program. By definition, a comprehensive program had 3 key components[4]:

1. It identified a skilled person to oversee infection control efforts.
2. It conducted organized surveillance and control activities.
3. It maintained a system for reporting findings back to stakeholders.[4]

Unfortunately, there are no similar data on HAIs in veterinary medicine. However, if these components are incorporated into veterinary infection control programs, one might expect a similar reduction in HAIs. In fact, there is a recognizable standard of practice with respect to veterinary infection control according to a recent consensus opinion of an international group of experts.[5] Appropriate effort must be given to the prevention of infectious disease transmission through the development and maintenance of an infection control program that is founded on results obtained through organized surveillance efforts.[5]

Infection control efforts should strive to minimize the negative impact of HAIs to patients and personnel, and ultimately to the hospital. Although hospital-associated outbreaks tend to garner much attention, the occurrence of epidemic disease really represents a small proportion of HAIs, the proverbial tip of the iceberg, due to unusual circumstances that have resulted in an extraordinary event. In truth, the baseline level or endemic rate actually accounts for the majority of HAIs.[6] It is this expected or endemic rate that should be the emphasis of ongoing surveillance efforts. By monitoring the endemic rate, facility managers can begin to understand and address factors contributing to HAIs in specific health care environments, thereby preventing an escalation to epidemic levels.

DEFINING SURVEILLANCE METHODS

Surveillance is the systematic collection, analysis, and interpretation of health events in a population to enable specific responses for the control of adverse outcomes. In other words, a surveillance program incorporates a monitoring system and a critical limit at which a predetermined action will be undertaken in an effort to mitigate an identified risk. There are many different methods that can be used for disease monitoring including active, passive, targeted, and syndromic surveillance. Although there is no definitively correct method, infection control programs are dynamic and should rely upon organized surveillance efforts in their development, implementation, and continued improvement.[5]

Active surveillance is conducted with the express purpose of finding outcomes or indicators of interest as part of a formal surveillance program, while passive surveillance uses information and/or samples collected for another purpose (eg, laboratory samples submitted for diagnostic purposes). As such, active surveillance provides a primary source of data, and may be more time consuming and expensive to collect, but typically yields much more complete data than passive surveillance, which depends upon the quality of a secondary data source. Targeted or risk-based surveillance tends to focus efforts on previously identified hazards or known risks factors for a particular outcome.[7] For example (see **Table 1** for an example surveillance

Table 1
Example[a] surveillance program for *Salmonella enterica* conducted at the James L. Voss Veterinary Teaching Hospital, Colorado State University

Components	Advantages	Disadvantages	Example(s)
Active surveillance	• Primary data source • Generally provides better quality and more complete data • Can be representative of specific patient groups of interest and the overall hospital population • Allows collection of data customized to address specific questions of interest	• Greater investments required ○ Time ○ Expense	1. Fecal sample culture[b] of all large animal inpatients on admission and twice weekly for the duration of hospitalization 2. Environmental culture[c] of approximately 60 sites throughout the small animal, equine, and livestock hospitals 3. Collection of information about risk factors and patient movements during hospitalization
Targeted surveillance	• Generally accurate • Represents population of concern, which is not necessarily representative of all patient groups of interest • Focuses on previously identified risk(s) • Less difficult and less expensive than larger active surveillance programs	• Greater investment than passive surveillance	1. Fecal sample culture[b] of all patients with 2 of 3 signs (fever, leukopenia, diarrhea) or developing diarrhea during hospitalization 2. Environmental culture[c] of select locations when an increase (above baseline) in positive patients or positive environmental samples is detected
Passive surveillance	• Easy • Relatively inexpensive	• Secondary data source • Limitations in data quality • Data are limited to that collected for other purposes (ie, not specifically to enhance surveillance efforts) • Study population generally not representative of patient groups of interest or the larger hospital population	1. All diagnostic samples culture positive for *Salmonella* from inpatients (small and large animal) are reported to biosecurity personnel 2. Laboratory, pharmacy, and financial databases
Syndromic surveillance	• Easy • Inexpensive	• No laboratory diagnosis • Nonspecific indicators of disease	1. 3–5 fecal cultures from all patients (small and large animal) developing GI disease (eg, diarrhea or colitis) during hospitalization

[a] Surveillance programs must be tailored to each facility's specific needs.
[b] 1-gram fecal sample for enriched culture.
[c] Collected using a Swiffer (Proctor & Gamble, Cincinnati, OH).[22]

program), a program may target surveillance for *Salmonella* toward patients with gastrointestinal (GI) disease or those with 2 of 3 signs commonly associated with *Salmonella* infection (eg, fever, diarrhea, and leukopenia), as these patients are known to have a greater likelihood of shedding.[8] In some situations, it may be possible to take effective actions even without a definitive diagnosis (ie, laboratory confirmation). In such instances, syndromic surveillance may be used.[9] This method focuses on nonspecific indicators of disease (eg, clinical indicators and other nonspecific indicators) that are often present before the determination of a definitive diagnosis can be made and may be used in lieu of establishing a diagnosis.[10] Many veterinary facilities conduct pathogen-specific, laboratory-confirmed surveillance (eg, *Salmonella* or methicillin-resistant *Staphylococcus aureus* [MRSA]), and relatively fewer facilities conduct formal clinical disease syndromic surveillance.[3] Recently, 4 small animal veterinary referral hospitals demonstrated the effective implementation of a standardized syndromic surveillance system to estimate health care-associated events among canine patients in critical care units.[9] Overall, the occurrence of any of 6 syndromes (intravenous catheter site inflammation, urinary tract inflammation, acute respiratory disorders, GI disorders, surgical site inflammation, and fever of unknown origin) were detected in 5.2 canine patients per 100 hospitalization days (95% confidence interval [CI] 4.6, 6.0), controlling for differences among veterinary hospitals.[9] This syndromic surveillance system was a simple 1-page survey that could be completed quickly, without exhausting available resources (including financial or personnel time), and worked well with different staffing and patient management structures. This is a nice example of employing a simple strategy across multiple institutions to try to gain perspective on the occurrence of HAIs in veterinary medicine.

SHOULD VETERINARY HEALTH CARE FACILITIES PERFORM SURVEILLANCE?

Will caring for the patient of today adversely affect the patients of tomorrow? In the practice of veterinary medicine, the goal is to provide optimal patient care. To attain this, one must take all reasonable precautions to prevent foreseeable risks associated with infectious disease transmission among patients and personnel (ie, health care-associated infections and zoonotic infections). But how do veterinary practitioners and hospitals demonstrate the provision of optimal patient care? By demonstrating that they can achieve optimal patient care outcomes (ie, the results of patient care and management).[11]

Surveillance is a means to that end. By performing routine surveillance, hospitals can establish the endemic or expected levels of a particular outcome or process, thereby informing infection prevention efforts and resource allocation. As veterinary medicine advances through more intensive patient management and more invasive procedures, the risks increase for the occurrence of HAIs. Determining which outcomes or processes are of greatest concern for a particular facility will shape the type of surveillance that may be conducted. Outcome-based surveillance provides rates for adverse outcomes (such as surgical site infections or catheter site infections) but may provide limited information regarding what factors actually contributed to this occurrence. An alternative can be to conduct process-based surveillance, focusing on factors known to contribute to the development of HAIs (eg, prophylactic antimicrobial use, catheter management procedures).[12] This type of surveillance may allow for the identification of protocol drift or the practice of risky behaviors before adverse outcomes are detected. For example, a surgical facility may determine that catheter-site inflammation is an important outcome and choose to conduct syndromic surveillance or monitor compliance with catheter management procedures to aid in prevention efforts. Alternatively, a tertiary care facility may determine that MRSA colonization among dermatologic patients presents a high risk and thus pursue active surveillance for this specific organism among this subpopulation of patients (ie, targeted surveillance for a specific organism of concern).

Findings from SENIC are clear; human health care facilities incorporating surveillance system(s) into infection prevention and control programs improve patient outcomes.[4] In order to provide optimal patient care, veterinary medicine must embrace the lessons learned. There is not only an ethical responsibility to do so, but as veterinary medicine advances, there is a legal responsibility to meet the minimum standard of practice with respect to veterinary infection prevention and control.

WHERE TO GO WITH SURVEILLANCE IN VETERINARY HOSPITALS?

There is no such thing as zero risk, and thus not all adverse outcomes are avoidable. However, the likelihood of occurrence can be minimized through coordinated prevention efforts, of which surveillance is an essential component. A surveillance program should strive to evaluate the effectiveness of infection control practices, assess compliance with established procedures, provide a foundation for infection control decisions, and enable the efficient use of resources.[13]

Every facility has unique physical attributes and organizational support (ie, financial and personnel); therefore infection control programs (including surveillance efforts) should be tailored for each facility; there is no "one size fits all." That said, there are key characteristics that each surveillance system should take into consideration during program development[11,13]:

- Delineate specific program objectives and identify methods to address each (eg, monitor surgical sites for inflammation or infection [SSI], calculate SSI rates, and compare to previously established baseline rates)
- Select and define outcomes or processes to be measured (eg, surgical site inflammation or infection rate as defined by redness, swelling, heat, or drainage at an incision site with laboratory confirmation)
- Define patient population(s) or risk-group(s) to be monitored (eg, all canine patients undergoing orthopedic surgery)
- Outline the data collection process, time period, and analytical methods (eg, active surveillance through postoperative follow-up phone calls and passive surveillance through recheck visits)
- Establish critical limits that will trigger action (eg, when the SSI rate exceeds a previously established baseline rate).
- Develop a mechanism for reporting results back to hospital personnel/stakeholders (eg, provide a monthly report of SSI rates to clinic personnel)
- Document the plan in writing

The patient population(s) to be monitored in a surveillance system will be derived from the specific program objectives. Although it is impractical to conduct global surveillance (ie, all patients, all outcomes) a facility may elect to monitor all inpatients but for a specific outcome, organism (eg, *Salmonella* or MRSA), or syndrome (eg, catheter site inflammation or diarrhea). Another option would be to perform targeted surveillance of a particular high-risk patient subgroup such as critical care patients or those with GI disease. Yet another possible method would be to perform environmental surveillance for microbial contamination, an indirect indicator of infectious disease presence, instead of (or in combination with) performing patient surveillance. Although hospitals should strive to develop comprehensive surveillance programs and often employ multiple methods to that end, history has shown that focused efforts on specific adverse outcomes (ie, surveillance by objective) can improve overall program success.[14]

There are many different secondary data sources available including the medical record, invoice, and pharmacy data. Electronic medical records systems (EMRs) offer a unique opportunity to automate data collection and create specific data entry/collection systems.[13,15] For example, at the Colorado State University Veterinary Teaching Hospital (CSU-VTH), the EMR has a section dedicated to monitoring for HAIs, specifically catheter site inflammation, urinary catheter inflammation, respiratory disease, GI disease, surgical site inflammation, fever of unknown origin, and septicemia. A detailed description of electronic surveillance program considerations has been provided elsewhere.[15] Keep in mind that although automatic data collection may improve efficiency, it does not necessarily improve accuracy. The EMR can also be used to create point-of-care reminders or flag patients with clinical presentations or infections that are of specific concern for the hospital (eg, nonhealing wounds, diarrhea, laboratory-confirmed MRSA infection), thus allowing appropriate surveillance and precautions to be implemented much earlier in the patient evaluation process and possibly on admission or readmission to the facility.

In a survey of veterinary hospitals accredited by the American Veterinary Medical Association, many employed some type of passive and/or active surveillance, including summaries of contagious diseases as reported by clinicians, compiling laboratory results from diagnostic samples (as opposed to surveillance samples), environmental sampling for bacterial culture, and patient sampling for contagious diseases of concern (eg, *Salmonella*, methicillin-resistant *Staphylococcus* species).[3] However, these surveillance efforts were not necessarily performed at a predetermined time interval (eg, monthly or quarterly). This lack of predetermination makes it difficult to establish an expected endemic rate, thereby precluding the ability of a facility to establish a benchmark to which future surveillance efforts can be compared. Although it is not necessary to conduct continuous on-going surveillance (some facilities may conduct intermittent, periodic surveillance), it is recommended to do so in a routine, predetermined manner (ie, at a defined time interval).

Fundamental to the reduction of adverse outcomes is the reporting of surveillance results back to hospital personnel.[14] Creating awareness can drive changes in behavior which in turn can lead to improved patient care. It is important to report stratum specific (eg, by patient type or hospital service) rates, controlling for intrinsic differences among patients and medical management that may influence infectious disease risk, which then allows for more meaningful comparisons and interventions.

Finally, a surveillance program should be written down to allow for consistency over time. This includes both creating standard definitions in data collection and standard processes that will ensure the same rigor in efforts. In addition, educational opportunities should be provided to personnel to facilitate compliance with processes and so that they may become knowledgeable about the program and its importance for protecting patients and personnel. In this way, facilities can gain an understanding of the endemic occurrence of the adverse outcome of interest; comparisons can be made over time, and programs can be adjusted to the ever-changing landscape of the veterinary hospital environment.

THE COSTS OF SURVEILLANCE

Unfortunately, hospitalization has with it an inherent risk of developing an HAI. Although it is impossible to reduce this risk to zero, efforts can focus on the proportion of HAIs that could be avoided with cost-effective prevention and control strategies—the preventable fraction.

In US hospitals, it is estimated that 5% of hospitalized people will develop an HAI during hospitalization, at a direct cost of $28 billion to $45 billion per year.[16,17] If one considers the results of a systematic review that estimated the preventable fraction of HAIs to be 20%, in light of current routine medical practices and technology in human medicine, an effective infection prevention and control program could represent a cost savings of approximately $5.6 to $9.0 billion per year.[18] Although there are no similar data in veterinary medicine, it is known that direct costs of $4.12 million were associated with a single large outbreak of salmonellosis in an equine hospital that was attributed to an ineffective infection control program.[19] It is difficult to know the true cost (both direct and indirect) of an outbreak avoided. What is the monetary value of a life or illness, of lost teaching and learning opportunities, and of the impact on public relations?

Although it is clear that every veterinary facility should base infection prevention and control strategies on organized surveillance efforts, every program will be unique. A balance must be found between surveillance efforts to obtain useful data and the operational limits, both financial and personnel, of the facility. The added benefit of an effective infection prevention and control program with a comprehensive surveillance system is that results can inform program refinements and help guide resource allocation in the future.

AN EXAMPLE SURVEILLANCE PROGRAM FOR METHICILLIN-RESISTANT *STAPHYLOCOCCUS PSEUDINTERMEDIUS* IN A SMALL ANIMAL VETERINARY HOSPITAL

Methicillin-resistant *Staphylococcus* species are newly emerging opportunistic pathogens in veterinary medicine. At the Colorado State University Veterinary Teaching Hospital (CSU-VTH), current infection prevention and control procedures rely upon passive surveillance (ie, laboratory samples submitted for diagnostic purposes rather than for surveillance) for the detection of patients colonized or infected with methicillin-resistant *Staphylococcus pseudintermedius* (MRSP). In North America, limited information suggests that MRSP colonization prevalence estimates among hospitalized dogs are approximately 2% to 6%.[20,21] Although there is not a prevalence estimate for patients admitted to CSU, subjectively (based on anecdotal evidence and passive surveillance), MRSP is a commonly identified organism among patients managed by the dermatologic and oncological specialty services, and it poses a potential infectious disease risk to other patients, including being a frequent cause of SSIs. To gain a better understanding of the epidemiology and prevalence (endemic colonization rate) among the CSU canine patient population, the authors began a short-term targeted surveillance program. This is an example of an active surveillance system and thus a primary data source, with patient samples being collected for this express purpose. The surveillance effort focuses on 2 high-risk groups, dermatologic and oncological canine patients. The data from this short term surveillance effort will be used to develop more specific infection prevention and control procedures and to tailor the surveillance system to effectively manage this risk within the CSU-VTH Small Animal Hospital.

REFERENCES

1. Langmuir AD. The surveillance of communicable diseases of national importance. N Engl J Med 1963;268:182–92.
2. Morley PS. Evidence-based infection control in clinical practice: if you buy clothes for the emperor, will he wear them? J Vet Intern Med 2013;27(3):430–8.

3. Benedict KM, Morley PS, Van Metre DC. Characteristics of biosecurity and infection control programs at veterinary teaching hospitals. J Am Vet Med Assoc 2008; 233(5):767–73.
4. Haley RW, Culver DH, White JW, et al. The efficacy of infection surveillance and control programs in preventing nosocomial infections in US hospitals. Am J Epidemiol 1985;121(2):182–205.
5. Morley P, Anderson M, Burgess B. Report of the third Havemeyer workshop on infection control in equine populations. Equine Vet J 2012;45:131–6.
6. Stamm WE, Weinstein RA, Dixon RE. Comparison of endemic and epidemic nosocomial infections. Am J Med 1981;70(2):393–7.
7. Stark KD, Regula G, Hernandez J, et al. Concepts for risk-based surveillance in the field of veterinary medicine and veterinary public health: review of current approaches. BMC Health Serv Res 2006;6:20.
8. Burgess BA. Epidemiology and prevention of *Salmonella* in veterinary hospitals. Colorado State University; 2014. Colorado State University Libraries, Fort Collins, CO.
9. Ruple-Czerniak A, Aceto HW, Bender JB, et al. Using syndromic surveillance to estimate baseline rates for healthcare-associated infections in critical care units of small animal referral hospitals. J Vet Intern Med 2013;27(6):1392–9.
10. Dorea FC, Sanchez J, Revie CW. Veterinary syndromic surveillance: current initiatives and potential for development. Prev Vet Med 2011;101(1–2):1–17.
11. Lee TB, Montgomery OG, Marx J, et al. Recommended practices for surveillance: Association for Professionals in Infection Control and Epidemiology (APIC), Inc. Am J Infect Control 2007;35(7):427–40.
12. Tokars JI, Richards C, Andrus M, et al. The changing face of surveillance for health care-associated infections. Clin Infect Dis 2004;39(9):1347–52.
13. Morley PS. Surveillance for nosocomial infections in veterinary hospitals. Vet Clin North Am Equine Pract 2004;20(3):561–76, vi–vii.
14. Haley RW. The scientific basis for using surveillance and risk factor data to reduce nosocomial infection rates. J Hosp Infect 1995;30(Suppl):3–14.
15. Woeltje KF, Lin MY, Klompas M, et al. Data requirements for electronic surveillance of healthcare-associated infections. Infect Control Hosp Epidemiol 2014; 35(9):1083–91.
16. Calfee DP. Crisis in hospital-acquired, healthcare-associated infections. Annu Rev Med 2012;63:359–71.
17. Scott RD. The direct medical costs of healthcare-associated infections in US hospitals and the benefits of prevention. 2009. Available at: http://www.cdc.gov/HAI/pdfs/hai/Scott_CostPaper.pdf. Accessed March 21, 2012.
18. Harbarth S, Sax H, Gastmeier P. The preventable proportion of nosocomial infections: an overview of published reports. J Hosp Infect 2003;54(4):258–66 [quiz: 321].
19. Dallap Schaer BL, Aceto H, Rankin SC. Outbreak of salmonellosis caused by *Salmonella enterica serovar* Newport MDR-AmpC in a large animal veterinary teaching hospital. J Vet Intern Med 2010;24(5):1138–46.
20. Hanselman BA, Kruth S, Weese JS. Methicillin-resistant staphylococcal colonization in dogs entering a veterinary teaching hospital. Vet Microbiol 2008;126(1–3):277–81.
21. Detwiler A, Bloom P, Petersen A, et al. Multi-drug and methicillin resistance of staphylococci from canine patients at a veterinary teaching hospital (2006–2011). Vet Q 2013;33(2):60–7.
22. Burgess BA, Morley PS, Hyatt DR. Environmental surveillance for *Salmonella enterica* in a veterinary teaching hospital. J Am Vet Med Assoc 2004;225(9): 1344–8.

Fighting Surgical Site Infections in Small Animals

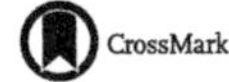

Are We Getting Anywhere?

Denis Verwilghen, DVM, MSc, PhD, DES[a,*], Ameet Singh, DVM, DVSc[b]

KEYWORDS

- Surgical site infections • Prevention • Compliance • Antimicrobial prophylaxis

KEY POINTS

- Surgical site infection (SSI) rates after surgery are still considerable, despite the array of preventive measures available.
- Hand hygiene, appropriate antimicrobial prophylaxis, careful selection of surgical patients, and surgical experience/technique are the preventive measures with highest preventive impact on SSIs.
- Compliance rates with known and established measures are dramatically low.
- Correct adherence to the current knowledge has the greatest potential in reducing SSIs.

INTRODUCTION

Surgical site infections (SSIs) are a burden of surgery. They lead to increased health care cost as a result of additional treatment, antimicrobial administrations, extended hospital stay, and patient morbidity/mortality. Further, these complications create emotional and financial distress for owners and drastically affect the animal's welfare. We are distant from the early days of surgery, when the treatment was worse than the disease. In those days, most surgical procedures failed because of infectious complications. In the early eighteenth century, pus was believed to be normal, even adequate, during the phases of wound healing. Discoveries made by Louis Pasteur showed the involvement of microbes in this process, and simultaneously, methods were established to focus on combating sepsis, ushering in the antisepsis era.

Before the antimicrobial era, the pioneering work of Semmelweis in the mid-1800s made us understand the critical role of the hands of health care workers in the

The authors have nothing to disclose.

[a] Department of Large Animal Sciences, University of Copenhagen, Hojbakkegaerd Allé 5, Taatsrup 2630, Denmark; [b] Department of Clinical Studies, Ontario Veterinary College, University of Guelph, 50 Stone Road East, Guelph, Ontario N1G 2W1, Canada
* Corresponding author.
E-mail address: dv@sund.ku.dk

Vet Clin Small Anim 45 (2015) 243–276
http://dx.doi.org/10.1016/j.cvsm.2014.11.001 **vetsmall.theclinics.com**
0195-5616/15/$ – see front matter

transmission of infections.[1] Soon after, and led by Pasteur's saying "Instead of fighting bacteria in wounds, would it not just be better not to introduce them?," surgeons like Koch, Lister, and Halstead developed the principles to avoid the development of sepsis; the principles of asepsis and aseptic technique were established. These discoveries, coupled with the understanding of the germ theory of disease and the development of aseptic techniques, may have had the greatest impact on patient survival with regard to infectious diseases or any other medical advancement. With the discovery of antimicrobials, many believed that infectious disease would become a thing of the past, and the focus on prevention measures may have lapsed because of the ease with which infections could seemingly be treated. However, in the late twentieth and early twenty-first centuries, with the effectiveness of the antimicrobial arsenal waning, infection prevention has come to the forefront once again. Considering that no pathogen has yet developed any resistance to aseptic technique, the saying by Pasteur is more pertinent than ever in our journey trying to chase zero infection rates.

DEFINITIONS

Surveillance of SSI rates, including feedback to the surgical team, has been shown to be an important and effective component of SSI reduction strategy in human medicine.[2–4] A successful surveillance program includes proper identification of the targeted risks and the use of universally accepted infection definitions.[5] Differentiating inflammatory processes, infections present on admission (POA), and other health care–associated infections (HAI) from SSI is, therefore, the cornerstone of a multimodal approach to SSI prevention. The US Centers for Disease Control and Prevention (CDC) has recently updated its documents *Surveillance Definitions for Specific Types of Infections*[6] and *Surgical Site Infection Event*[7] (**Table 1**).

At its most basic level, an SSI is an infection that is associated with a particular operative procedure and the facility in which that procedure was performed.[7] An operative procedure is defined as a procedure in which at least 1 incision is made through the skin or mucous membrane or reoperation is performed via an incision made during a previous operative procedure. Primary incisional closure is not part of the operative procedure definition, and infections occurring in wounds that have not been closed by primary intention (packed with gauze, covered with adhesive plastic) are, therefore, included in SSI surveillance.[7] The duration of the operative procedure is defined as the interval in hours and minutes between the start and the end of the procedure. The start of the procedure is defined as the moment when the incision is made. The procedure ends when all instruments and sponge counts are completed, all radiologic studies to be performed in the operating room (OR) are completed, all dressings and drains are secured, and the surgeon has completed all procedure-related activities on the patient.[7]

SSIs are classified according to superficial, deep, or organ/space infections (see **Table 1**). The combined interpretation of clinical and laboratory data allows identification of an SSI in one of these categories.

EPIDEMIOLOGY

Surgical Site Infection Incidence

SSIs account for as many as one-fourth of all HAIs (nosocomial infections) and are the most common cause of infections in human surgical patients.[9] The rate of SSIs is highly dependent on the type of surgery.[10] Several veterinary studies have reported SSI rates, including overall infection and procedure-specific infections (**Table 2**). Most of these studies are limited by the lack of use of appropriate SSI definitions, absence

Table 1
SSI definitions according to CDC

SSI	Definition	Criteria (≥1 Should Be Met)
Superficial incisional infections	Infection occurring within 30 d of a surgical procedure involving only the skin and subcutaneous tissues of the incision	Purulent drainage from the superficial incision Organisms isolated from an aseptically obtained culture of fluid or tissue from the superficial incision Superficial incision that is deliberately opened and patient has ≥1 of the following signs or symptoms of infection: pain or tenderness; localized redness; swelling; or heat, unless incision is cultured negative Diagnosis of superficial incision infection by the attending surgeon
Deep incisional infection	Infection occurs within 30 or 90 d (depending on procedure) involving deep soft tissues of the incision (within a year after implant placement and infection seems to be related to surgical procedure in veterinary medicine[8])	Purulent drainage from the deep incision Deep incision that spontaneously dehisces or is deliberately opened by a surgeon and is cultured positive or not cultured but patient has signs of fever, localized pain and tenderness, unless the site is cultured negative An abscess or other evidence of infection involving the deep incision that is detected on direct examination, during invasive procedure, or by histopathologic or imaging examination Diagnosis of deep incision infection by the attending surgeon
Organ/space infections	Infection occurring within 30 or 90 d (depending on procedure) of the operative procedure (within a year after implant placement and infection seems to be related to surgical procedure in veterinary medicine[8])	Infection involving any part of the body, excluding skin incision, fascia or muscle layer that is opened or manipulated during the operative procedure, and The patient has at least a purulent drainage from a drain that is placed in the organ/space, organisms isolated from an aseptically obtained culture of fluid or tissue from the organ/space, or an abscess or other evidence of infection involving the organ/space that is detected on direct examination, during invasive procedure, or by histologic or imaging examination Diagnosis of organ/space infection by the attending surgeon

Adapted from Centers for Disease Control. CDC/NHSN Surveillance Definitions for Specific types of Infections. Atlanta: CDC; 2014.

Table 2
Reported SSI rates grouped by type of surgery in small animal practice

Surgical Procedure	Sample Size (n)	SSI Incidence (%)	Reference
All surgical procedures	846	3.0	Turk et al,[8] 2014
All surgical procedures	1010	3.0	Eugster et al,[11] 2004
All surgical procedures	1574	5.5	Brown et al,[12] 1997
All surgical procedures	2063	5.1	Vasseur et al,[13] 1988
Clean-contaminated surgical wounds	239	5.9	Nicholson et al,[14] 2002
Clean surgical wounds	777	4.8	Beal et al,[15] 2000
Clean surgical wounds	863	4.5	Heldmann et al,[16] 1999
Clean surgical wounds	128	0.8	Vasseur et al,[17] 1985
Clean, elective orthopedic surgical procedures	112	7.1	Whittem et al,[18] 1999
Clean, elective orthopedic surgical procedures	60	3.3	Holmberg,[19] 1985
Laparoscopy and VATS	179	1.7	Mayhew et al,[20] 2012
TPLO	226	13.3	Nazarali et al,[21] 2014
TPLO	208	21.3	Solano et al,[22] 2014
TPLO		8.8	Etter et al,[23] 2013
TPLO	2739	3.8	Savicky et al,[24] 2013
TPLO	282	7.4	Gallagher & Mertens,[25] 2012
TPLO	476	2.9	Gatineau et al,[26] 2011
TPLO	1146	6.6	Fitzpatrick & Solano,[27] 2010
Extracapsular stifle stabilization and TPLO	902	6.1	Frey et al,[28] 2010

Abbreviations: TPLO, tibial plateau leveling osteotomy; VATS, video-assisted thoracic surgery.
Data from Refs.[8,11–28]

of proper prospective surveillance programs, and small sample size. In retrospective studies, many infections, particularly more superficial ones, may never be reported, because they may be treated by veterinarians other than the primary surgeon or not be reported in the medical record at the surgical facility. Therefore, retrospective studies likely provide an underestimation of true SSI rates. In human surgery, in which surveillance programs are more rigorous, the overall SSI rate is ~5% but is still considered largely underestimated because of the reasons outlined earlier.

Common Pathogens Recovered from Canine Surgical Site Infections

A variety of pathogens can result in SSIs in dogs; however, bacteria are most common and are the focus of this section (**Table 3**). Staphylococci are most commonly cultured from canine SSI,[8,21,24,27] likely because of their commensal and opportunistic nature. Before 2007, *Staphylococcus intermedius* was believed to be the major canine staphylococcal pathogen, but molecular reclassification studies have shown that this bacterium is *Staphylococcus pseudintermedius*.[29] This species has rapidly emerged as the most common cause of canine SSI worldwide, with a recent concerning trend being an apparent marked increase in methicillin and multidrug resistance.[8,30,31] Methicillin resistance confers resistance against all β-lactam antimicrobials, in addition to other commonly used antimicrobials, which poses a tremendous treatment challenge.

Table 3
Common pathogens found in canine SSI

Pathogen	Notes
Staphylococcus pseudintermedius	Formerly known as *S intermedius* Commensal organism of canines Biofilm-forming ability Most commonly found pathogen of canine SSI Limited zoonotic potential Methicillin and multidrug resistance common
Staphylococcus aureus	Commensal organism of humans Biofilm-forming ability Infrequent cause of canine SSI Greater zoonotic potential Methicillin and multidrug resistance common
Coagulase-negative staphylococci (CONS)	Comprises several species, including *S epidermidis, S schleiferi schleiferi, S haemolyticus, S lentus, S capitus* Commensal organism in a variety of animals Methicillin and multidrug resistance variable Uncommon cause of SSI Can be contaminants Commonly found in immunocompromised patients
Pseudomonas spp	Thrive in moist conditions allowing for environmental persistence Biofilm-forming ability High-level multidrug resistance can occur
Enterococci	Commensal of gastrointestinal tract in a variety of animals High-level multidrug resistance can occur Resistant to a variety of drug classes Ability to persist in host for long periods Usually of limited virulence but can be difficult to treat when disease is present
Extended spectrum β-lactamase (ESBL) producing Enterobacteriaceae	Includes *E coli, Enterobacter,* and *Klebsiella* spp Seem to be an emerging problem in veterinary medicine High-level multidrug resistance can occur

Adapted from Weese JS, van Duijkeren E. Methicillin-resistant Staphylococcus aureus and Staphylococcus pseudintermedius in veterinary medicine. Vet Microbiol 2010;140(3–4):418–29; and Weese JS. A review of multidrug resistant surgical site infections. Vet Comp Orthop Traumatol 2008;21(1):1–7.

S aureus, the human counterpart to *S pseudintermedius*, is the leading cause of human SSIs and is a cause of SSIs in dogs, albeit less frequently than *S pseudintermedius*.[32–35] The incidence of methicillin-resistant *S pseudintermedius* (MRSP) SSI is increasing, which is of great concern, because this bacterium has wide multidrug resistance, even greater than methicillin-resistant *S aureus* (MRSA).[30,35,36] In addition, *S pseudintermedius* has strong biofilm-forming ability, which can further complicate treatment, especially in implant-associated SSI.[37] *S pseudintermedius* has lower zoonotic potential compared with *S aureus*; however, zoonotic infections have been reported.[35] In an investigation into bacterial load and type on veterinary surgeons hands, 5% of small animal veterinarians were determined to be carriers of *S pseudintermedius*, whereas no other group of veterinary or human health care workers carried this bacterium,[38] underlining the dissemination of this bacterium in small animal practice. For additional information on staphylococcal pathogens in dogs see the article entitled “Hospital-associated infections in small animal practice” by Stull, elsewhere in this issue.

CHALLENGES AND RISKS

The source of bacterial contamination in a surgical wound can be endogenous and exogenous. The endogenous sources of contamination come from the patient's commensal microbiota at the surgical site or distant body sites (eg, skin, oropharynx, gastrointestinal tract). The exogenous sources of contamination are those originating from the surgical team, the environment, and the materials and instruments used. By carefully selecting (eg, avoid operating on a patient with remote infections) and preparing the patient, endogenous sources of contamination can be reduced; exogenous factors are likely the biggest challenges. Reported risk factors for SSI in small animal surgery are listed in **Table 4**.

Table 4
Reported risk factors associated with small animal surgical procedures

Risk Factor for SSI	Protective Factor For SSI	Reference
Hypotension, surgical wound classification and implant	None identified	Turk et al,[8] 2014
Anesthesia time	Postoperative administration of antimicrobials	Nazarali et al,[21] 2014
Use of a nonlocking plate in TPLO	Postoperative administration of antimicrobials	Solano et al,[22] 2014
None identified	Staples vs suture for skin closure	Etter et al,[23] 2013
Synthes implant in TPLO	None identified	Savicky et al,[24] 2013
Hair clipped at surgical site >4 h Surgical time	None identified	Mayhew et al,[20] 2012
None identified	Postoperative administration of antimicrobials	Gatineau et al,[26] 2011
TPLO vs extracapsular stifle stabilization	Suture for skin closure Postoperative administration of antimicrobials	Frey et al,[28] 2010
Increasing body weight Intact male	Postoperative administration of antimicrobials Labrador retriever	Fitzpatrick & Solano,[27] 2010
Duration of surgery Increasing number of persons in the OR Dirty surgical wound classification	Antimicrobial prophylaxis	Eugster et al,[11] 2004
Intact males Concurrent endocrinopathy Duration of surgery Duration of anesthesia time	None identified	Nicholson et al,[14] 2002
Duration of anesthesia	None identified	Beal et al,[15] 2000
Use of propofol for anesthetic induction	None identified	Heldmann et al,[16] 1999
Antimicrobial prophylaxis not administered	Antimicrobial prophylaxis	Whittem et al,[18] 1999
Duration of surgery Time of preoperative clipping	None identified	Brown et al,[12] 1997
Postoperative rectal temperature Duration of surgery	Antimicrobial prophylaxis	Vasseur et al,[13] 1988

Data from Refs.[8,11–16,18,20–24,26,27]

Surgical asepsis prevents wound contamination from microorganisms that originate from the patient, the OR personnel, and the environment. The methods and practices that prevent contamination are defined in part by surgical technique and are described in the prevention section of this article. Proper prevention measures are not an individual action but involve adequate preparation of the surgical facility and the environment, surgical site, surgical and anesthesia team, and surgical equipment. Basic rules are straightforward and simple to implement but are often not followed. Every member of a health care setting, including the surgeon, assistants, cleaning staff and the management team, carries responsibility for the achievement of aseptic procedures and the corresponding success of surgeries. Adhering to all these practices builds the basis of **surgical and OR team conscience**. To deliver quality patient care, all members of the surgical team must possess honesty and moral integrity enough to be able to perform their required duties to the best of their ability, as well as recognize, report, and correct breaks in aseptic technique. There must not be any hesitation to carry out this duty. In this aspect, denial is our biggest enemy.

Compliance as a Risk Factor

Risk factors for various surgical procedures have been established in human medicine and include the patient's health status (eg, diabetes, nicotine use, alcoholism, obesity, malnutrition) and potential bacterial carriage (eg, MRSA). The type of surgical procedure, surgical environment, surgical expertise, and postoperative care all contain risk factors for the development of SSI in humans. Many of these factors are probably also applicable in veterinary medicine. Risk factors reported in veterinary surgery are listed in **Table 4**. Like in human surgery, duration of the procedure both in surgery and anesthesia time is a consistent finding in risk analysis. Nevertheless, many identified risk factors can be attributed to our own behavior, and **the prime and most threatening factor for development of SSI is probably ourselves.**

In humans, SSIs are considered the most preventable of all the HAIs. Yet, despite the available literature and the many guidelines that are accessible, compliance rates remain unsatisfactory.[39] In a survey performed in human surgeons,[40] 63% did not comply with the current recommended guidelines on preoperative bathing, hair removal, antimicrobial prophylaxis (AMP), and intraoperative skin preparation. In comparison, an observational study in companion animal clinics reported inconsistent and often poor compliance to well-established surgical preparation practices.[41] Recommended times for antiseptic soap during patient surgical site and surgeon hand preparation are at least 2 minutes; however, observations made in the study[41] reported that these times can be as low as 10 and 7 seconds, respectively.[41] Further, this study reported that nonsterile contact with the previously aseptically prepared surgical site occurs in at least 36% of cases.[41] Many similar examples are available in human surgery,[42] and the example most difficult to understand is probably that of hand hygiene. Although Semmelweis's discovery was regarded as controversial at the time, this simple, cheap, and efficient method of SSI prevention is recognized as a pioneering and key infection prevention element.[43] Considering that, in addition to patient care concerns, animal health care workers are also exposed to zoonotic disease risks, it is difficult to understand why reported compliance rates with hand hygiene are so low. In a recent observational study of small animal veterinarians,[44] it was shown that compliance rate was only 14%, and that only 3% performed a hand wash before and after patient contact. In a human study, more extensive hygienic measures than recommended did not have a significant impact on SSI; however, failing to comply with principles of asepsis showed a 3.5 times increase in risk for SSI development.[45]

Tibial Plateau Leveling Osteotomy

Tibial plateau leveling osteotomy (TPLO) is one of the most commonly performed surgical techniques to stabilize a cranial cruciate insufficient stifle joint in dogs.[46] It is classified as a clean, orthopedic surgical procedure but is associated with an unusually higher incidence of SSI compared with other clean surgical procedures.[21–24,27] Multiple factors have been suggested for this situation, including prolonged surgical and anesthesia times, aggressive periosteal dissection of the proximal tibia, thermal injury from the osteotomy saw, reduced soft tissue coverage of the proximal tibia, and use of an implant.[27] However, many of these factors are present in non-TPLO orthopedic surgical procedures, such as fracture fixation, corrective osteotomy, and total joint replacement, yet, SSI incidence is lower than for TPLO. Similarly, in humans, a high tibial wedge valgization osteotomy procedure is performed for treatment of unicompartment stifle osteoarthritis,[47–49] with infection rates ranging from 0.5% to 4.7%, which is within the reported range for clean surgical procedures.[47,48] The reason for the high incidence of SSI after TPLO remains unknown but is likely complex and multifactorial.

Risk factors associated with TPLO SSI reported in the veterinary literature are listed in **Table 4**. In many institutions, humans undergoing elective orthopedic surgery are screened to determine whether they are carriers of MRSA, because it is the leading cause of SSI.[32,33] It has been shown in numerous studies that the risk of MRSA SSI significantly increases in humans who are nasal carriers of MRSA.[50–53] Based on these findings, many institutions perform eradication protocols in nasal carries of MRSA, most commonly with topical mupirocin. Although less thoroughly studied, a similar role of preoperative colonization with MRSP as a risk factor for MRSP TPLO infections has recently been reported.[54] The overall prevalence of MRSP carriage in dogs at time of admission was 4.4%, and MRSP SSI rate was 2.2%. Preoperative carriers of MRSP were 14 times more likely (odds ratio = 14.8; $P<.0001$; 95% confidence interval, 4.0–54.7) to develop MRSP SSI after TPLO.[54] Although only a small percentage of dogs presenting for TPLO were carriers of MRSP, the association with MRSP SSI deserves further consideration, because the impacts of TPLO SSI can be devastating.[55] In humans presenting for elective orthopedic surgery, a rapid polymerase chain reaction–based test is available to determine MRSA carrier status within a few hours. This test allows for decision making regarding surgery (eg, postpone surgery until decolonized if carrier, alterations in AMP, prescribe decolonization therapy) to occur the same day. In veterinary medicine, a universally used in-house assay for detection of MRSP is not available that would ideally allow surgeons to determine MRSP carrier status at time of consultation with the dog owner, allowing for immediate decision making depending on carrier status. A 48-hour to 72-hour delay for swab results is required, which is not practical in veterinary medicine. Diribe and colleagues[56] developed a rapid loop-mediated amplification procedure for nucleic acid detection for *S pseudintermedius*, with 94.6% sensitivity in ~15 minutes. It remains to be determined whether this rapid detection method of *S pseudintermedius* will gain widespread use in combination with an eradication protocol in dogs carrying MRSP before undergoing TPLO.

To provide further emphasis on the consequences of TPLO SSI, Nicoll and colleagues[55] recently reported the economic impact of TPLO SSI. Postoperative treatment costs associated with TPLO SSI ranged from CAD $145 to $5022 and dogs with SSI returned for a mean of 4.1 ± 2.9 (range 1–13) postoperative visits for additional evaluation related to SSI. The mean duration of final case closure from the day of surgery was significantly longer in SSI dogs (194 days ± 158) compared with control dogs (71 days ± 51). The investigators concluded that the costs for TPLO SSI can be tremendous, emphasizing the need for a thorough, multimodal SSI prevention program.

In humans, antimicrobials are generally not administered more than 24 hours postoperatively, because this practice may contribute to antimicrobial resistance, results in increased patient morbidity, and is not associated with a reduced incidence of SSI.[57–59] Recently, several reports[21,22,26–28] have shown a protective effect of postoperative administration antimicrobials against SSI in dogs undergoing TPLO. The most common antimicrobial prescribed for postoperative administration is cephazolin, a first-generation cephalosporin, which is also most frequently used for perioperative AMP. MRSP is inherently resistant to all β-lactam antimicrobials, yet, it is unknown why postoperative administration of cefazolin is protective against SSI after TPLO in dogs. With evidence from multiple studies[21,22,26–28] showing protection against SSI, postoperative administration of antimicrobials in dogs undergoing TPLO is becoming less controversial and is standard of care at our institutions. Future study into this association is required in a prospective, randomized fashion to ascertain the minimum amount of time of antimicrobial administration required to maintain a protective effect to limit morbidities and development of antimicrobial resistance.

Bacterial Biofilms

Biofilm can be defined as a "microbial derived sessile community characterized by cells that are irreversibly attached to a substratum, embedded in a matrix of extracellular polymeric substance (EPS) that they have produced, and exhibit an altered phenotype with respect to growth rate and gene transcription."[60] Biofilm formation confers a survival advantage that allows persistence of bacteria in a community-based lifestyle compared with a nomadic existence. It has become apparent that bacterial biofilms are implicated in, and complicate, the treatment of SSIs.[60–63] It is suggested that they are involved in 80% of chronic microbial infections in humans.[64] *S pseudintermedius*, the most common bacterial pathogen found in canine SSIs, has been shown to have strong biofilm-forming potential.[37] Embracing and understanding the biofilm theory is essential for veterinarians who may be faced with treating SSIs.

Biofilm lifecycle

Initially, planktonic bacteria reversibly attach to a conditioned surface (eg, suture, implant,). If disruption does not occur, irreversible attachment proceeds, and bacteria replicate and promote cell-to-cell adhesion, allowing biofilm maturation. A key event is the shift of the bacteria from planktonic to sessile (metabolically quiescent), with dramatic reduction in metabolic activity. Commonly used antimicrobials attacking the cell wall of rapidly dividing cells are rendered ineffective. In multilayered biofilm community, the embedded cells are able to communicate with each other through a complex mechanism, allowing the community to make group decisions and promote survival. When reaching a critical point in a particular environment, cells at the edge of the biofilm revert back to a planktonic stage and disperse, initiating the life cycle again.[60,61,65,66]

Diagnosis

Recovering biofilm-embedded cells using standard wound swab cultures is challenging.[67,68] It frequently results in negative cultures on agar media, because of the metabolically quiescent nature of biofilm-embedded bacteria.[67,68] In chronic/persistent soft tissue wounds or implant-associated SSIs, only planktonic bacteria can be cultured using standard microbiological techniques for investigation (wound swab).

The organism identified and results of susceptibility testing may not be representative of the biofilm, and caution must be exercised when interpreting these data, because treatment may fail if based on these results.[60,67]

The challenges associated with diagnosis of biofilm infections in humans have led to the creation of guidelines to aid clinicians (**Box 1**) and can probably be applied in veterinary medicine.

Treatment

Therapy for biofilm-associated infections in veterinary medicine is limited. Minimum inhibitory concentration (MIC) of biofilm-embedded bacteria can be up to 400 times the MIC of planktonic bacteria,[69] and biofilm MIC-based treatment could result in systemic toxicity in the patient. Antimicrobial therapy may suffice for treatment of the clinical signs associated with planktonic infection. However, clinical signs often recur after cessation of therapy.

When dealing with infected fracture-fixation devices, antimicrobial therapy can be performed until radiographic evidence of fracture consolidation has occurred, at which time the implant can be removed.[68] A recent case report[70] described maintenance of a prosthetic hip (cementless) in a dog diagnosed with an implant-associated SSI.

In chronic soft tissue wounds, debridement is considered the treatment of choice for disrupting and removing biofilms.[62,63] Debridement can be performed using hydrosurgical techniques or sharply with a scalpel blade and is believed to disrupt the biofilm. Disruption and dispersal of the biofilm may render it susceptible to the activity of systemic or local antimicrobials. However, chronic wound biofilms can rapidly recover (~24 hours) from debridement, providing only a small window for antimicrobial therapy.[62,63] Based on the properties of a biofilm, it is obvious that current treatment options, such as antimicrobial therapy, are futile, and investigation into novel therapies directed at biofilms is required.

Novel therapies

The architecture of a biofilm has been considered a potential therapeutic target. DispersinB is a naturally occurring *N*-acetylglucosaminidase enzyme produced by *Aggregatibacter actinomycetemcomitans*.[71] It was shown to prevent biofilm formation and disperse a preexisting biofilm by targeting polysaccharides in the glycocalyx.[71] Preliminary in vitro investigation in *S pseudintermedius* has shown that DispersinB is

Box 1
Guidelines for diagnosis of biofilm-associated infections

Microbiological evidence of localized chronic or foreign body–associated infection

Microscopic evidence of aggregated microorganisms

Medical history of biofilm predisposing condition (eg, implanted medical device, cystic fibrosis, infective endocarditis)

Recurrence of infection, particularly if same organism found at various time points

Antibiotic failure or persistent infection despite appropriate selection

Evidence of local or systemic signs that resolve with antibiotic therapy that recur after therapy completed

Adapted from Hall-Stoodley L, Stoodley P, Kathju S, et al. Toward diagnostic guidelines for biofilm-associated infections. FEMS Immunol Med Microbiol 2012;65(2):127–45; with permission.

effective at preventing biofilm formation and eradicating established biofilms.[72] This enzyme may be used in combination with an antimicrobial, because DispersinB renders biofilm-associated cells out of the protective glycocalyx and makes them susceptible to antimicrobials and the host immune response.

Coating implants with a variety of antibiofilm molecules has garnered tremendous interest in the area of biomedical engineering.[65] Coatings such as silver and titanium nanoparticles, antimicrobials, antimicrobial peptides, and various other materials prevent bacterial adhesion and subsequent biofilm formation. Further evaluation of implant coatings with veterinary-specific pathogens is required.

PREVENTION

Current widespread recommendations to reduce SSI in humans are supported by a variable level of evidence. Most of the rules and habits originated in intellectual rationales and expert opinions rather than scientific grounds. Three preventive measures are considered to have a high level of evidence (grade IA) in humans, according to evidence-based guidelines[73]: surgical hand preparation, appropriate AMP, and postponing elective surgeries in cases of active remote infections. Although included in the 1999 CDC guidelines, clipping hair before surgery is now a debatable measure.[73] Similar high-evidence studies are not available in the veterinary literature. Therefore, we have to base ourselves on evidence from human literature. Surgical etiquette, comprising common sense based on theoretic rationale, is still valid, because many standard practices (eg, wearing gloves, gown, masks, and caps) are unlikely to ever be tested in controlled studies, because of the ethics of including a control group. However, it should not be forgotten that the absence of proof is not the proof of absence.[74]

Based on human data, it is said that approximately half of all the identified SSI risk factors are endogenous (eg, age, systemic disease, history of previous surgery) and difficult to modify in the direct preoperative and perioperative periods.[73] However, the other half are exogenous (change of surgeon during surgery, visitors during surgery, hair removal methods) factors that can be adapted easily. Past experience has shown that simple and low-cost interventions have the best chance of having an impact on reduction of HAI.

Evidence-Based and Preventive Measures with High Efficacy

Hand hygiene

According to the World Health Organization, the simple act of hand hygiene is considered a pillar for prevention of spread of infectious disease,[43] and, although lacking strict randomized trials of surgeries with and without previous hand asepsis preparation, it is probably the most important SSI prevention strategy.[73] Knowledge about correct surgical hand preparation is low in both human[42] and veterinary surgeons (Verwilghen and colleagues, unpublished data, 2014). A 2008 Cochrane review addressed the issue of preoperative surgical hand preparation.[75] Alcohol-based waterless formulations are considered as effective as scrubbing.[75] However, considering the numerous advantages of hydroalcoholic solutions (HAS),[76] like rapid antimicrobial action, wider spectrum of activity, fewer side effects, lower potential for resistance development, and the absence of recontamination risk with rinsing water, this method is recommended over traditional hand scrubbing in both human and veterinary surgery.[77–81] Despite, and in contradiction with their own stated beliefs that HAS are superior for hand asepsis, 66% of respondents to a survey of American and European College of Veterinary Surgeons specialists do not follow these recommendations.[82] This finding confirms that surgeons' behavior in the operating theater does not necessarily correlate with their scientific knowledge,[42] and that even compliance with established protocols is low,[41] underlining ourselves as one of the main risk factors in the occurrence of SSI.

In addition, outside the closed environment of the OR, transmission of microbial pathogens by the hands of health care workers during patient care plays a crucial role in the occurrence of SSIs. Hand hygiene is therefore regarded as one of the most effective measures to contain SSIs, particularly superficial SSIs.[83] Several reports have shown a temporal association between interventions to improve hand hygiene measures, compliance rates, or reduced infection rates. A recent British report evaluating the *Clean Your Hands* campaign[84] showed that in the 4-year study period, the alcohol use per bed day increased more than 2-fold simultaneously with a 2-fold decrease in MRSA bacteremia and *Clostridium difficile* infections, strongly emphasizing the importance of these measures. To achieve these results, compliance with hand hygiene measures should be improved. The weakest link seems to be the surgeons and physicians, because compliance in these groups seems to be more difficult to obtain than from the nursing staff.[85,86] The introduction of HAS and improving the accessibility of materials have been identified as associated with higher hand hygiene compliance rates.[87,88] For additional information on hand hygiene, see the article entitled "Contact precautions and hand hygiene in veterinary clinics" by Anderson, elsewhere in this issue.

Appropriate antimicrobial prophylaxis

General principles

SSI risk is based on the equation shown in **Fig. 1**. Bacterial contamination occurs in each surgical wound and can progress to SSI if the host defense response is overwhelmed. Foreign material in a wound can further potentiate infection.[89] Zimmerli and colleagues[90] showed that nonphagocytosable material in surgical wounds induces a defect in granulocytes, which could allow for SSI to develop even in the face of strict aseptic technique. To reduce bacterial contamination to a level that the host defense response can prevent SSI development, prophylactic administration of antimicrobials is frequently performed in human and veterinary medicine (see **Fig. 1**). AMP, performed in the absence of established infection, is indicated in surgical procedures with the wound classification clean-contaminated or contaminated, because of the heightened risk of SSI. The use of AMP in clean wounds is controversial in both human and veterinary medicine. This wound classification is associated with a low incidence of SSI; however, many elective orthopedic procedures in veterinary surgery (eg, TPLO, total hip replacement) are classified as a clean surgical wound, yet, SSI development can result in devastating consequences. For this reason, in veterinary medicine, AMP has become standard practice for most elective orthopedic surgery or any procedures involving implant placement or when SSI development would be catastrophic, despite the clean wound classification.

In 2002, the CDC and Centers for Medicare and Medicaid Services developed the Surgical Care Improvement Project (SCIP) in a joint effort to reduce SSI incidence in humans.[91] Within this comprehensive project, 3 measures relating to AMP were developed: (1) selection of antimicrobials based on expected pathogens, (2) appropriate

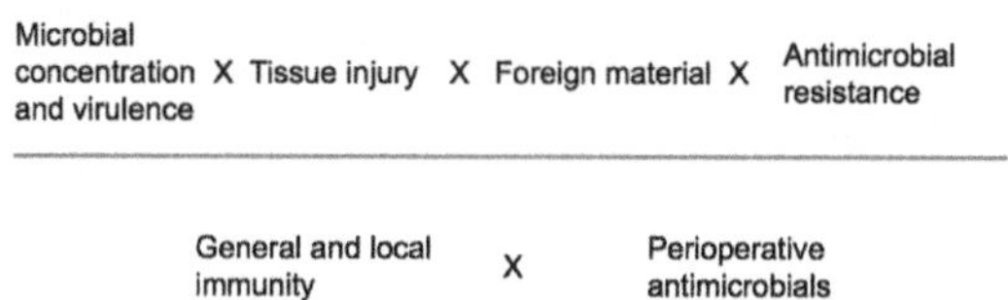

Fig. 1. Risk of SSIs.

timing of antimicrobial administration to ensure peak serum concentration at time of incision, and (3) discontinuation of prophylactic antimicrobials within 24 hours postoperatively.[91] A fourth factor discussed by others is appropriate intraoperative redosing of antimicrobials.[92] These guidelines have reduced morbidity and mortality associated with SSI in humans.[93–96] Guidelines for AMP use have not been established in veterinary medicine; however, current recommendations are extrapolated from human medicine and are likely transferrable across species. Several veterinary studies have shown that the use of AMP reduces SSI in certain cases, depending on surgical wound classification.[11,12,17,18] AMP complements meticulous aseptic surgical technique and appropriate infection control strategies and is not a reason to compromise in these areas.

Selection of antimicrobials

The surgeon must be knowledgeable about the anticipated pathogen(s) to be encountered, depending on the surgical procedure. Empirically selecting antimicrobials with a narrow spectrum of activity is recommended to preserve the patient's normal flora and reduce development of antimicrobial resistance. Surgical procedures, anticipated pathogen(s), and recommended antimicrobial(s) are listed in **Table 5**.

Table 5
List of small animal surgical procedures, anticipated pathogen(s), and recommended antimicrobial(s)

Procedure	Anticipated Pathogen(s)	Recommended Antimicrobial
Skin and reconstructive surgery	*Staphylococcus* spp (*S pseudintermedius* most common)	Cefazolin
Head and neck surgery	*Staphylococcus* spp, *Streptococcus* spp, anaerobes	Clindamycin or cefazolin
Orthopedic and Neurologic		
Elective procedures, closed fractures, spinal decompression	*Staphylococcus* spp	Cefazolin
Open fractures	*Staphylococcus* spp, *Streptococcus* spp, anaerobes	Cefazolin
Cardiothoracic surgery	*Staphylococcus* spp	Cefazolin
GI		
Hepatobiliary surgery	*Clostridia* sp, gram-negative bacilli, anaerobes	Cefoxitin
Upper GI	Gram-positive cocci, enteric gram-negative bacilli	Cefazolin
Lower GI	Enterococci, gram-negative bacilli, anaerobes	Cefoxitin
Ruptured bowel	Enteric gram-negative bacilli, enterococci, anaerobes, gram-positive cocci	Ampicillin + fluoroquinolone
Abdominal surgery	*Staphylococcus* spp	Cefazolin
Urogenital surgery	*Escherichia coli*, *Streptococcus* spp, anaerobes	Cefazolin or ampicillin

Abbreviation: GI, gastrointestinal.

Timing of administration of antimicrobial prophylaxis

This subject has received considerable attention in human medicine, because timing of administration may be one of the most critical aspects of AMP. Current established guidelines for humans, established by the CDC as part of the SCIP, include administration of an appropriately selected antimicrobial within 60 minutes of surgical incision, readministration every 2 half-lives to maintain therapeutic concentrations, and then, discontinuing antimicrobial administration within 24 hours postoperatively.[97,98] Despite the reported reduction in morbidity and mortality associated with SCIP guidelines for timing of administration of AMP,[93–96] compliance is poor in human medicine. Bratzler and colleagues[99] showed that only 55.7% of 34,133 surgical patients received antibiotics within 60 minutes of incision. In a study evaluating AMP and the risk of SSI after total hip replacement in 1922 patients,[100] the highest odds ratio for SSI was found in patients who received AMP after incision.

Guidelines based on recommendations in humans for timing of administration of AMP are also followed in veterinary medicine yet have undergone little scrutiny.[21,101] Nazarali and colleagues[21] retrospectively evaluated AMP practices in 226 cases of TPLO at a single institution. Only 42.5% of dogs met SCIP guidelines for timing of AMP and dose.[21] Although this finding was not statistically associated with SSI in this study, prolonged time from administration of antimicrobial to incision was trending toward increased SSI risk. A similar association was seen with increased SSI risk when intraoperative dosing was delayed or not given at all.[21] The lack of statistical significance between lack of compliance with timing of AMP administration and SSI could be a true association, which has been found in several human studies,[102,103] or it may have been a result of reduced statistical power. Regardless, all efforts should be made to ensure appropriate timing of administration of AMP.

Postoperative administration of antimicrobials

Human guidelines[98] recommend cessation of AMP within 24 hours postoperatively. In human studies,[57–59] continuing AMP beyond this point has not shown a beneficial effect in reducing SSI and may contribute to antimicrobial resistance. Guidelines for postoperative use of AMP in veterinary medicine do not exist; however, extrapolation from human medicine is common. The 1 surgical procedure exception is TPLO, for which several reports[21,22,26–28] have documented the protective effect of postoperative administration of antimicrobials against SSI development. It is assumed that only a few days of postoperative antimicrobial administration is required, because if the SSI pathogens remain in the wound beyond this time, extending therapy to 14 days is not of any further benefit. Further investigation into this association is required to determine the ideal length of time of postoperative administration of antimicrobials to reduce TPLO SSI risk as well as limit the development of antimicrobial resistance and patient morbidity.

Postponing elective surgeries in case of remote infection or systemic disease

Although lacking any randomized trials, this issue is regarded as high evidence by the CDC guidelines[104] and is supported by numerous retrospective reports, in which remote infections were found to be significant risk factors in the development of SSI.[105–107] The most common origin of remote site infections are the lungs and gastrointestinal and urinary tracts.[108,109]

The preoperative systemic inflammatory status of the patient has also been correlated with increased risk,[110,111] as have several factors like obesity, smoking, diabetes, and nutritional status of the patient and intake of certain medication.[104] In veterinary patients, wound and skin infections are likely both of greatest occurrence and greatest risk, and postponing elective surgery in patients with those conditions is a prudent approach.

Active and postdischarge surveillance programs

Surveillance has a dramatic impact on reduction of HAI, including SSI,[112] and surveillance has now become an essential part of SSI prevention.[113] Active surveillance (**Table 6**) programs may have an impact on SSI rate decrease merely by reporting without any other formal form of intervention.[114] Nevertheless, SSI data collection allows for calculation of risk-specific infection rates and can be used by the local hospital and entire health care system to set priorities in infection control programs, review of protocols, and evaluation of the effectiveness of their efforts.[115] In one of the first large-scale reports from US hospitals published in 1985,[112] it was estimated that 32% of hospital-associated infections could be avoided by the implementation of a program, and a specific surgical wound program in the same period[3] showed that SSI rates declined from 3.5% to less than 1% after implementation of a surveillance program.

Implementation of surveillance programs first requires the use of standardized definitions, allowing comparison within and among veterinary health care institutions. Further, putting these strategies into practice is complex and requires engineering changes in behavioral and logistical aspects[116,117] and often becomes frustrating for driving forces behind the program. It may require several years to reach full effectiveness, but powerful impacts ranging from a 25% to 50% decrease in SSI rates within 4 to 6 years can be achieved.[118,119] Recently, the crucial importance of including active postdischarge surveillance (PDS) in these programs has become clear,[73] considering that 20% to 94% of SSIs are diagnosed only after discharge,[10,120,121] and statistically higher SSI rates are reported when PDS is applied,[122] particularly in cases of superficial SSI, which may not be serious enough to warrant readmission to a hospital.[122] In the sole report of prospective SSI surveillance in veterinary medicine, active follow-up of SSI cases and scrutiny of medical records have shown that approximately 35% of SSIs are not reported in the medical record system,[8] underlining the importance of prospective data collection.

Surgical experience, technique, and operating room etiquette

Many surgeons rightly consider that the most critical factor in the prevention of SSI (although one that is difficult to measure scientifically) is the sound judgment and proper technique of the surgeon and surgical team.[122] It is impossible to perform randomized trials of this subjective area. An excellent surgical technique with strict adherence to Halsted principles is believed to reduce SSI. Maintaining adequate hemostasis and preserving blood supply, gentle handling of the tissues, removal of devitalized tissue, eradication of dead space, and appropriate management of the postoperative incision are all gestures and actions that can be learned and for which experience increases performance[123] and reduces complications. This statement is supported by several human and veterinary studies,[124,125] in which the experience of the surgeon,

Table 6
Active versus passive surveillance

Passive Surveillance	Active Surveillance
Routine reporting of cases by health care providers; no special effort is made to identify cases	Routine reporting of cases by health care providers in addition to active contact by infection control team with surgeons and nursing team in order to identify cases

both in general and for a particular procedure, was associated with lower SSI, wound complications, or even patient survival. Studies[126,127] have also reported a higher incidence of wound dehiscence in abdominal procedures when closure was performed by a trainee rather than an attending surgeon. Similar findings were reported in a veterinary study in which closure of the abdominal wound by first-year and second-year residents was considered a significant risk factor for development of SSI.[128] Considering that surgical and anesthesia time is often reported as a crucial risk factor in complication development, it is easy to relate inexperience with longer surgery. However, in the veterinary study mentioned earlier, surgery and anesthesia time were not different in level of experience,[128] probably indicating that several other factors, such as technique, sound judgment, and adherence to aseptic principles contribute to a greater extent in unexperienced surgeons. Relating to our personal experience, confidence with procedures increases with the years and number of procedures performed, reducing stress and improving decision making and concentration on the task. It is probable, therefore, that similar to the preparation of professional sportsmen, some recommend the inclusion of mental/cognitive training into the curriculum of surgeons.[123,129]

Longer wound exposure times and longer tissue manipulation provide more opportunities for pathogens to seed into the wound and cause SSI, allowing for a greater chance of wound desiccation or other forms of damage. Although surgeon experience can be 1 factor in extending operation time, time spent in surgery is dictated by the entire surgical team. Surgical planning, availability of appropriate instrumentations, delivery of requested disposals in an efficient way, coordination with diagnostic imaging, and myriad other factors can reduce surgical time. Hospitals in which surgical, anesthesia, and nursing teams are unfamiliar with their role and communication function have been shown to prolong teamwork intervals, resulting in higher than usual SSI rates.[130]

The establishment of proper OR etiquette receives little attention in the veterinary community, and its importance is likely underestimated. Although probably a surrogate outcome to assess behavior of the surgical team, noise level in the surgical theater has been significantly correlated with higher SSI rates in human medicine.[131] Noise leads to a significant decrease in concentration capacity[131] and in a significant increase in errors[132] performed during the surgery. Talking about non–surgery-related topics has not only been shown to reduce concentration to the task but is significantly associated with higher sound levels.[131] Potentially, noise could also be a proxy for more or louder talking, corresponding to greater aerosolization of pathogens in the OR.

One of the most interesting articles on the subject that should remind us that our daily work involves variable issues that affect outcomes is a study on the impact of intraoperative behavior on SSIs.[45] This prospective investigation of more than 1000 procedures showed clearly that lapses in discipline by the surgical team were an independent risk factor for development of SSIs. Increased movement in the theater, exchange of surgical team members, noise, and the presence of visitors in the OR all independently contributed to an increase in infection rates. Considering that the implementation of checklists into surgical routine was shown to decrease surgical complications of all sorts significantly,[133] improving OR discipline may also be able to reduce morbidities other than purely SSI.

> Surgical technique is one of the primary factors in preventing wound infection.
>
> Poor surgical technique cannot be overridden by the use of antibiotics or any other method.

Table 7
Low evidence–based but commonly accepted measures for prevention of SSI

	Human Evidence and Recommendations	Veterinary Evidence
Preoperative Patient Preparation		
	SURGICAL SITE PREPARATION: HAIR REMOVAL	
	• Clipping superior to shaving • Timing hair removal no effect Hair removal only if it interferes with surgical site	• No randomized controlled trial or valuable studies available • Presence of hair does not reduce ability of antiseptics to reduce bacterial flora in sites for arthrocentesis in horses[134] • Clipping before induction vs after increases SSI risk[12]
Veterinary recommendations	• Removing of hair mostly indicated unless in nonhaired to very poor haired regions • Use clippers, not razors for hair removal • Remove hair immediately before surgery/after induction of anesthesia • Start with clean patient/groom outside the surgery ward	
	SURGICAL SITE PREPARATION: DISINFECTION	
	• Little evidence for superior method • Use of 0.5% or 2% chlorhexidine with methylated considered superior[73,135]; however, latest trial no difference with iodine-based alcohol[136] • Alcohol-based products probably more efficient and longer lasting than aqueous-based solutions[137] • Investigation into new methods that target high bacterial load into hair follicles[138] • Cyanoacrylate microbial sealants: small positive difference in SSI rates but still weak evidence[139] No particular recommendations	• No randomized controlled trial available • Number of studies available[140–149] but conflicting results and no evidence for superior method • Most studies look at bacterial reduction and not SSI end point
Veterinary recommendations	• Prepare surgical site immediately before surgery with aqueous-based or alcohol-based biocide • Chlorhexidine and povidone iodine are suitable	

(continued on next page)

Table 7
(*continued*)

	Human Evidence and Recommendations	Veterinary Evidence
	SURGICAL SITE PREPARATION: PREOPERATIVE BATHING OR SHOWERING WITH SKIN ANTISEPTICS	
	There is no evidence for benefit of preoperative bathing or showering with chlorhexidine over other wash products to reduce SSI[150]	• No studies in this field available
Veterinary recommendations	For maximum efficacy of the product and to reduce spreading of large quantities of active ingredient of biocides (potential for chlorhexidine resistance development[151]) in the environment, gross decontamination with a neutral soap wash of the surgical area is advised before starting the aseptic skin preparation procedure	
	SURGICAL SITE PREPARATION: DRAPING	
	• Little evidence investigating various drape types • Use of drapes based on theoretic rationale of reducing contamination of surgical site by surrounding area • Disposable provides highest cost/benefit ratio[152] and is more efficient in reducing SSI than reusable[153] • One randomized trial (low number of patients) showing clear superiority of single use compared with reusable in reducing SSI[154]	• Retrospective study found no difference in SSI using disposable vs drapes[155] • Cost-effectiveness of single use probably same as in humans
Veterinary recommendations	• Draping the surgical site is advised • Best practice: use of impervious single-use disposable drapes[156]	
	SURGICAL SITE PREPARATION: INCISE FILMS	
	• No effect[157,158] of incise drapes on reduction of SSI rate, non–iodophore-impregnated incise drapes may even increase the risk of SSIs,[157,158] because of higher bacterial regrowth under the drape[158] • Application technique is important, lifting of the edges of adhesive drapes may enhance bacterial contamination[159] If used, use iodophore impregnated with proper application technique	• No trial available
Veterinary recommendations	Do not use routinely; if used, use iodophore impregnated with proper application technique	

	SURGICAL SITE PREPARATION: PLASTIC BUSTER-TYPE DRAPES	
	• Pure plastic draping is not used in human medicine; no trials available	Plastic buster-type drapes are widely used in veterinary medicine. Although there are no trials available either on the difference between SSI rates or on the bacterial growth potential underneath buster-type plastic drapes and conventional woven reusable or disposable drapes, evidence from human medicine shows substantial increase in bacterial regrowth under plastic drapes. Increased moisture retention near the skin could facilitate bacterial growth.[158] Clinical experience shows that patients often sweat profusely under these drapes. Plastic buster drapes are therefore not recommended
Veterinary recommendations	• Until further evidence with regards to their safety is available, their use should be abandoned	
Preparation of the Surgical Team		
	MASKS AND CAPS	
	• No difference between masked/capped and unmasked/uncapped procedures[160] • Bacterial contamination of the operative field has shown to be reduced[156]	• No studies available
Veterinary recommendations	Scrubbed personnel should always wear masks and caps. Considering that face masks and head caps contribute to theater discipline and are therefore beneficial in reducing SSI in other ways, it remains advised for all people in the surgical room to wear them	
	GOWNS	
	• Strong theoretic rationale for reducing bacterial count[161] • Reduced SSI with single-use gowns and impervious material shown in nonrandomized trial[162] • Randomized studies no significant difference[156] • Bacterial strike-through found in 26 of 27 cloth gowns tested compared with 0 of 27 paper gowns. There is a 4-fold higher level of baseline bacterial contamination on cloth gowns sleeves than in paper gowns[161]	• No evidence specific to veterinary medicine
Veterinary recommendations	Wear of sterile gowns is recommended for all surgical procedures. As per European standard, the use of single-use disposable gowns is recommended.[156] Pure plastic gowns are not recommended for similar reasons to those mentioned above for plastic draping	

(*continued on next page*)

Table 7
(continued)

	Human Evidence and Recommendations	Veterinary Evidence
	GLOVES	
	• Gloving based on theoretic rational of reducing bacterial contamination originating from hands. No randomized controlled trial with and without wear of surgical gloves. Historical benefit shown • High rate of glove puncture depending on procedure. ≤80% of punctures go unnoticed[163,164] • Importance of good hand preparation independently of wear of surgical gloves, because higher SSI rates reported because of glove punctures[165] • Bacterial passage is reported in approximately 5% of perforations[166] • Recommended timing for glove change is variable and depending on procedure, range from 60 to 150 min,[167] but significantly more punctures have been found 90 min within surgery[164] • Puncture risk increases by 1.12 per 60 min of surgery	• Glove perforation shown to vary from 10% to 26%[168–170] • Most prevalent in index finger nondominant hand[169,170] • Significantly more punctures in orthopedic vs soft tissue surgery[168–170] • Most punctures occur in procedures lasting >60 min[168–170]
Veterinary recommendations	• Use of sterile gloves is always needed • Good hand preparation independently of use of sterile gloves • Change gloves after 60–90 min	
	DOUBLE GLOVING	
	• From low-powered studies, there is no evidence that double gloving reduces SSI; however, a second pair of gloves significantly reduces perforations to the innermost gloves[171,172] • Perforation indicators result in significantly more detection of perforations[171] • Change outer glove before handling implants because of increased bacterial load on outer glove[161]	• No studies available
Veterinary recommendations	• Use double gloving for draping and discard outer pair for the surgical procedure • Use double gloving for implant related procedures or procedures with high risk of glove perforation • Use double gloving, special orthopedic gloves or indicator gloves for orthopedic procedures or procedures lasting >60 min • Change outer glove when handling implants	

Intraoperative Measures		
	DEBRIDEMENT	
	• There is a lack of randomized controlled trials comparing the effect of debridement and different debridement methods[173]	• No studies available
Veterinary recommendations	Debridement of contaminated wounds remains a key factor in reducing the bacterial and foreign body load, both factors known to increase the risk of SSI. However, the method of debridement should be chosen based on situation and surgeon's preference	
	WOUND DRESSING	
	• Following the conclusions of a recent Cochrane review, there is no evidence to suggest that covering surgical wounds healing by primary intention with wound dressings reduces the risk for SSI or that any wound dressing is more effective than others. Based on small poor-quality trials[174]	• No randomized trial or meta-analysis available • Some equine studies show the protective effect of belly bands or stents bandage in reducing SSI risk[175,176] • All available studies are small, with considerable bias
Veterinary recommendations	Although evidence is confusing, the covering of the surgical site has many advantages to improve healing of the surgical site. Considering the environment in which our veterinary patients reside and considering their tendency to lick and bite their surgical wounds, independently of the scientific evidence, wound protection remains advised	
	SUTURE CHOICE	
	• Monofilament sutures are less prone to potentiate infections than multifilament sutures, because of decreased bioadherence and improvement of phagocytic cells to reach bacteria on or within sutures[159] • Continuous sutures of the same material are associated with fewer infections than interrupted sutures, possibly because of reduction of tissue necrosis at suture site and more even distribution of tension and reduced suture material[159] • Stapled wounds in orthopedic surgery are more at risk of infection than sutured wounds[177] • Different studies show decrease in SSI rates with the use of antimicrobial-impregnated sutures[159]	• Triclosan-impregnated sutures did not decrease infection in TPLO surgeries[23] • No beneficial effect of triclosan in equine abdominal wall closure[178] • Inconclusive evidence for staples vs sutures
Veterinary recommendations	• Suture choice is important • Antimicrobial-impregnated sutures may be of some benefit based on theoretic rational, but they have not been tested sufficiently in well-controlled studies. Their widespread use is therefore not recommended	

Table 8
Promising avenues in prevention of SSI and future research

Screening for multiresistant staphylococci carriage on admission	The rationale behind this approach is to reduce SSI by detection of resistant bacteria carriers before the incision and to administer prophylaxis or decolonize before surgery. In human settings, some before and after studies have shown a benefit, whereas other crossover design trials have failed to show a decrease in SSI.[73] In veterinary settings, dogs undergoing surgery have been shown to be at significant risk of contracting *S pseudintermedius* colonization during their hospitalization.[180] Some studies have found MRSP carriage to be a significant risk factor for SSI[54]; however, other veterinary studies found no association between colonization status and infections.[181] Final outcome remains debatable, and further studies are warranted
Screening for nasal *S aureus* colonization and decolonization	Screening for nasal *S aureus* colonization in humans with subsequent decolonization can significantly reduce hospital-acquired *S aureus*[182] colonization; however, they generally fail or show limited potential in reduction of SSI rates.[73] Nasal colonization of MRSA is less frequent in animals
Intraoperative hypothermia	Hypothermia increases the risk for development of wound infections, because of the adverse effects on immunologic and physiologic functions necessary to kill bacterial contamination.[159] The primary beneficial effect of normorthermia is mediated through increased blood flow and oxygenation tension at the tissue levels Hypothermia affects molecular interactions and cellular functions of numerous systems, including coagulation, viscosity, packed cell volume, and the immune and endocrine system.[73] One veterinary study[15] investigating the effects of hypothermia during surgery in dogs did not find that mild hypothermia was correlated with higher SSI incidence. This finding is clearly in controversy with human data, in which several studies have shown high relative risks for postoperative wound infection in nonwarmed patients vs warmed[73,159]
Glucose control	Although dogs with concurrent endocrinopathy have been shown to be 8.2 times more likely to develop infections, none of the animals in that study had diabetes,[14] and a study on intraocular infections after cataract surgery failed to show animals with diabetes to be at increased risk[183] Nevertheless, human patients with diabetes have long been shown to be at risk for increased incidence of several surgery-associated complications. Independently, there are numerous adverse effects of hyperglycemia, separately from diabetes, on the immune system, and hyperglycemia during surgery has been shown to be an independent risk factor for SSI.[73] Recording glycemia levels during surgery and relating them to SSI would be an interesting further research topic in veterinary medicine

Oxygenation	Low concentrations of oxygen at wound sites impair antibacterial function of neutrophils and promote the development of SSI.[159] Intraoperative administration of inspired oxygen of <50% was identified as an independent risk factor for SSI[184]; however the results of other studies investigating intraoperative oxygen administration are variable, ranging from a highly significant reduction over no effect to significant increased infection rates.[73] Most likely, this situation is caused by other factors altering the effectiveness of hyperoxia and consequently tissue Po_2, like body temperature, blood pressure, type of anesthesia, fluid management, use of vasopressors, and tissue handling. From a theoretic and physiologic point of view, SSI reduction with supplemental oxygen is believed to be related to low Po_2 in surgical wounds and enhanced oxidative kill of leukocytes with oxygen supply.[73] Supplemental O_2 should start with induction; however, optimal concentration and duration of therapy have not been established. Current human data suggest that it should at least be given for $\geq$2 h after wound closure[159]
Blood transfusion	Although blood transfusions have obvious beneficial effects, including reversal of shock and improved patient survival after acute hemorrhage, blood transfusion is also associated with alterations in numerous immunologic responses and has been identified as a risk factor for SSI.[185] Multifactorial analysis of human studies and experimental trials performed in animal models have shown a clear relationship between blood transfusion and the development of infections. The effect seems to increase with the number of transfusions given, and some evidence suggests that early leukocyte reduction by filtration partially reduces the effect on wound infections[159]
Fluid management	All factors decreasing the delivery of oxygen to a wound can increase the incidence and severity of infection. Although the need for fluid administration during surgery cannot be debated, type, volume, and duration have been put in relationship with SSI development. Restrictive fluid administration during many surgeries may be beneficial compared with liberal fluid administration, as shown in a prospective randomized study showing a significant decrease in SSI with restricted fluids.[186] Ringer solutions as a sole means of fluid may reduce oxygen tension for $\geq$24 h[187]

Low Evidence-Based but Commonly Accepted Measures for Prevention of Surgical Site Infections

Table 7 provides an overview of measures based on knowledge from the human literature that are known to affect the SSI rates, with variable degrees of evidence. The main data reported are based on Cochrane reviews combined with high-evidence supportive trials if available. The veterinary column provides an overview of available studies in the veterinary sector. Recommendations provided are based on current knowledge and expert opinion.

Promising Avenues in Prevention and Future Research

The intraoperative period is important in terms of SSI prevention and leaves room for measures not targeting the transmission of pathogens but rather enhancing the host's immunity. **Table 8** provides an overview of such factors for the prevention of SSI. Although few are based on the veterinary literature and some may seem to be contradictory to some extent, these measures represent possibilities to be implemented in our veterinary surgical routine and used for future research and development. Some of these points, like intraoperative hypothermia, glucose control, and fluid management, clearly underline the multidisciplinary effort needed to reduce SSIs. The role of the anesthesiologist cannot be underestimated in many aspects,[179] including the preparation and administration of drugs. In a veterinary study,[16] the administration of propofol was significantly linked to the development of SSI, likely because of the ease with which this lipid-based emulsion can become contaminated with bacteria. This finding stresses the importance of adhering to good hand hygiene by all members of staff involved.

SUMMARY: MULTIMODAL INTERVENTIONS = CONVERTING THEORY INTO PRACTICE

The development of SSIs is a dynamic process involving several factors, in which the patient, the procedure, and the health care infrastructure and personnel play a role. Optimal SSI prevention is possible only by a multidisciplinary and multimodal approach, in which the most important factor is the consciences of every individual involved. Enhancing compliance with best practice requires an ownership from all concerned. Only when all players realize that they share responsibility for the contribution to success or failure of a surgical procedure will our ambition to reach zero rate SSI come to a reality. Some have therefore postulated that if current guidelines are complied with, surgical infections could decrease lower than 0.5% in clean, 1% in clean-contaminated and less than 2% in highly contaminated wounds.[159] Until then, the human sector has chosen to introduce health care bundles, incorporating validated methods and measures to prevent infection, which are rigorously policed and audited.[122] Although some local regulators have now set mandatory hygiene protocols for veterinary health care settings,[88] in general, it looks like the entire veterinary sector still believes that the emperor is dressed.[188]

REFERENCES

1. Best M, Neuhauser D. Ignaz Semmelweis and the birth of infection control. Qual Saf Health Care 2004;13(3):233–4.
2. Awad SS. Adherence to surgical care improvement project measures and postoperative surgical site infections. Surg Infect (Larchmt) 2012;13(4):234–7.
3. Condon RE, Schulte WJ, Malangoni MA, et al. Effectiveness of a surgical wound surveillance program. Arch Surg 1983;118(3):303–7.

4. Mu Y, Edwards JR, Horan TC, et al. Improving risk-adjusted measures of surgical site infection for the national healthcare safety network. Infect Control Hosp Epidemiol 2011;32(10):970–86.
5. Gibbons C, Bruce J, Carpenter J, et al. Identification of risk factors by systematic review and development of risk-adjusted models for surgical site infection. Health Technol Assess 2011;15(30):1–156, iii–iv.
6. (Center of Disease Control and Prevention) CfDCaP. CDC/NHSN surveillance definitions for specific types of infections. In: DCDC, editor. Atlanta (GA): CDC; 2014.
7. (Center of Disease Control and Prevention) CfDCaP. Surgical site infection (event). In: CDC, editor. Atlanta (GA): CDC; 2014.
8. Turk R, Singh A, Weese JS. Prospective surgical site infection surveillance in dogs. Vet Surg 2014. [Epub ahead of print].
9. Cheadle WG. Risk factors for surgical site infection. Surg Infect (Larchmt) 2006; 7(Suppl 1):S7–11.
10. Staszewicz W, Eisenring MC, Bettschart V, et al. Thirteen years of surgical site infection surveillance in Swiss hospitals. J Hosp Infect 2014;88(1):40–7.
11. Eugster S, Schawalder P, Gaschen F, et al. A prospective study of postoperative surgical site infections in dogs and cats. Vet Surg 2004;33(5):542–50.
12. Brown DC, Conzemius MG, Shofer F, et al. Epidemiologic evaluation of postoperative wound infections in dogs and cats. J Am Vet Med Assoc 1997;210(9):1302–6.
13. Vasseur PB, Levy J, Dowd E, et al. Surgical wound infection rates in dogs and cats. Data from a teaching hospital. Vet Surg 1988;17(2):60–4.
14. Nicholson M, Beal M, Shofer F, et al. Epidemiologic evaluation of postoperative wound infection in clean-contaminated wounds: a retrospective study of 239 dogs and cats. Vet Surg 2002;31(6):577–81.
15. Beal MW, Brown DC, Shofer FS. The effects of perioperative hypothermia and the duration of anesthesia on postoperative wound infection rate in clean wounds: a retrospective study. Vet Surg 2000;29(2):123–7.
16. Heldmann E, Brown DC, Shofer F. The association of propofol usage with postoperative wound infection rate in clean wounds: a retrospective study. Vet Surg 1999;28(4):256–9.
17. Vasseur PB, Paul HA, Enos LR, et al. Infection rates in clean surgical procedures: a comparison of ampicillin prophylaxis vs a placebo. J Am Vet Med Assoc 1985;187(8):825–7.
18. Whittem TL, Johnson AL, Smith CW, et al. Effect of perioperative prophylactic antimicrobial treatment in dogs undergoing elective orthopedic surgery. J Am Vet Med Assoc 1999;215(2):212–6.
19. Holmberg DL. The use of prophylactic penicillin in orthopedic surgery. A clinical trial. Vet Surg 1985;14:160–5.
20. Mayhew PD, Freeman L, Kwan T, et al. Comparison of surgical site infection rates in clean and clean-contaminated wounds in dogs and cats after minimally invasive versus open surgery: 179 cases (2007-2008). J Am Vet Med Assoc 2012;240(2):193–8.
21. Nazarali A, Singh A, Weese JS. Perioperative administration of antimicrobials during tibial plateau leveling osteotomy. Vet Surg 2014;43(8):966–71.
22. Solano MA, Danielski A, Kovach K, et al. Locking plate and screw fixation after tibial plateau leveling osteotomy reduces postoperative infection rate in dogs over 50 kg. Vet Surg 2014. [Epub ahead of print].
23. Etter SW, Ragetly GR, Bennett RA, et al. Effect of using triclosan-impregnated suture for incisional closure on surgical site infection and inflammation following

tibial plateau leveling osteotomy in dogs. J Am Vet Med Assoc 2013;242(3): 355–8.

24. Savicky R, Beale B, Murtaugh R, et al. Outcome following removal of TPLO implants with surgical site infection. Vet Comp Orthop Traumatol 2013;26(4):260–5.
25. Gallagher AD, Mertens WD. Implant removal rate from infection after tibial plateau leveling osteotomy in dogs. Vet Surg 2012;41(6):705–11.
26. Gatineau M, Dupuis J, Plante J, et al. Retrospective study of 476 tibial plateau levelling osteotomy procedures. Rate of subsequent 'pivot shift', meniscal tear and other complications. Vet Comp Orthop Traumatol 2011;24(5):333–41.
27. Fitzpatrick N, Solano MA. Predictive variables for complications after TPLO with stifle inspection by arthrotomy in 1000 consecutive dogs. Vet Surg 2010;39(4): 460–74.
28. Frey TN, Hoelzler MG, Scavelli TD, et al. Risk factors for surgical site infection–inflammation in dogs undergoing surgery for rupture of the cranial cruciate ligament: 902 cases (2005-2006). J Am Vet Med Assoc 2010;236(1):88–94.
29. Sasaki T, Kikuchi K, Tanaka Y, et al. Reclassification of phenotypically identified *Staphylococcus intermedius* strains. J Clin Microbiol 2007;45(9):2770–8.
30. Perreten V, Kadlec K, Schwarz S, et al. Clonal spread of methicillin-resistant *Staphylococcus pseudintermedius* in Europe and North America: an international multicentre study. J Antimicrob Chemother 2010;65(6):1145–54.
31. Weese JS, Faires MC, Frank LA, et al. Factors associated with methicillin-resistant versus methicillin-susceptible *Staphylococcus pseudintermedius* infection in dogs. J Am Vet Med Assoc 2012;240(12):1450–5.
32. Bengtsson S, Hambraeus A, Laurell G. Wound infections after surgery in a modern operating suite: clinical, bacteriological and epidemiological findings. J Hyg (Lond) 1979;83(1):41–57.
33. Norton TD, Skeete F, Dubrovskaya Y, et al. Orthopedic surgical site infections: analysis of causative bacteria and implications for antibiotic stewardship. Am J Orthop (Belle Mead NJ) 2014;43(5):E89–92.
34. Si D, Rajmokan M, Lakhan P, et al. Surgical site infections following coronary artery bypass graft procedures: 10 years of surveillance data. BMC Infect Dis 2014;14:318.
35. Weese JS, van Duijkeren E. Methicillin-resistant *Staphylococcus aureus* and *Staphylococcus pseudintermedius* in veterinary medicine. Vet Microbiol 2010; 140(3-4):418–29.
36. Osland AM, Vestby LK, Fanuelsen H, et al. Clonal diversity and biofilm-forming ability of methicillin-resistant *Staphylococcus pseudintermedius*. J Antimicrob Chemother 2012;67(4):841–8.
37. Singh A, Walker M, Rousseau J, et al. Characterization of the biofilm forming ability of *Staphylococcus pseudintermedius* from dogs. BMC Vet Res 2013;9:93.
38. Thorup S. An investigation into bacterial type and load in on veterinary compared to human healthcare workers. Copenhagen (Denmark): Department of Large Animal Sciences, University of Copenhagen; 2014.
39. Leaper DJ, Tanner J, Kiernan M, et al. Surgical site infection: poor compliance with guidelines and care bundles. Int Wound J 2014. [Epub ahead of print].
40. Davis PJ, Spady D, de Gara C, et al. Practices and attitudes of surgeons toward the prevention of surgical site infections: a provincial survey in Alberta, Canada. Infect Control Hosp Epidemiol 2008;29(12):1164–6.
41. Anderson ME, Foster BA, Weese JS. Observational study of patient and surgeon preoperative preparation in ten companion animal clinics in Ontario, Canada. BMC Vet Res 2013;9:194.

42. Umit UM, Sina M, Ferhat Y, et al. Surgeon behavior and knowledge on hand scrub and skin antisepsis in the operating room. J Surg Educ 2014;71(2):241–5.
43. World Health Organization. WHO guidelines on hand hygiene in health care. Geneva (Switzerland): World Health Organization; 2009. p. 270.
44. Anderson ME, Sargeant JM, Weese JS. Video observation of hand hygiene practices during routine companion animal appointments and the effect of a poster intervention on hand hygiene compliance. BMC Vet Res 2014;10:106.
45. Beldi G, Bisch-Knaden S, Banz V, et al. Impact of intraoperative behavior on surgical site infections. Am J Surg 2009;198(2):157–62.
46. Kim SE, Pozzi A, Kowaleski MP, et al. Tibial osteotomies for cranial cruciate ligament insufficiency in dogs. Vet Surg 2008;37(2):111–25.
47. Anagnostakos K, Mosser P, Kohn D. Infections after high tibial osteotomy. Knee Surg Sports Traumatol Arthrosc 2013;21(1):161–9.
48. Reischl N, Wahl P, Jacobi M, et al. Infections after high tibial open wedge osteotomy: a case control study. Arch Orthop Trauma Surg 2009;129(11):1483–7.
49. von Eiff C, Becker K, Machka K, et al. Nasal carriage as a source of *Staphylococcus aureus* bacteremia. Study Group. N Engl J Med 2001;344(1):11–6.
50. Awad SS, Palacio CH, Subramanian A, et al. Implementation of a methicillin-resistant *Staphylococcus aureus* (MRSA) prevention bundle results in decreased MRSA surgical site infections. Am J Surg 2009;198(5):607–10.
51. Chen AF, Wessel CB, Rao N. *Staphylococcus aureus* screening and decolonization in orthopaedic surgery and reduction of surgical site infections. Clin Orthop Relat Res 2013;471(7):2383–99.
52. Kim DH, Spencer M, Davidson SM, et al. Institutional prescreening for detection and eradication of methicillin-resistant *Staphylococcus aureus* in patients undergoing elective orthopaedic surgery. J Bone Joint Surg Am 2010;92(9):1820–6.
53. Pofahl WE, Goettler CE, Ramsey KM, et al. Active surveillance screening of MRSA and eradication of the carrier state decreases surgical-site infections caused by MRSA. J Am Coll Surg 2009;208(5):981–6 [discussion: 986–8].
54. Nazarali A, Singh A, Weese JS. Evaluation of the impact of preoperative carriage of methicillin-resistant *Staphylococcus pseudintermedius* (MRSP) on MRSP surgical site infection following tibial plateau leveling osteotomy in dogs. Presented at: European College of Veterinary Surgeons Annual symposium; 2014. Copenhagen, Denmark, 2-4 July, 2014.
55. Nicoll C, Singh A, Weese JS. Economic impact of tibial plateau leveling osteotomy surgical site infection in dogs. Vet Surg 2014;43(8):899–902.
56. Diribe O, North S, Sawyer J, et al. Design and application of a loop-mediated isothermal amplification assay for the rapid detection of *Staphylococcus pseudintermedius*. J Vet Diagn Invest 2014;26(1):42–8.
57. McDonald M, Grabsch E, Marshall C, et al. Single- versus multiple-dose antimicrobial prophylaxis for major surgery: a systematic review. Aust N Z J Surg 1998;68(6):388–96.
58. Slobogean GP, Kennedy SA, Davidson D, et al. Single- versus multiple-dose antibiotic prophylaxis in the surgical treatment of closed fractures: a meta-analysis. J Orthop Trauma 2008;22(4):264–9.
59. Terpstra S, Noordhoek GT, Voesten HG, et al. Rapid emergence of resistant coagulase-negative staphylococci on the skin after antibiotic prophylaxis. J Hosp Infect 1999;43(3):195–202.
60. Donlan RM, Costerton JW. Biofilms: survival mechanisms of clinically relevant microorganisms. Clin Microbiol Rev 2002;15(2):167–93.

61. Donlan RM. Biofilms: microbial life on surfaces. Emerg Infect Dis 2002;8(9): 881–90.
62. James GA, Swogger E, Wolcott R, et al. Biofilms in chronic wounds. Wound Repair Regen 2008;16(1):37–44.
63. Percival SL, Hill KE, Williams DW, et al. A review of the scientific evidence for biofilms in wounds. Wound Repair Regen 2012;20(5):647–57.
64. Minutes of the National Advisory Dental and Craniofacial Research Council - 153rd Meeting. National Institutes of Health 1997, September 9. Available at: http://www.nidcr.nih.gov/AboutNIDCR/CouncilAndCommittees/NADCRC/Minutes/Minutes153.htm
65. Arciola CR, Campoccia D, Speziale P, et al. Biofilm formation in *Staphylococcus* implant infections. A review of molecular mechanisms and implications for biofilm-resistant materials. Biomaterials 2012;33(26):5967–82.
66. Dunne WM Jr. Bacterial adhesion: seen any good biofilms lately? Clin Microbiol Rev 2002;15(2):155–66.
67. Stoodley P, Kathju S, Hu FZ, et al. Molecular and imaging techniques for bacterial biofilms in joint arthroplasty infections. Clin Orthop Relat Res 2005;(437):31–40.
68. Trampuz A, Zimmerli W. Diagnosis and treatment of implant-associated septic arthritis and osteomyelitis. Curr Infect Dis Rep 2008;10(5):394–403.
69. Patel R. Biofilms and antimicrobial resistance. Clin Orthop Relat Res 2005;(437): 41–7.
70. Dan BJ, Kim SE, Pozzi A. Management of an infected cementless cup with prosthetic retention and antibiotic therapy in a dog. J Small Anim Pract 2014;55(11):585–8.
71. Gawande PV, Clinton AP, LoVetri K, et al. Antibiofilm efficacy of DispersinB((R)) wound spray used in combination with a silver wound dressing. Microbiol Insights 2014;7:9–13.
72. Turk R, Singh A, Rousseau J, et al. In vitro evaluation of DispersinB on methicillin-resistant *Staphylococcus pseudintermedius* biofilm. Vet Microbiol 2013;166(3–4):576–9.
73. Uckay I, Harbarth S, Peter R, et al. Preventing surgical site infections. Expert Rev Anti Infect Ther 2010;8(6):657–70.
74. Smith GC, Pell JP. Parachute use to prevent death and major trauma related to gravitational challenge: systematic review of randomised controlled trials. BMJ 2003;327(7429):1459–61.
75. Tanner J, Swarbrook S, Stuart J. Surgical hand antisepsis to reduce surgical site infection. Cochrane Database Syst Rev 2008;(1):CD004288.
76. Verwilghen D, Grulke S, Kampf G. Presurgical hand antisepsis: concepts and current habits of veterinary surgeons. Vet Surg 2011;40(5):515–21.
77. Widmer AF, Rotter M, Voss A, et al. Surgical hand preparation: state-of-the-art. J Hosp Infect 2010;74(2):112–22.
78. Nthumba PM, Stepita-Poenaru E, Poenaru D, et al. Cluster-randomized, crossover trial of the efficacy of plain soap and water versus alcohol-based rub for surgical hand preparation in a rural hospital in Kenya. Br J Surg 2010;97(11):1621–8.
79. Widmer AF. Surgical hand hygiene: scrub or rub? J Hosp Infect 2013;83(Suppl 1):S35–9.
80. Pittet D, Allegranzi B, Boyce J. The World Health Organization guidelines on hand hygiene in health care and their consensus recommendations. Infect Control Hosp Epidemiol 2009;30(7):611–22.
81. Verwilghen DR, Mainil J, Mastrocicco E, et al. Surgical hand antisepsis in veterinary practice: evaluation of soap scrubs and alcohol based rub techniques. Vet J 2011;190(3):372–7.

82. Verwilghen D, Findji S, Weese JS, et al. Evidence based hand hygiene in veterinary surgery: what is holding us back? Presented at: Annual symposium of the American College of Veterinary Surgeons. San Antonio, TX, 24-26 October, 2013.
83. Thu LT, Dibley MJ, Van Nho V, et al. Reduction in surgical site infections in neurosurgical patients associated with a bedside hand hygiene program in Vietnam. Infect Control Hosp Epidemiol 2007;28(5):583–8.
84. Stone SP, Fuller C, Savage J, et al. Evaluation of the national Cleanyourhands campaign to reduce *Staphylococcus aureus* bacteraemia and *Clostridium difficile* infection in hospitals in England and Wales by improved hand hygiene: four year, prospective, ecological, interrupted time series study. BMJ 2012;344: e3005.
85. Costers M, Viseur N, Catry B, et al. Four multifaceted countrywide campaigns to promote hand hygiene in Belgian hospitals between 2005 and 2011: impact on compliance to hand hygiene. Euro Surveill 2012;17(18).
86. Asensio A, de Gregorio L. Practical experience in a surgical unit when changing from scrub to rub. J Hosp Infect 2013;83(Suppl 1):S40–2.
87. Erasmus V, Daha TJ, Brug H, et al. Systematic review of studies on compliance with hand hygiene guidelines in hospital care. Infect Control Hosp Epidemiol 2010;31(3):283–94.
88. Bergstrom A, Gronlund U. A pre- and post-intervention study of infection control in equine hospitals in Sweden. Acta Vet Scand 2014;56:52.
89. Elek SD, Conen PE. The virulence of *Staphylococcus pyogenes* for man: a study of the problems of wound infection. Br J Exp Pathol 1957;38(6):573–86.
90. Zimmerli W, Waldvogel FA, Vaudaux P, et al. Pathogenesis of foreign body infection: description and characteristics of an animal model. J Infect Dis 1982; 146(4):487–97.
91. Bratzler DW, Hunt DR. The surgical infection prevention and surgical care improvement projects: national initiatives to improve outcomes for patients having surgery. Clin Infect Dis 2006;43(3):322–30.
92. Goede WJ, Lovely JK, Thompson RL, et al. Assessment of prophylactic antibiotic use in patients with surgical site infections. Hosp Pharm 2013;48(7):560–7.
93. Cataife G, Weinberg DA, Wong HH, et al. The effect of Surgical Care Improvement Project (SCIP) compliance on surgical site infections (SSI). Med Care 2014;52(2 Suppl 1):S66–73.
94. Crolla RM, van der Laan L, Veen EJ, et al. Reduction of surgical site infections after implementation of a bundle of care. PLoS One 2012;7(9):e44599.
95. Prospero E, Barbadoro P, Marigliano A, et al. Perioperative antibiotic prophylaxis: improved compliance and impact on infection rates. Epidemiol Infect 2011;139(9):1326–31.
96. van der Slegt J, van der Laan L, Veen EJ, et al. Implementation of a bundle of care to reduce surgical site infections in patients undergoing vascular surgery. PLoS One 2013;8(8):e71566.
97. Classen DC, Evans RS, Pestotnik SL, et al. The timing of prophylactic administration of antibiotics and the risk of surgical-wound infection. N Engl J Med 1992; 326(5):281–6.
98. Bratzler DW, Houck PM, Surgical Infection Prevention Guidelines Writers, et al. Antimicrobial prophylaxis for surgery: an advisory statement from the National Surgical Infection Prevention Project. Clin Infect Dis 2004;38(12):1706–15.
99. Bratzler DW, Houck PM, Richards C, et al. Use of antimicrobial prophylaxis for major surgery: baseline results from the National Surgical Infection Prevention Project. Arch Surg 2005;140(2):174–82.

100. van Kasteren ME, Mannien J, Ott A, et al. Antibiotic prophylaxis and the risk of surgical site infections following total hip arthroplasty: timely administration is the most important factor. Clin Infect Dis 2007;44(7):921–7.
101. Weese JS, Halling KB. Perioperative administration of antimicrobials associated with elective surgery for cranial cruciate ligament rupture in dogs: 83 cases (2003-2005). J Am Vet Med Assoc 2006;229(1):92–5.
102. Hawn MT, Richman JS, Vick CC, et al. Timing of surgical antibiotic prophylaxis and the risk of surgical site infection. JAMA Surg 2013;148(7):649–57.
103. Lee FM, Trevino S, Kent-Street E, et al. Antimicrobial prophylaxis may not be the answer: surgical site infections among patients receiving care per recommended guidelines. Am J Infect Control 2013;41(9):799–802.
104. Mangram AJ, Horan TC, Pearson ML, et al. Guideline for prevention of surgical site infection, 1999. Hospital Infection Control Practices Advisory Committee. Infect Control Hosp Epidemiol 1999;20(4):250–78 [quiz: 279–80].
105. Pruzansky JS, Bronson MJ, Grelsamer RP, et al. Prevalence of modifiable surgical site infection risk factors in hip and knee joint arthroplasty patients at an urban academic hospital. J Arthroplasty 2014;29(2):272–6.
106. Velasco E, Thuler LC, Martins CA, et al. Risk factors for infectious complications after abdominal surgery for malignant disease. Am J Infect Control 1996;24(1): 1–6.
107. Kessler B, Sendi P, Graber P, et al. Risk factors for periprosthetic ankle joint infection: a case-control study. J Bone Joint Surg Am 2012;94(20):1871–6.
108. Uckay I, Luebbeke A, Emonet S, et al. Low incidence of haematogenous seeding to total hip and knee prostheses in patients with remote infections. J Infect 2009;59(5):337–45.
109. David TS, Vrahas MS. Perioperative lower urinary tract infections and deep sepsis in patients undergoing total joint arthroplasty. J Am Acad Orthop Surg 2000;8(1):66–74.
110. Mohri Y, Miki C, Kobayashi M, et al. Correlation between preoperative systemic inflammation and postoperative infection in patients with gastrointestinal cancer: a multicenter study. Surg Today 2014;44(5):859–67.
111. Udofia AA, Oyetunji T, Fossett D. 115 risk factors for laminectomy surgical site infection in a majority minority patient population. Neurosurgery 2014; 61(Suppl 1):196–7.
112. Haley RW, Culver DH, White JW, et al. The efficacy of infection surveillance and control programs in preventing nosocomial infections in US hospitals. Am J Epidemiol 1985;121(2):182–205.
113. Anderson DJ, Kaye KS, Classen D, et al. Strategies to prevent surgical site infections in acute care hospitals. Infect Control Hosp Epidemiol 2008;29(Suppl 1):S51–61.
114. Astagneau P, L'Heriteau F, Daniel F, et al. Reducing surgical site infection incidence through a network: results from the French ISO-RAISIN surveillance system. J Hosp Infect 2009;72(2):127–34.
115. Emori TG, Culver DH, Horan TC, et al. National nosocomial infections surveillance system (NNIS): description of surveillance methods. Am J Infect Control 1991;19(1):19–35.
116. Gould D. Infection control practice: interview with 20 nurses reveals themes of rationalising their own behaviour and justifying any deviations from policy. Evid Based Nurs 2014. [Epub ahead of print].
117. Pittet D. The Lowbury lecture: behaviour in infection control. J Hosp Infect 2004; 58(1):1–13.

118. Brandt C, Sohr D, Behnke M, et al. Reduction of surgical site infection rates associated with active surveillance. Infect Control Hosp Epidemiol 2006; 27(12):1347–51.
119. Rioux C, Grandbastien B, Astagneau P. Impact of a six-year control programme on surgical site infections in France: results of the INCISO surveillance. J Hosp Infect 2007;66(3):217–23.
120. Mannien J, Wille JC, Snoeren RL, et al. Impact of postdischarge surveillance on surgical site infection rates for several surgical procedures: results from the nosocomial surveillance network in the Netherlands. Infect Control Hosp Epidemiol 2006;27(8):809–16.
121. Limon E, Shaw E, Badia JM, et al. Post-discharge surgical site infections after uncomplicated elective colorectal surgery: impact and risk factors. The experience of the VINCat Program. J Hosp Infect 2014;86(2):127–32.
122. Humphreys H. Preventing surgical site infection. Where now? J Hosp Infect 2009;73(4):316–22.
123. Aggarwal R, Darzi A. Symposium on surgical simulation for training and certification. World J Surg 2008;32(2):139–40.
124. Wurtz R, Wittrock B, Lavin MA, et al. Do new surgeons have higher surgical-site infection rates? Infect Control Hosp Epidemiol 2001;22(6):375–7.
125. Wormstrand BH, Ihler CF, Diesen R, et al. Surgical treatment of equine colic–a retrospective study of 297 surgeries in Norway 2005-2011. Acta Vet Scand 2014;56:38.
126. Carlson MA. Acute wound failure. Surg Clin North Am 1997;77(3):607–36.
127. Webster C, Neumayer L, Smout R, et al. Prognostic models of abdominal wound dehiscence after laparotomy. J Surg Res 2003;109(2):130–7.
128. Torfs S, Levet T, Delesalle C, et al. Risk factors for incisional complications after exploratory celiotomy in horses: do skin staples increase the risk? Vet Surg 2010;39(5):616–20.
129. Aggarwal R, Warren O, Darzi A. Mental training in surgical education: a randomized controlled trial. Ann Surg 2007;245(6):1002.
130. Campbell DA, Henderson WG, Englesbe MJ, et al. Surgical site infection prevention: the importance of operative duration and blood transfusion–results of the first American College of Surgeons–National Surgical Quality Improvement Program best practices initiative. J Am Coll Surg 2008;207(6):810–20.
131. Kurmann A, Peter M, Tschan F, et al. Adverse effect of noise in the operating theatre on surgical-site infection. Br J Surg 2011;98(7):1021–5.
132. Moorthy K, Munz Y, Undre S, et al. Objective evaluation of the effect of noise on the performance of a complex laparoscopic task. Surgery 2004;136(1):25–30 [discussion: 31].
133. Haynes AB, Weiser TG, Berry WR, et al. A surgical safety checklist to reduce morbidity and mortality in a global population. N Engl J Med 2009;360(5): 491–9.
134. Hague BA, Honnas CM, Simpson RB, et al. Evaluation of skin bacterial flora before and after aseptic preparation of clipped and nonclipped arthrocentesis sites in horses. Vet Surg 1997;26(2):121–5.
135. Dumville JC, McFarlane E, Edwards P, et al. Preoperative skin antiseptics for preventing surgical wound infections after clean surgery. Cochrane Database Syst Rev 2013;(3):CD003949.
136. Charehbili A, Swijnenburg RJ, van de Velde C, et al. A retrospective analysis of surgical site infections after chlorhexidine-alcohol versus iodine-alcohol for preoperative antisepsis. Surg Infect (Larchmt) 2014;15(3):310–3.

137. Hemani ML, Lepor H. Skin preparation for the prevention of surgical site infection: which agent is best? Rev Urol 2009;11(4):190–5.
138. Ulmer M, Lademann J, Patzelt A, et al. New strategies for preoperative skin antisepsis. Skin Pharmacol Physiol 2014;27(6):283–92.
139. Lipp A, Phillips C, Harris P, et al. Cyanoacrylate microbial sealants for skin preparation prior to surgery. Cochrane Database Syst Rev 2013;(8):CD008062.
140. Coolman BR, Marretta SM, Kakoma I, et al. Cutaneous antimicrobial preparation prior to intravenous catheterization in healthy dogs: clinical, microbiological, and histopathological evaluation. Can Vet J 1998;39(12):757–63.
141. Dorey-Phillips CL, Murison PJ. Comparison of two techniques for intravenous catheter site preparation in dogs. Vet Rec 2008;162(9):280–1.
142. Evans LK, Knowles TG, Werrett G, et al. The efficacy of chlorhexidine gluconate in canine skin preparation–practice survey and clinical trials. J Small Anim Pract 2009;50(9):458–65.
143. Gibson KL, Donald AW, Hariharan H, et al. Comparison of two pre-surgical skin preparation techniques. Can J Vet Res 1997;61(2):154–6.
144. Lambrechts NE, Hurter K, Picard JA, et al. A prospective comparison between stabilized glutaraldehyde and chlorhexidine gluconate for preoperative skin antisepsis in dogs. Vet Surg 2004;33(6):636–43.
145. Osuna DJ, DeYoung DJ, Walker RL. Comparison of three skin preparation techniques. Part 2: Clinical trial in 100 dogs. Vet Surg 1990;19(1):20–3.
146. Osuna DJ, DeYoung DJ, Walker RL. Comparison of three skin preparation techniques in the dog. Part 1: experimental trial. Vet Surg 1990;19(1):14–9.
147. Rochat MC, Mann FA, Berg JN. Evaluation of a one-step surgical preparation technique in dogs. J Am Vet Med Assoc 1993;203(3):392–5.
148. Stubbs WP, Bellah JR, Vermaas-Hekman D, et al. Chlorhexidine gluconate versus chloroxylenol for preoperative skin preparation in dogs. Vet Surg 1996; 25(6):487–94.
149. Zimmerman FC. Comparison of three skin preparation techniques in the dog. Vet Surg 1990;19(6):405.
150. Webster J, Osborne S. Preoperative bathing or showering with skin antiseptics to prevent surgical site infection. Cochrane Database Syst Rev 2012;(9):CD004985.
151. Lepainteur M, Royer G, Bourrel AS, et al. Prevalence of resistance to antiseptics and mupirocin among invasive coagulase-negative staphylococci from very preterm neonates in NICU: the creeping threat? J Hosp Infect 2013;83(4):333–6.
152. Baykasoglu A, Dereli T, Yilankirkan N. Application of cost/benefit analysis for surgical gown and drape selection: a case study. Am J Infect Control 2009; 37(3):215–26.
153. Moylan JA, Fitzpatrick KT, Davenport KE. Reducing wound infections. Improved gown and drape barrier performance. Arch Surg 1987;122(2):152–7.
154. Showalter BM, Crantford JC, Russell GB, et al. The effect of reusable versus disposable draping material on infection rates in implant-based breast reconstruction: a prospective randomized trial. Ann Plast Surg 2014;72(6):S165–9.
155. Billings L, Vasseur PB, Fancher C, et al. Wound infection rates in dogs and cats after use of cotton muslin or disposable impermeable fabric as barrier material: 720 cases (1983-1989). J Am Vet Med Assoc 1990;197(7):889–92.
156. McHugh SM, Corrigan MA, Hill AD, et al. Surgical attire, practices and their perception in the prevention of surgical site infection. Surg J R Coll Surg Edinb Irel 2014;12(1):47–52.
157. Webster J, Alghamdi A. Use of plastic adhesive drapes during surgery for preventing surgical site infection. Cochrane Database Syst Rev 2013;(1):CD006353.

158. Falk-Brynhildsen K, Soderquist B, Friberg O, et al. Bacterial recolonization of the skin and wound contamination during cardiac surgery: a randomized controlled trial of the use of plastic adhesive drape compared with bare skin. J Hosp Infect 2013;84(2):151–8.
159. Alexander JW, Solomkin JS, Edwards MJ. Updated recommendations for control of surgical site infections. Ann Surg 2011;253(6):1082–93.
160. Lipp A, Edwards P. Disposable surgical face masks for preventing surgical wound infection in clean surgery. Cochrane Database Syst Rev 2014;(2):CD002929.
161. Ward WG, Cooper JM, Lippert D, et al. Glove and gown effects on intraoperative bacterial contamination. Ann Surg 2014;259(3):591–7.
162. Moylan JA, Kennedy BV. The importance of gown and drape barriers in the prevention of wound infection. Surg Gynecol Obstet 1980;151(4):465–70.
163. Naver LP, Gottrup F. Incidence of glove perforations in gastrointestinal surgery and the protective effect of double gloves: a prospective, randomised controlled study. Eur J Surg 2000;166(4):293–5.
164. Partecke LI, Goerdt AM, Langner I, et al. Incidence of microperforation for surgical gloves depends on duration of wear. Infect Control Hosp Epidemiol 2009; 30(5):409–14.
165. Misteli H, Weber WP, Reck S, et al. Surgical glove perforation and the risk of surgical site infection. Arch Surg 2009;144(6):553–8 [discussion: 558].
166. Harnoss JC, Partecke LI, Heidecke CD, et al. Concentration of bacteria passing through puncture holes in surgical gloves. Am J Infect Control 2010;38(2):154–8.
167. Harnoss JC, Kramer A, Heidecke CD, et al. What is the appropriate time-interval for changing gloves during surgical procedures. Zentralbl Chir 2010;135(1): 25–7 [in German].
168. Hayes GM, Reynolds D, Moens NM, et al. Investigation of incidence and risk factors for surgical glove perforation in small animal surgery. Vet Surg 2014; 43(4):400–4.
169. Character BJ, McLaughlin RM, Hedlund CS, et al. Postoperative integrity of veterinary surgical gloves. J Am Anim Hosp Assoc 2003;39(3):311–20.
170. Burrow R, Pinchbeck G. Study of how frequently surgeons' gloves are perforated during operations. Vet Rec 2006;158(16):558–61.
171. Tanner J, Parkinson H. Double gloving to reduce surgical cross-infection. Cochrane Database Syst Rev 2006;(3):CD003087.
172. Thomas S, Agarwal M, Mehta G. Intraoperative glove perforation–single versus double gloving in protection against skin contamination. Postgrad Med J 2001; 77(909):458–60.
173. Smith F, Dryburgh N, Donaldson J, et al. Debridement for surgical wounds. Cochrane Database Syst Rev 2013;(9):CD006214.
174. Dumville JC, Walter CJ, Sharp CA, et al. Dressings for the prevention of surgical site infection. Cochrane Database Syst Rev 2011;(7):CD003091.
175. Tnibar A, Grubbe Lin K, Thuroe Nielsen K, et al. Effect of a stent bandage on the likelihood of incisional infection following exploratory coeliotomy for colic in horses: a comparative retrospective study. Equine Vet J 2013;45(5):564–9.
176. Smith LJ, Mellor DJ, Marr CM, et al. Incisional complications following exploratory celiotomy: does an abdominal bandage reduce the risk? Equine Vet J 2007;39(3):277–83.
177. Smith TO, Sexton D, Mann C, et al. Sutures versus staples for skin closure in orthopaedic surgery: meta-analysis. BMJ 2010;340:c1199.
178. Bischofberger AS, Brauer T, Gugelchuk G, et al. Difference in incisional complications following exploratory celiotomies using antibacterial-coated suture

material for subcutaneous closure: prospective randomised study in 100 horses. Equine Vet J 2010;42(4):304–9.
179. Gifford C, Christelis N, Cheng A. Preventing postoperative infections: the anaesthetist's role. Continuing Education in Anaesthesia, Critical Care & Pain Advances 2011;11:151–6.
180. Bergstrom A, Gustafsson C, Leander M, et al. Occurrence of methicillin-resistant staphylococci in surgically treated dogs and the environment in a Swedish animal hospital. J Small Anim Pract 2012;53(7):404–10.
181. Vanderhaeghen W, Van de Velde E, Crombe F, et al. Screening for methicillin-resistant staphylococci in dogs admitted to a veterinary teaching hospital. Res Vet Sci 2012;93(1):133–6.
182. Bode LG, Kluytmans JA, Wertheim HF, et al. Preventing surgical-site infections in nasal carriers of *Staphylococcus aureus*. N Engl J Med 2010;362(1):9–17.
183. Taylor MM, Kern TJ, Riis RC, et al. Intraocular bacterial-contamination during cataract-surgery in dogs. J Am Vet Med Assoc 1995;206(11):1716–20.
184. Maragakis LL, Cosgrove SE, Martinez EA, et al. Intraoperative fraction of inspired oxygen is a modifiable risk factor for surgical site infection after spinal surgery. Anesthesiology 2009;110(3):556–62.
185. Triulzi DJ, Blumberg N, Heal JM. Association of transfusion with postoperative bacterial infection. Crit Rev Clin Lab Sci 1990;28(2):95–107.
186. Brandstrup B, Tonnesen H, Beier-Holgersen R, et al. Effects of intravenous fluid restriction on postoperative complications: comparison of two perioperative fluid regimens: a randomized assessor-blinded multicenter trial. Ann Surg 2003; 238(5):641–8.
187. Lang K, Boldt J, Suttner S, et al. Colloids versus crystalloids and tissue oxygen tension in patients undergoing major abdominal surgery. Anesth Analg 2001; 93(2):405–9, 403rd contents page.
188. Morley PS. Evidence-based infection control in clinical practice: if you buy clothes for the emperor, will he wear them? J Vet Intern Med 2013;27(3):430–8.

Patient Management

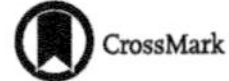

Lynn Guptill, DVM, PhD

KEYWORDS

- Infection control • Patient management • Risk assessment • Barrier nursing
- Isolation

KEY POINTS

- Patient management includes risk assessment and routine practices, in addition to enhanced precautions (barrier nursing, strict isolation), all of which are designed to minimize transmission of infectious disease pathogens.
- Protocols for barrier nursing and strict isolation, including clear guidelines and strong support for implementation, are needed for every veterinary hospital.
- Patient management guidelines and practices should be regularly audited and updated to ensure that the most relevant and effective practices are being used.

INTRODUCTION

Keeping patients healthy is a primary goal of all practicing veterinarians. To minimize the incidence of hospital-associated infections (HAIs) in animal patients, and to protect veterinary staff, volunteers, and animal owners from acquiring infectious diseases from animal patients or the environment, veterinary hospitals must develop and implement guidelines for patient management. These guidelines should contain specific protocols for patient admission, housing, diagnostic procedures, and treatment, so that the cycle of pathogen transmission is effectively interrupted. Guidelines must be regularly updated, and clinics should provide ongoing education of staff and animal owners regarding the guidelines. There has been progress in developing evidence-based guidelines and resources for management of animals with infectious diseases in veterinary hospitals in recent years, although in large part, the veterinary industry still depends on studies carried out in human medicine for guidance. Several comprehensive documents are available to assist veterinary hospitals in this area, including, the *Compendium of Veterinary Standard Precautions for Zoonotic Disease Prevention in Veterinary Personnel*, provided by the National Association of State Public Health Veterinarians,[1] and the *Infection Prevention and Control Best Practices for Small Animal Veterinary Clinics* provided by the Canadian Committee on

The author has nothing to disclose.

Small Animal Internal Medicine, Department of Veterinary Clinical Sciences, Purdue University, 625 Harrison Street, West Lafayette, IN 47907, USA
E-mail address: guptillc@purdue.edu

Vet Clin Small Anim 45 (2015) 277–298
http://dx.doi.org/10.1016/j.cvsm.2014.11.010 vetsmall.theclinics.com
0195-5616/15/$ – see front matter

Antibiotic Resistance (CCAR).[2] Please see section on additional resources for further suggested readings in this area. Key components of patient management include risk assessment and routine practices for handling patients considered at risk for transmitting or acquiring infectious agents when they are presented to the veterinary hospital. Such routine practices include, but are not limited to, admission processes, protocols for housing and caring for these animals once they are admitted, how to move these animals between hospital service areas (eg, from their cages to diagnostic imaging or surgery areas), including management of housing and examination areas (traffic flow, cleaning and disinfection protocols). Clear protocols for each component and ongoing staff education facilitate successfully implementing patient management strategies.

RISK ASSESSMENT

Definition and Factors to Consider

Globally, infection control risk assessment for small animal practices is the process of calculating the likelihood that contagious infectious diseases will enter or be disseminated in a veterinary hospital and the consequences of such an event. General guidelines provided by the Association for Professionals in Infection Control and Epidemiology[3] include evaluating what patient population(s) a hospital serves and identifying the most common diagnoses encountered, the most frequently performed invasive procedures (eg, surgery, endoscopy), and the most frequently used treatments. Medical and financial records may be reviewed to assist in gathering these data. The information is used to help determine which patients may increase the risk of transmitting infections, which patients are at increased risk for acquiring infections, and which treatments and interventions are most likely to increase infection risks for patients. Hospital-wide risk assessment should be a nonbiased assessment that identifies successful processes, areas for improvement, and what changes are most practical, applicable, and economically viable. All practice staff should be involved in, and educated about, risk assessment and the policies and procedures in place to minimize, or manage, risks relevant to the practice.[3,4]

Regular audits (checking current practices against published standards of practice) of infection control practices at a clinic help to maintain good infection control practices and ensure that the most effective plans for patient management are in place.[5] The Iowa State University Center for Food Security and Public Health and the CCAR publications provide tools for performing clinic audits for infection control practices and staff education. Audits should include observation of daily practices by hospital staff and assessment of their knowledge of infection control principles and policies, evaluation of the physical facilities, and review of the hospital's written infection control and patient management protocols. Observations made in audits are then compared with standards, for assessment of adherence to standards and identifying areas in which change is needed. The final step in any audit is planning and implementing changes that will improve practice and commending areas in which infection control principles and practices are implemented well. Communicating audit findings to clinic staff in group meetings is an effective means of keeping everyone invested and working together to maintain good infection control practices.

Assessing Risk at the Patient Level

Assessing whether a patient is at risk of, or poses a risk for, pathogen transmission is a multifaceted process. At the most basic level, this assessment involves evaluating an animal's clinical signs and history to determine the risk for transmission of an infectious agent (syndromic screening). For example, an unvaccinated puppy with a fever and hemorrhagic diarrhea is considered at risk for transmitting canine parvovirus. A dog with acute renal failure, a fever, and icterus may be considered at risk for transmitting *Leptospira*. An animal that comes directly from an animal shelter may be considered at risk for potential transmission of infectious agents, particularly when there are clinical signs, such as nasal or ocular discharge, a cough, a fever, or diarrhea.

Providing veterinary staff members with a simple rubric for determining which animals pose a risk for transmission of infectious agents is a vital step. All personnel who work or volunteer in a veterinary hospital must be involved. Receptionists, other front office staff, and volunteers could all be exposed to zoonotic pathogens or play roles in the infection control program and therefore need a clear understanding of which animals are at risk or pose a risk for others. In this way, such animals may be prevented from coming into contact with other patients in reception and waiting areas or otherwise contaminate or be placed at risk from other common areas (eg, multipurpose examination and procedure rooms). Personnel in these positions are usually the first to encounter owners and animals coming in to a facility, and therefore, education regarding how to assess whether a patient is likely to transmit a contagious infectious disease is vital for them. Staff members responsible for making appointments should have a simple list of questions to ask owners who come in with ill pets, so that they may more easily assess the likelihood that an animal has a contagious infectious disease (**Box 1**). As appropriate, alternative entrances, waiting/examination locations, or

Box 1
Questions to ask when making appointments for ill patients to help determine whether additional precautions should be used[a]

- Age of patient
- Vaccination history
- Recent history: has the pet been to a boarding kennel, dog park, day care facility, animal shelter, or other similar venue in the past month? Travel to another area or country? Are other pets in the household ill?
- Acute vomiting?
- Acute diarrhea? (Defined as 3 or more loose stools during the past 24 hours, or episodes of bloody diarrhea)
- Acute coughing?
- Acute sneezing?
- Fever? (Client may not know the answer to this)

If the patient is not vaccinated, is less than 2 years old, has a recent history of exposure to other animals, and is acutely coughing, sneezing, vomiting or having diarrhea, ± a fever, the pet should not enter the reception area. Evaluate such animals before entry into the building or immediately transport them to a dedicated examination or isolation room depending on clinic policy.
If hospital records indicate that the pet has a multiple-drug–resistant infection, the pet should not enter the reception area.

[a] Patients fitting these criteria should not enter the reception area. Meet owners outside and escort them in via a separate entrance, or use a carrier or gurney to transport the pet through the reception area if necessary. Use alternative waiting/examination locations or use of barrier precautions based on the initial risk assessment. Clean and disinfect any waiting or examination locations occupied before using those areas again for other animals.

barrier precautions should be used based on the initial risk assessment. It is important to inform owners of concerns and precautions that will be taken to minimize potential pathogen transmission (alternative entry/examination area/barrier precautions), and to reassure them that if their pet is critically ill, hospital staff will attend to them immediately on their arrival.

ROUTINE PRACTICES

Approach/Goals

Risk assessment helps to shape routine practices for managing patients to minimize the risk of infectious agent transmission. Providing easily accessible standard protocols in an infection control plan or manual greatly enhances infection control efforts (see the article by Stull and Weese on "Hospital associated infections in small animal practice" elsewhere in this issue for more details).[1] Ongoing review and updating of protocols allows integration of new findings from risk assessment and keeps infection control routine practices relevant. Hospital owners, administrators, and staff must support (financially and philosophically) the infection control program,[6,7] and there must be personnel dedicated to the implementation of the program, often referred to as infection control practitioners (ICPs) (see the article by Stull and Weese on "Hospital associated infections in small animal practice" elsewhere in this issue for more details). The ICPs manage the day-to-day issues in infection control. This may be their only job responsibility, or this may be only 1 aspect of their duties, depending on the size and scope of the hospital. The responsibilities may be shared among people who work various shifts in 24-hour facilities, or among people working in different departments of large hospitals. This strategy provides someone consistently in place to help with implementation of patient management practices. These staff members serve as resources and support for hospital staff to assist with decisions about patient management (eg, level of personal protective equipment (PPE) required, where patients are housed) to make it as easy as possible to meet infection control standards. Ideally, they also provide regular surveillance reports to hospital staff (see the article by Morley and Burgess on "Surveillance for hospital-associated infections" elsewhere in this issue for more information). In this article, routine practices in patient management designed to minimize transmission of infectious disease agents are discussed.

General Hospitalization Routines

Management of animals that are confirmed or strongly suspected of having a contagious disease or harboring a concerning pathogen requiring barrier nursing or full isolation is discussed in the following section. Standard practices that minimize the likelihood of pathogen transmission (eg, hand washing, contact precautions, cohorting patients) should be used in all areas of the hospital. There is little research in veterinary medicine to directly support many specific practices; this is also a concern for human medicine.[8,9]

Most veterinary pathogens are transmitted primarily via 1 of 4 common routes: aerosol, droplet, contact, or vector-borne.[2] Airborne transmission of infectious agents is uncommon in veterinary medicine, but some agents such as *Yersinia pestis* (pneumonic form) may be transmitted this way. Transmission may occur from patients with signs of disease; however, animals colonized with transmissible pathogens without clinical signs may also transmit pathogens, complicating disease prevention efforts. Standard precautions, involving routine cleaning and disinfection of facilities and vigilance in identifying and eliminating arthropod and other vectors, are therefore key hospital routines for minimizing pathogen transmission (see other articles elsewhere in this issue by Aceto H and Traverse M in article "Environmental cleaning and disinfection" for more information). Clinic pets (cats, dogs, or other animals belonging to the veterinary hospital that roam freely in parts of the hospital) are a potential source of pathogen transmission and environment contamination, and should not be kept in veterinary hospitals.[10] Similarly, staff pets should not be permitted to roam freely in the hospital. When hospitals allow staff members to bring their pets to work, clear guidelines are needed regarding whether these pets are confined to a staff member's office or housed in a clinic cage or kennel. These animals should be appropriately vaccinated and dewormed and should receive other necessary preventive health care and medications. Staff pets that are in a hospital for nonmedical reasons should not have contact with hospitalized patients. Veterinary hospitals that also offer boarding and grooming services should maintain separate facilities for animals using those services and should use standard precautions in handling those animals.

Admission, Patient Food, and Belongings

Syndromic screening of patients at the time of scheduling and handling of patients suspected of having contagious infectious disease at arrival was discussed earlier. Owners should be discouraged from allowing animals to interact in waiting areas, for safety reasons in addition to infection control concerns. At the time of admission, owners should be requested to keep collars, leashes, toys, bedding, and any other personal items, because these items may be contaminated if an animal has or develops a contagious infectious disease. In addition, such items may become contaminated if used in the hospital, because they may come into contact with contaminated hospital surfaces.[11,12] If such items are not left with the owner, they can be placed in a sealed plastic bag labeled with the owner/patient name, stored in a designated area (preferably away from wards and treatment areas), and returned to the owner at the time of discharge. The owner should be provided with instructions for decontamination of the items if the animal is suspected or proved to have a contagious infectious disease. All animals should be inspected for the presence of external parasites before hospitalization, and infested animals treated appropriately to eliminate these disease vectors, before admission if possible. Vaccination history should be verified and travel history investigated. The value of screening patients via culture for certain pathogens at admission (eg, methicillin-resistant *Staphylococcus*) is debated and not yet verified to be of more use than cohorting, syndromic screening, and diligent use of standard precautions.[8,9] Physical examination and complete history information are used to make a final determination regarding animal housing and precautions needed.

Patient food is best provided by the hospital, unless a specialized diet, necessary for the animal's well-being, is needed and not available at the hospital. Food should be stored in 1 designated area of the hospital, outside of the wards, and animal and human food stored separately. Different refrigerators should be used for human food, patient food, patient specimens, and patient medications. When possible, use disposable food bowls. Used food dishes and unfinished food should be promptly removed from patient cages. Water dishes should be made of an impervious material, such as stainless steel. Reusable dishes should be carefully cleaned of all organic debris, then washed and rinsed with hot water, ideally using a dishwasher with high water temperature. Raw diets should not be used in veterinary hospitals (**Box 2**) unless for specific patients (some exotic species). These diets commonly contain viable pathogens, which may contaminate the environment and pose a hazard to veterinary health care workers preparing food for hospitalized animals.[13–15] Viable pathogens

Box 2
Example of raw food policy

Animals admitted to ______________________ may not be fed diets containing raw meat products and by-products while hospitalized.

Any foods containing meat or meat products must be cooked thoroughly before delivery to the hospital. No uncooked or undercooked meats will be accepted, and it is the pet owner's responsibility to provide any requested information regarding the content and preparation of diets brought in with pets.

Most hospitalized pets will be fed foods supplied by the hospital. When it is necessary for owners to bring food, any food delivered by clients for feeding to their pets while hospitalized will be inspected by the admitting clinician to ascertain that there are not raw meat components in the foods. Any foods containing raw or undercooked meat or meat products will be returned to the client or discarded. Any food about which there is any question or concern regarding preparation will be returned to the client or discarded.

The only exceptions made to this policy will be for exotic animals that are admitted by clinicians trained to handle those species. Any foods for exotic animals will be inspected by the admitting clinician and those containing raw meat will be stored exclusively in the freezer and refrigerator in the exotics ward. This food will be handled according to the Standard Operating Procedure on file in the exotics area, and anyone handling the food will be trained by the clinicians in charge of the exotics area.

Modified from Purdue University Veterinary Teaching Hospital Infection Control Committee materials.

may be shed in the feces of animals fed raw diets for a period after ingestion; *Salmonella* was shed in feces of dogs fed contaminated raw diets for 1 to 7 days after ingestion.[16] The feces of animals fed raw diets may present a risk for exposure of staff to pathogens and for environmental contamination; therefore, appropriate standard precautions should be used when housing and handling these animals. If animals fed raw diets have signs of gastrointestinal disease (eg, diarrhea, vomiting), they should be housed in isolation.

HOUSING AND EXAMINATION AREAS

Basic Housing

All hospitalized patients should be housed in clean, dry, disinfected cages (see the article "Environmental cleaning and disinfection" by Aceto H and Traverse M elsewhere in this issue). Ideally, cages should not be placed across from each other and animals not moved from cage to cage during hospitalization, unless absolutely necessary. Standard operating procedures for cleaning and disinfection should be posted in all wards and treatment areas, so that appropriate cleaning of these areas may be accomplished by any member of the hospital staff. It is important to monitor for evidence of rodent or insect infestations in the environment and promptly address these as needed.

Cohorting

Cohorting of patients may be used to help minimize pathogen transmission. Cohorting refers to grouping animals that are infected or colonized with similar or the same organism(s) in the same area or ward of a hospital. This practice is used in human health care facilities to help minimize occurrence or spread of HAIs. A cohort is created based on several variables, including clinical diagnosis (established using factors such as history and physical examination findings), microbiology laboratory data, knowledge of the epidemiology/transmission of the suspected or confirmed infectious agent, and knowledge of the health status of the patient. Cohorting has been successfully used in human health care facilities for management of outbreaks of multiple drug–resistant organism bacterial infections and some viral infections.[17,18] Cohorting of patients may at first seem complex and not easily applied to veterinary medicine. However, this technique is applied in several general ways. Healthy and sick animals may be housed separately, and dogs and cats housed separately. Other examples are cohorting of patients entering the hospital from a shelter to minimize the likelihood that these animals will introduce pathogens to the general hospital environment; housing oncology patients in a ward separate from general wards to minimize the exposure of these immunocompromised patients to pathogens; housing dermatology patients separately from other animals; and housing surgical patients separately from other animals. Patients in various cohorts may be identified by the likelihood of disease transmission. Some hospitals use color-coding systems, including placement of colored dots on cage cards, or placement of colored identification bands on patients. One example is a 3-color system, in which green indicates no concern for disease transmission, yellow indicates suspicion that a patient is at risk for pathogen acquisition, or is suspected of being infected, and red identifies patients known to be infected with highly contagious pathogens.[19] Another example is a 2-color system of identification bands (P. Gomes, personal communication, May, 2014), in which a green band indicates no concern, and a yellow identification band indicates that caution is advised (the patient is known or suspected to be infected with a contagious pathogen). When the banding system is used, the pathogen is written on the band.

Cohorting may also be applied to those who care for patients (eg, assigning only certain staff members to care for a particular group of patients). This aspect of cohorting may be difficult to implement in veterinary medicine, because of the small staff size of many veterinary hospitals. However, some aspects of this practice (eg, limiting contact with a patient in isolation to the clinician assigned to that patient or limiting staff who handle that patient to 1 staff member per shift) may be possible in veterinary health care.

Traffic patterns

Traffic patterns in veterinary hospitals should be studied as part of the risk assessment process and establishment of routines. Surgery suites should be used only for sterile surgical procedures, and not as treatment rooms when not in use for surgery. Areas designated for surgery or other invasive procedures, critical care, isolation, or barrier nursing should not be in areas of the hospital with high traffic flow. Ideally, a specific area is designated for working with hospitalized patients with known or suspected infectious diseases; this includes bandage changes or wound care for contaminated wounds. Ideally, wound care that requires lavage is not performed in the same bathtub area that is used for bathing other patients. Careful cleaning and disinfection of such areas is vital to help minimize the establishment of biofilms of resistant bacteria. Multiple hospital entrances are helpful and may be used to help segregate patients with known or suspected infectious disease on entry to the facility.

Examination Areas

Physical environment

It is important to keep animal housing and examination areas free of clutter. Schedule and conduct daily environmental cleaning, and terminal cleaning when appropriate, according to established hospital protocols (see the article "Environmental cleaning and disinfection" by Aceto H and Traverse M elsewhere in this issue). Do not store equipment in wards and treatment areas, unless it is kept in cabinets or closets with clearly labeled closed doors and drawers. The daily routine in examination areas should include cleaning and disinfection of examination tables and equipment shared among patients after each use. Be sure that protocols and materials for cleaning and disinfecting common equipment, such as clippers, blood pressure monitors, fluid pumps, otoscopes and ophthalmoscopes, are readily available for all staff (**Table 1**). Probe covers should be routinely used for thermometers, carefully discarding the

Table 1
Considerations for items used in day-to-day patient management

Device	Risk for Contamination	Intervention
Thermometer	High	Use probe cover or provide separate thermometers for each patient. Animals in barrier nursing or isolation have individual thermometers that are discarded at discharge.
Clippers	High	Clean and disinfect blades after each use, wipe down body.
Blood pressure monitor, fluid pump, ophthalmoscope, transilluminator	Moderate	Clean and disinfect probes or cuffs after each use; wipe down remainder of instrument.
Otoscope	High	Clean and disinfect cones after each use; wipe down instrument; consider use of disposable otoscope cones.
Bandage scissors, suture scissors, reflex hammers, penlights, stethoscope, hand lens	Moderate to high	Clean and disinfect after each use
Cell phones, pagers, tablets and stylus, other personal electronic equipment, computer keyboards and mice	High	Perform hand hygiene before and after using; do not use while wearing gloves or working with patients. Avoid contact with patients. Use protective sleeves that can be cleaned and disinfected. Follow manufacturer directions for cleaning and disinfection.
Animal leashes	High	Soak at least daily in appropriate disinfectant (follow manufacturer directions). Dry overnight. If possible, provide a separate leash for each patient, making sure the leash remains with the patient. Any animal in barrier nursing or isolation must have a dedicated leash.
Medical records, pens, pencils	Moderate to high	Perform hand hygiene before and after using; do not use while wearing gloves. Avoid contact of these items with patients or patient care surfaces.
Hospital outerwear	Moderate to high	Change when obviously soiled. Change at least daily when there is animal contact. Change at least weekly when there is no animal contact. Do not wear hospital outerwear outside the hospital.

covers after use, followed by cleaning and disinfecting the thermometer. For animals hospitalized in critical care units, it is advisable to have a thermometer for each patient (purchased by the owner), which is cleaned and disinfected after each use. Stethoscopes and any instrument (eg, reflex hammer, bandage scissors, suture scissors) used for a patient should be cleaned and disinfected after each use. These devices harbor pathogens, and isopropanol, or other disinfectants determined safe by the manufacturer, are effective for cleaning such equipment.[20–24] Hospital leashes should be cleaned and disinfected at least once daily, or provide a new leash (which stays with the patient) for each patient on arrival at the hospital. Cloth leashes may be soaked in an accelerated hydrogen peroxide disinfectant, following manufacturer directions, then hung up to dry overnight. Grooming equipment should be cleaned and disinfected between patients.

Staff equipment and procedures

Recently, personal electronic equipment, such as pagers, cell phones, and tablets, have become an integral part of patient management routines. These devices should be handled only after washing hands and should not come into contact with animals. Several studies have reported high-level contamination of these devices with pathogens, and support cleaning of the devices regularly.[25–28] Covers are available for smartphones and tablets to make them water resistant or waterproof, washable, and to allow disinfection.

Similarly, medical records and pens are a potential source of pathogen transmission.[29–31] Physical medical records may become contaminated via contact with contaminated hands, placement on patient contact surfaces (examination tables, the floor), or via direct contact with patients. Computer keyboards and mice need regular cleaning and disinfection, because they are also readily contaminated as hospital personnel making entries into electronic medical records handle this equipment during patient care.[12,32] Contamination of medical records, electronic devices, and other equipment serves as a reminder of the importance of adherence to hand-hygiene protocols and other standard precautions.

Hospital attire (laboratory coats, smocks, other outerwear) used during patient care should be changed whenever obviously soiled, and at least daily after animal contact, to minimize the likelihood of contaminated clothing serving as a fomite. Wearing hospital attire home, or into public places outside the hospital, could increase the likelihood that pathogens from the hospital will be transferred to the community environment, household pets, or to human members of veterinary staff households. A recent review of literature from the human medical community[33] provided expert guidance on the topic of health care personnel attire outside operating rooms: hospital protective outerwear should be laundered after daily use if it comes into contact with patients or patients' environment, but if not, then launder white coats no less frequently than once a week and when visibly soiled. Bearman and colleagues[33] note that it remains unclear whether attire such as white coats should be laundered at the facility or home-laundered. If self-laundering is expected, then best practices would include removing the outerwear before leaving the hospital, placing it in a plastic bag, and laundering it separately at home using a protocol designed to minimize pathogen persistence. Based on their review of the literature, Bearman and colleagues[33] stated that if nonsurgical hospital attire is laundered at home, a hot-water wash cycle (ideally with bleach) followed by a cycle in the dryer is preferable. Please see the article, "Environmental cleaning and disinfection" by Aceto H and Traverse M elsewhere in this issue, for more information about hospital laundry.

Patient care

Clear protocols for placement of intravenous and urethral catheters, wound care, bandage changes, and other procedures that may introduce pathogens should be available as standard operating procedures (**Boxes 3** and **4**). Routine patient management procedures should be designed to minimize the likelihood of certain high-risk patients acquiring HAIs (**Table 2**).

The use of multiple-dose vials of medications, and the use of other materials (eg, eye lubricants, other lubricants, ear cleaning solutions) for more than 1 patient should be carefully examined. Multiple-dose vials and multiple-use medications have been found to be contaminated with pathogens in human and veterinary medicine,[36,37] emphasizing the need for careful attention to technique when using such medications. Apothecary jars and similar containers used for storage and dispensing of items such as cotton balls, cotton-tipped applicators, and tongue depressors are easily contaminated. If used, these containers should be cleaned and disinfected at least weekly.

Housing Animals with Confirmed or Suspected Infectious Disease

Barrier nursing and isolation are key means of managing patients with contagious infectious diseases. Most small animal practices in 1 recent survey[38] reported always using barrier or isolation methods for patients that were confirmed or suspected to have an infection considered zoonotic. Another survey,[39] not specifically investigating methods used to limit zoonotic pathogens, found that only 35% of responding clinics had separate isolation units, and only 69% of those isolation units were used

Box 3
Placing and maintaining peripheral intravenous catheters

1. Clip hair from the proposed site of catheter insertion.
2. Perform hand hygiene and don clean examination gloves.
3. Use sterile gauze sponges, sterile saline, and chlorhexidine scrub diluted with sterile saline to between 0.5% and 2% chlorhexidine,[34] to prepare the catheter site (≥3 scrubs with each solution).
4. Perform hand hygiene and don sterile or clean gloves to insert the catheter. Do not reuse a catheter after a failed attempt.
5. Attach a catheter cap, T set, or suitable extension set to the catheter, and flush the catheter with sterile saline solution. Carefully secure the catheter with tape and cover it with sterile bandage materials. Povidone iodine ointment may be applied at the site of entry into the skin.
6. Examine the catheter site at least 2 times daily. Palpate for pain and evaluate for evidence of swelling or thrombophlebitis. If the bandage is not clean and dry, replace the bandage. If there is any evidence of thrombophlebitis and the catheter is still necessary, replace the catheter in a different site.
7. When intravenous lines are disconnected (eg, to take a dog for a walk), the sites of connection should be cleaned with isopropyl alcohol single-use wipes and capped with injection caps. Do not reuse injection caps.
8. Intravenous tubing used for fluid administration should be changed every 72 hours. The intravenous tubing used for total parenteral nutrition (TPN) administration should be changed every time a new bag of TPN is placed, or every 24 hours, whichever is more frequent.

Modified from Purdue University Veterinary Teaching Hospital Infection Control Committee materials.

Box 4
Placing and managing indwelling urethral catheters

For all site cleansing, wear examination gloves, and use sterile gauze sponges to cleanse, alternating between chlorhexidine scrub diluted with sterile saline to 0.5% to no more than 2% chlorhexidine, and sterile saline.

Dogs

- Clip hair on prepuce and surrounding ventral abdomen to a distance of 5 cm (dogs) or 2 to 3 cm (cats) from the preputial opening (males) or the perineal area to 5 cm (dogs) or 2 to 3 cm (cats) from the vulva (females). Shorten nearby long hair so that none overlaps the clipped area
- Cleanse the area, using at least 3 scrubs with each solution.

Males:

- Dogs: flush the prepuce 3 to 5 times with 2 to 12 mL of dilute iodine solution (1:200 povidone iodine/sterile saline; volume depends on size of dog) using a sterile syringe.
- Assistant wearing clean examination gloves should exteriorize the penis. Cleanse of any gross exudate, then cleanse the entire area, using at least 3 scrubs with each solution.
- Flush the penis with 2 to 5 mL of dilute betadine solution.

Females:

- Cleanse vulva and perivulvar area, using at least 3 scrubs with each solution.
- Flush the vaginal vault 3 to 5 times with 0.5 to 12 mL of dilute iodine solution (volume depends on size of animal) using a sterile syringe.

All:

- Place a sterile fenestrated drape over the work area.
- Perform hand hygiene and don sterile gloves.
- Test the bulbs of Foley catheters before placement.
- Coat the distal catheter with sterile lubricating jelly from a single-use packet and place the catheter using sterile technique.
- Immediately connect a sterile closed collection system.
- Anchor the catheter to prevent displacement and place an Elizabethan collar on the animal.

Daily maintenance of indwelling catheters

Perform hand hygiene and don sterile gloves. Clean at the junction of the patient and the external portion of the catheter every 24 hours with sterile gauze sponges, alternating between dilute chlorhexidine scrub and sterile saline ($\geq$3 scrubs with each solution).

Managing the closed collection system:

Do not administer prophylactic antimicrobials; these increase the risk of hospital-acquired resistant infections, and have not been shown to prevent infection. Give antimicrobials only for documented infection.

Position collection bags lower than the animal to allow urine to flow by gravity. Prevent retrograde flow of urine from the collection bag back into the patient, because this may cause iatrogenic urinary tract infection with resistant organisms. The collection system clamp mechanism should be closed when the patient is moved or walked and immediately reopened once the collection bag is again lower than the patient. Check patency of the tubing hourly.

Culture the urine via cystocentesis at the time of catheter removal. Urine culture results drawn from indwelling catheters (not recommended) should be interpreted with caution. Do not culture the tip of a removed catheter.[35]

Modified from Purdue University Veterinary Teaching Hospital Infection Control Committee materials.

Table 2
Patient care procedures to reduce risks for HAIs

HAI category[a]	Patient Procedure
Catheter-associated urinary tract infections	Aseptic technique during placement and maintenance of urethral catheters Avoid urinary catheter retrograde urine flow Avoid urinary catheterization unless necessary At least daily reassessment of whether urinary catheterization still required
Aspiration pneumonia	Elevate cranial portion of the body if patient is recumbent, sedated, debilitated, or has megaesophagus, a nasogastric/nasoesophageal tube, or tracheal intubation
Bloodstream infection	Aseptic technique for intravenous catheter placement (eg, appropriate skin preparation, hand hygiene immediately before placement, minimal contact with the catheter site) and daily catheter maintenance Use single-use containers of sterile sponges and scrub/sterile saline for preparing catheter insertion sites
Infectious diarrhea	Identify patients at high risk for shedding enteropathogens (eg, cats and dogs that recently consumed raw [or undercooked] meat/egg products; young animals with diarrhea and a fever) Handle animals with signs of gastrointestinal disease not attributed to a known noninfectious cause as suspected to have infectious diarrhea Standard infection control practices (eg, isolation, PPE, strict hand hygiene) for patients with known/suspected infectious diarrhea

[a] Surgical site infections are covered in the article "Surgical site infections" by Verwilghen D and Singh A elsewhere in this issue.

exclusively for patients with infectious disease. All practices should designate an area for infectious disease isolation, or at a minimum, use barrier nursing, to minimize HAIs. Whether an animal is managed solely using barrier precautions or is housed in full isolation depends in part on what facilities and support staff are available in a veterinary facility, the condition of the patient, and on the pathogen(s) involved.

Barrier nursing

Barrier nursing is primarily used for animals infected with pathogens for which the route of transmission indicates that contact precautions are sufficient. Animals requiring barrier nursing should ideally be placed in cages or runs at the end of a ward, and separated from other animals by keeping the cages or runs immediately surrounding the animal empty. If cages are stacked, place the animal requiring contact precautions in the lower cage. If possible, house animals requiring barrier nursing in a separate ward. A laminated sign should be placed on the cage to notify staff members that barrier nursing is in use and should identify the known or suspected pathogen (**Fig. 1**). Supplies needed include PPE, including gowns and gloves, sometimes boots or shoe covers, and a thermometer dedicated to use for that animal. It is important to store supplies and the patient chart or treatment sheet near the patient (eg, in a cage above or near the patient), but not on the floor or cage door. Once working with the patient, it is important that staff do not leave the area until all PPE are removed and hand hygiene performed; planning ahead or use of other noncontaminated personnel is important to reduce inadvertent pathogen spread. Staff should not touch treatment sheets while handling the patient or while wearing gloves after handling the patient. All

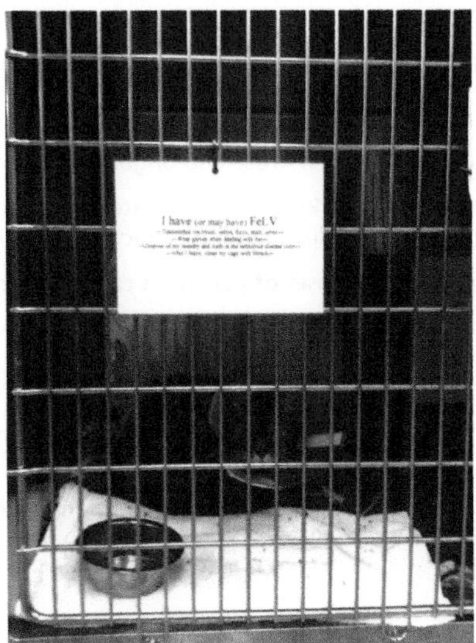

Fig. 1. Example of cage sign identifying infectious disease and summarizing precautions needed when handling the patient.

chart and treatment sheet entries should be made and telephones, pagers, or similar devices used only after removing all PPE and washing hands.

All regularly used equipment, such as stethoscopes and thermometers, should be dedicated to use with the animal in barrier nursing, remain with the animal, and be disinfected between uses. Carrying or using a gurney to transport animals to be weighed, followed by immediate disinfection of the scale, is important. The floor near the cage or run, and any examination table used, should be cleaned immediately after the animal is handled. In most cases, animals in barrier nursing may be taken outside if transported on a gurney or carried. They should use only a small, preferably fenced, area that is labeled as having been used by a patient with an infectious disease, and other patients should not use the same area. Grassy or gravel areas should be in sunny, well-drained areas. Concrete runs can be cleaned and disinfectant applied after use.

Containers for waste generated by patients in barrier nursing should be readily available and clearly labeled. Whenever possible, minimize the use of blankets and cloth towels and use disposable materials for bedding. Line waste containers with biohazard bags, and do not fill to more than one-half to two-thirds full. When full, remove bags and tie or close with large twist ties, and label with the name of the pathogen. Before removal from the area, the bags should be placed, with the help of a second person, into another clear clean bag, and if needed, the outside of that bag should be sprayed with disinfectant. These bags may then be placed outside the barrier area for transport for disposal according to institution or local regulations. Place any laundry generated by patients in barrier areas in biohazard bags labeled with the name of the pathogen, and, as done for waste, place the bags outside the barrier area for transport to the hospital laundry area.

Full isolation

Animals that must be housed in full isolation vary to some degree, depending on the hospital's facilities and personnel. Syndromic classification is commonly used to determine which animals should be housed in isolation, in the absence of diagnostic test results (**Box 5**). In most cases, animals acutely ill with confirmed or suspected

Box 5
Selected syndromes and infectious agents for which housing in isolation is recommended

Syndromes

Acute gastrointestinal tract signs (sudden onset and ongoing vomiting, diarrhea)

Recent exposure to other animals, lack of, inappropriate, or outdated vaccination history, young age, presence of fever add to likelihood of infectious enteric disease

Acute respiratory tract signs (sudden onset of persistent coughing, sneezing, nasal or ocular discharge)

Recent exposure to other animals, lack of, inappropriate, or outdated vaccination history, young age, presence of fever add to likelihood of infectious respiratory disease

Clinical (neurologic) signs consistent with rabies combined with potential exposure to rabid or suspected rabid animal

Combination of neurologic, respiratory, or gastrointestinal signs consistent with canine distemper or feline panleukopenia, combined with poor vaccination history, young age, and exposure to other animals

Infectious agents

Bordetella bronchiseptica

Chlamydophila species

Salmonella species

Yersinia pestis

Some multiple-drug–resistant bacterial infections if difficult to manage (eg, draining wounds or copious respiratory secretions with an enhanced risk of aerosolization)

Canine distemper virus

Canine influenza virus

Canine parvovirus

Feline panleukopenia virus

Feline herpesvirus I

Feline calicivirus

Microsporum canis

Rabies virus

infectious agents that are spread by aerosol or by difficult to control secretions/excretions such as vomitus, diarrhea, or saliva are housed in isolation. Animals that are considered rabies suspects should always be isolated. Laboratory data provide important additional information. There are some patients for which isolation is not feasible, even although it may be appropriate because of the pathogen involved. This situation may occur when an animal is critically ill, and isolation facilities are not located in a place where appropriate support and monitoring can be reasonably provided. When this is the case, strict barrier nursing should be used in the critical care ward or other treatment area. For animals infected with pathogens transmitted by the aerosol route, this practice presents an especially difficult situation, and hospital staff must take precautions to prevent pathogen transmission to other patients. An oxygen cage with high-efficiency particulate air filtration can help to minimize the spread of such pathogens. The cage must be disassembled and thoroughly cleaned and disinfected before housing another patient.

Isolation rooms should have negative pressure air handling, but it is recognized that many hospitals may not have this available. When possible, isolation areas should have an exit to the outside as well as access from inside the hospital, to facilitate entry to and discharge from the facility. Isolation facilities should be identified by prominent signs, and instructions for entry and exit from the facility should be posted where they can be easily read (**Box 6**). Ideally, isolation areas have an anteroom in which staff may keep patient charts and treatment log sheets, wash hands and don PPE (barrier gowns, shoe covers, gloves, and eye/face protection if needed) before entering the isolation room. Health care workers should remove clinic outerwear, pagers, cell phones, and other similar devices and leave them outside the isolation anteroom before entry. If an anteroom is not available, then, an area outside the isolation facility should be provided, such as a cart or cabinet. The necessary PPE is stored here, patient charts and treatment sheets posted here, and it provides an area to store clinic outerwear, personal electronic equipment, stethoscopes, and other required items.

Disposable supplies needed for animals in the isolation facility may be stored in the anteroom and carried into the isolation area when needed there. However, this area

Box 6
Example of instructions for use at isolation areas

Entering and exiting isolation rooms

1. Before entering the isolation area, remove your clinic outerwear (eg, smock, laboratory coat) and any equipment (stethoscope, scissors, thermometer, watch, cell phone, pager) and place it on a hook in the hallway outside the isolation anteroom.
2. Gather any necessary supplies and medications before donning PPE.
3. Wash your hands or use alcohol hand rub, then put on booties, gown, and gloves before entering the isolation room.
4. Attend to the patient in isolation as needed. DO NOT bring treatment sheets or pens into the isolation room.
5. Clean and disinfect any equipment used while caring for the patient.
6. Before leaving the isolation room, remove gown by grasping the shoulders and tearing it off. Place used gown in the trash container lined with a biohazard bag in the isolation room. DO NOT SAVE THE GOWN FOR REUSE.
7. Remove gloves and discard them into the trash container lined with a biohazard bag inside the isolation room.
8. Remove booties as you step out of the room; avoid touching the outer surface of the boots. Discard the boots into the trash container lined with a biohazard bag inside the isolation room. Avoid contact with external portions of the door when exiting the isolation room.
9. Wash hands, then disinfect any surfaces (eg, door knobs) that may have accidentally been contaminated when the room was exited. Make any needed chart entries. Wash hands again before leaving the anteroom.
10. See the Standard Operating Procedures Manual and Infection Control Manual about any specific procedures in isolation. The infection control practitioner can also be contacted for assistance or questions.

Phone number ________________ pager ________________.

Keep the area clean and neat. Dispose of all single-use material promptly after use. See posted cleaning and disinfection protocols.

Modified from Purdue University Veterinary Teaching Hospital Infection Control Committee materials.

should not be heavily stocked; only enough supplies sufficient for 1 to 2 days are needed. Storing larger quantities of supplies increases the potential for supplies to become outdated before use and for supplies to become contaminated. Although anterooms are considered clean areas, with no contact with patients, the potential exists for materials in these areas to become contaminated. Ideally, once animals are discharged from isolation, all remaining disposable single-use supplies (eg, 4 x 4 sponges, bandaging material, catheters and caps, syringes and needles) in the anteroom are discarded to minimize the potential for transmission of infectious agents.

Isolation areas need running water for cleaning and hand washing. Dedicated clippers, stethoscopes, and scales should be provided, so that these items are not regularly taken in and out of the area. Each patient in isolation should have its own thermometer, which is disinfected after each use and discarded when the patient is discharged. It is imperative that all shared equipment is cleaned of gross contamination before taking it out of isolation, then placed inside plastic bags for transport to the area of the hospital where final cleaning and disinfection takes place. The bag should be clearly labeled with the name of the known or suspected pathogen, and the outside of the bag must not be contaminated before leaving isolation. A telephone or intercom should be located in isolation rooms, so that staff may call for assistance if needed. If this facility is not possible, then another staff member should be nearby in case assistance is needed. Video and audio monitors are an excellent means of providing communication with the isolation area and allowing patient observation without staff entry into the isolation unit.

Considerations common to barrier nursing and isolation

There are several considerations that apply to procedures for animals whether they are in barrier nursing circumstances or in full isolation, and these are summarized here. It is important to limit the number of hospital staff caring for patients in isolation or under barrier nursing protocols to as few as possible. In teaching hospitals, only students directly involved with the patient should handle these patients. Schedule care of patients with infectious diseases at the end of hourly treatment cycles when possible. Movement to other areas of the hospital for procedures that cannot be performed in the isolation unit should be via gurneys or in carriers, using appropriate PPE. All instruments, equipment, and surfaces that contact the patients should be cleaned and disinfected. If possible, schedule procedures for these animals at the end of the day, or when the pathway and desired location are minimally populated, so that terminal cleaning may be performed before other animals are treated in the same hospital area. Notify personnel in other areas of the hospital and the ICP of the infectious agent suspected before moving the patient, to ensure that appropriate precautions are taken. Any specimens from patients in barrier nursing or isolation that are submitted to diagnostic laboratories should be clearly marked with the name of the pathogen suspected. No medications, fluids, or bandage materials from these animals should be returned to hospital stock. Animals under barrier precautions or in isolation should have limited owner visits. Ideally, client visits are not allowed for these pets. In reality, some of these animals are critically ill, and owners may need to visit to be able to make informed decisions about ongoing care for their pets. When owners visit, they must don the same PPE that health care workers wear and perform hand hygiene when the visit is completed. These visits can be short ($\leq$10 minutes).

When patients are discharged from isolation or barrier nursing, provide written information describing the infectious disease and detailed instructions about how to minimize transmission to other animals, and to people, in the case of zoonotic pathogens. Owners should be immediately notified when a zoonotic disease is identified; modes of transmission should be explained, and owners should be advised of potentially increased risk for developing disease for immunocompromised individuals. Written information about the zoonotic agents should always be provided for the owners to read. Providing trusted Internet sources of information for owners is also beneficial. Owners should be counseled to seek the advice of their physicians for any questions about human health.

The concern that isolation protocols may diminish patient care is often expressed in veterinary medicine. This concern has been validated in the human medical field.[40,41] Patients report perceiving a lower quality of care, and objective outcome measures validate that patients in isolation may receive a lower quality or lower frequency of care. However, until other effective means of preventing in-hospital spread of highly transmissible pathogens are clearly identified, isolation and barrier precautions remain important and necessary. In some hospitals, baby monitors can provide a means of improved monitoring of patients in isolation areas. Monitors featuring video and 2-way communication are the most useful, but monitors that transmit sound only out of the isolation area are also helpful. The physical facility must be such that the monitor transmits across the necessary distance. Wireless surveillance cameras with 2-way communication capability that are monitored on computers in the hospital are an excellent option for providing improved patient monitoring and communication with personnel in the isolation area. Veterinary health care workers must remain mindful to provide excellent patient care while implementing needed infection control practices. Using remote monitors and maintaining clear schedules for care of isolated patients helps to ensure high-quality care along with effective infection control.

Another concern about barrier nursing and isolation protocols is the increased cost of patient care. Costs include those of disposable items, costs associated with hospital design and repurposing or renovation to enable improved implementation of barrier nursing and isolation protocols, and costs associated with additional personnel who may be needed for better implementation of these protocols. A recent survey of veterinarians and horse owners at the University of Florida[42] showed that referring veterinarians and clients agreed that it was very important (10 on a scale of 1–10) for a hospital to operate a surveillance and infection control program. Most (428/572, 75%) clients responded that some additional cost involved in surveillance was not considered expensive. Notwithstanding, there is concern that the increased cost of isolation may keep veterinarians from using it when necessary. In some cases, hospitals distribute the increased costs of isolation across all patient fees, effectively removing cost as an obstacle to placing a patient in isolation or barrier nursing (J. Sykes, personal communication, June, 2014).

Taken together, the concern for adequate patient care, perceived inconvenience, and increased cost, along with the increased risk of disease transmission that these patients may create for the veterinary clinic, support the importance of clearly established clinic guidelines indicating which patients should be housed in isolation or under barrier nursing. These guidelines should serve as the default placement in all cases. When a clinician has an adequate reason to deviate from this default placement, the ICP (or an appropriately designated staff member) should be consulted to discuss this deviation and provide optimal infection control and patient care.

Non–personal protective equipment barriers

In some hospitals, footbaths and disinfectant-impregnated foot mats are used in an effort to minimize pathogen transmission from areas that house animals with contagious infectious diseases. The data regarding efficacy of these interventions to decrease contamination of hospital floors are not clear. Although 2 limited studies of footwear after use of foot mats containing peroxygen disinfectant showed decreased bacteria on footwear immediately after use of the foot mats,[43,44] another study found no effect of foot mat use over a 7-month period on contamination of hospital floors.[45] When footbaths or foot mats are used, they must be carefully maintained to ensure that the disinfectant remains effective. Appropriate maintenance depends to some degree on the disinfectant used, but in general, the disinfectant in footbaths is replaced at least daily or whenever visibly soiled. Disinfectants used must be formulated to be efficacious in the presence of organic material, but even those products cannot remain effective in the presence of large amounts of organic debris. Boots or shoes should be cleaned of gross debris before the footbath is used.[43] When foot mats are used, carefully follow manufacturer recommendations for use. There is some danger that footbaths may pose a risk for slips and falls resulting from people walking on to smooth floor surfaces with wet shoes after walking in footbaths or on foot mats. If foot mats and footbaths are used, caution is needed to avoid injury from slips and falls.

More research is needed before routine use of footbaths or foot mats for most small animal hospital applications can be recommended. An effective alternative to footbaths/foot mats is the use of disposable foot covers (see the sections on barrier nursing and isolation in this article; also the article "Hand hygiene and contact precautions" by Anderson M elsewhere in this issue). When used properly, these covers provide the needed barrier protection, without the concerns listed earlier.

Maintaining physical space between patients helps to minimize pathogen transmission. Most droplet particles do not travel more than approximately 0.9 to 1.2 m (3–4 ft); however, recent data suggest that depending on the force of particle expulsion, greater distances may be attained.[46] Aerosolized particles may travel further and may also become embedded with dust particles and thereby travel greater distances (as airborne transmission). Therefore, animals infected with pathogens transmitted by these routes are best housed in isolation units with negative pressure ventilation. If this practice is not possible, then maintaining a distance of at least 1.5 to 1.8 m (5 – 6 ft) between patients, and providing adequate numbers of air exchanges, in addition to using PPE and other standard barrier precautions, can help to minimize transmission.

SUMMARY

Patient management is integrated with the many other facets of infection control programs. All aspects of infection control programs must undergo continual reevaluation and modification. What is recommended will change in the future, as more data are collected and knowledge of the epidemiology and biology of infectious diseases evolves. The patient management guidelines provided here are meant to be implemented in individual veterinary hospitals according to their individual risk assessments and within the physical constraints of each facility. The hallmark of a strong infection control program is its malleability, and the willingness of all stakeholders to regularly reassess progress in multiple fields, including infectious disease medicine, infection control, epidemiology, and microbiology. Better understanding of pathogen transmission, pathogen biology, and relationship with hosts, along with ongoing objective evaluation of the efficacy of infection control methodology, will inform and improve current patient management protocols. Members of the veterinary medicine team continually address transmission of pathogens among veterinary patients and between animals and the human beings with whom they live and interact. Basic evidence-based patient management guidelines, implemented in a commonsense manner and adjusted as new information becomes available, remain a cornerstone of infection control.

ACKNOWLEDGMENTS

Thanks to Melissa Dunning, BS, RN, for thoughtful discussions and for reviewing the article. Information in boxes 2, 3, 4 and 6 is modified from Purdue University Veterinary Teaching Hospital Infection Control Committee materials.

REFERENCES

1. Scheftel J, Elchos B, DeBess EE, et al. Compendium of veterinary standard precautions for zoonotic disease prevention in veterinary personnel: National Association of State Public Health Veterinarians Veterinary Infection Control Committee 2010. J Am Vet Med Assoc 2010;237:1403–22. Available at: http://www.nasphv.org/Documents/VeterinaryPrecautions.pdf.
2. Canadian Committee on Antibiotic Resistance: infection prevention and control best practices for small animal veterinary clinics. Available at: http://ovc.uoguelph.ca/sites/default/files/users/ovcweb/files/GuidelinesFINALInfectionPreventionDec2008.pdf. Accessed August 29, 2014.
3. Lee TB, Montgomery OG, Marx J, et al. Recommended practices for surveillance: Association for Professionals in Infection Control and Epidemiology (APIC), Inc. Am J Infect Control 2007;35:427–40.
4. Steneroden K. Biological risk management for veterinary clinics–key points, March, 2005. Center for Food Security and Public Health. Available at: http://www.cfsph.iastate.edu. Accessed August 29, 2014.
5. Khamis N, van Knippenberg-Gordebeke G. Audits in infection prevention and control. Chapter 6. In: Friedman C, Newsom W, editors. IFIC Basic Concepts of Infection Control. Portadown, N Ireland, UK: International Federation of Infection Control (IFIC); 2011. p. 71–80.
6. Morley P. Evidence-based infection control in clinical practice: if you buy clothes for the emperor, will he wear them? J Vet Intern Med 2013;27:430–8.
7. Dowd K, Taylor M, Toribio JA, et al. Zoonotic disease risk perceptions and infection control practices of Australian veterinarians: call for change in work culture. Prev Vet Med 2013;111:17–24.
8. Septimus E, Weinstein RA, Perl TM, et al. Approaches for preventing healthcare-associated infections: go long or go wide? Infect Control Hosp Epidemiol 2014;35:797–801.
9. Weese JS. Infection control and biosecurity in equine disease control. Equine Vet J 2014. http://dx.doi.org/10.1111/evj.12295.
10. Ghosh A, KuKanich K, Brown CE, et al. Resident cats in small animal veterinary hospitals carry multi-drug resistant enterococci and are likely involved in cross-contamination of the hospital environment. Front Microbiol 2012;3:62.
11. Murphy CP, Reid-Smith RJ, Boerlin P, et al. *Escherichia coli* and selected veterinary and zoonotic pathogens isolated from environmental sites in companion animal veterinary hospitals in southern Ontario. Can Vet J 2010;51:963–72.
12. Hoet AE, Johnson A, Nava-Hoet RC, et al. Environmental methicillin-resistant *Staphylococcus aureus* in a veterinary teaching hospital during a non-outbreak period. Vector Borne Zoonotic Dis 2011;11:609–15.
13. Strohmeyer RA, Morley PS, Hyatt DR, et al. Evaluation of bacterial and protozoal contamination of commercially available raw meat diets for dogs. J Am Vet Med Assoc 2006;228:537–42.

14. Lefebvre SL, Reid-Smith R, Boerlin P, et al. Evaluation of the risks of shedding Salmonellae and other potential pathogens by therapy dogs fed raw diets in Ontario and Alberta. Zoonoses Public Health 2008;55:470–80.
15. Lenz J, Joffe D, Kauffman M, et al. Perceptions, practices, and consequences associated with foodborne pathogens and the feeding of raw meat to dogs. Can Vet J 2009;50:637–43.
16. Finley R, Ribble C, Aramini J, et al. The risk of salmonellae shedding by dogs fed *Salmonella*-contaminated commercial raw food diets. Can Vet J 2007;48:69–75.
17. Sehulster L, Chinn RY. Center for Disease Control and Prevention, HICPAC. Guidelines for environmental infection control in healthcare facilities: recommendations of CDC and the Healthcare Infection Control Practice Advisory Committee (HICPAC). MMWR Recomm Rep 2003;52:1–42.
18. Palmore TN, Henderson DK. Managing transmission of carbapenem-resistant enterobacteriaceae in healthcare settings: a view from the trenches. Clin Infect Dis 2013;57:1593–9.
19. Weese JS. Barrier precautions, isolation protocols, and personal hygiene in veterinary hospitals. Vet Clin North Am Equine Pract 2004;20:543–59.
20. Cohen SR, McCormack DJ, Youkhana A, et al. Bacterial colonization of stethoscopes and the effect of cleaning. J Hosp Infect 2003;55:236–7.
21. Bandi S, Uddin L, Milward K, et al. How clean are our stethoscopes and do we need to clean them? J Infect 2008;57:355–6.
22. Bandi S, Conway A. Question 2. Does regular cleaning of stethoscopes result in a reduction in nosocomial infections? Arch Dis Child 2012;97:175–7.
23. Messina G, Ceriale E, Lenzi D, et al. Environmental contaminants in hospital settings and progress in disinfecting techniques. Biomed Res Int 2013;429780. http://dx.doi.org/10.1155/2013/429780.
24. Littman Company website. Available at: http://www.littmann.com/wps/portal/3M/en_US/3M-Littmann/stethoscope/littmann-learning-institute/about-stethoscopes/stethoscope-cleaning/. Accessed August 29, 2014. Provides information about cleaning stethoscopes.
25. Beer D, Vandermeer B, Brosnikoff C, et al. Bacterial contamination of health care workers' pagers and the efficacy of various disinfecting agents. Pediatr Infect Dis J 2006;25:1074–5.
26. Ustun C, Cihangiroglu M. Health care workers' mobile phones: a potential cause of microbial cross-contamination between hospitals and community. J Occup Environ Hyg 2012;9:538–42.
27. Walia SS, Manchanda A, Narang RS, et al. Cellular telephone as reservoir of bacterial contamination: myth or fact. J Clin Diagn Res 2014;8:50–3.
28. Albrecht U-V, von Jan U, Sedlacek L, et al. Standardized, app-based disinfection of iPads in a clinical and nonclinical setting: comparative analysis. J Med Internet Res 2013;15:e176.
29. Panhotra BR, Saxena AK, Al-Mulhim AS. Contamination of patients' files in intensive care units: an indication of strict handwashing after entering case notes. Am J Infect Control 2005;33:398–401.
30. Chen KH, Chen LR, Wang YK. Contamination of medical charts: an important source of potential infection in hospitals. PLoS One 2014;9(2):e78512. http://dx.doi.org/10.1371/journal.pone.0078512.
31. Halton K, Arora V, Singh V, et al. Bacterial colonization on writing pens touched by healthcare professionals and hospitalized patients with and without cleaning the pen with alcohol-based hand sanitizing agent. Clin Microbiol Infect 2011;17:868–9.

32. Weese JS, Lowe T, Walker M. Use of fluorescent tagging for assessment of environmental cleaning and disinfection in a veterinary hospital. Vet Rec 2012;171:217.
33. Bearman G, Bryant K, Leekha S, et al. Healthcare personnel attire in non-operating-room settings. Infect Control Hosp Epidemiol 2014;35:107–21.
34. Bajaj TI, Loh C, Borgstrom D. Diluting chlorhexidine gluconate: one scrub or two? Surg Infect (Larchmt) 2014;15:544–7.
35. Smarick SD, Haskins SC, Aldrich J, et al. Incidence of catheter-associated urinary tract infection among dogs in a small animal intensive care unit. J Am Vet Med Assoc 2004;224:1936–40.
36. Rahman MQ, Tejwani D, Wilson JA, et al. Microbial contamination of preservative free eye drops in multiple application containers. Br J Ophthalmol 2006;90:139–41.
37. Sabino CV, Weese JS. Contamination of multiple-dose vials in a veterinary hospital. Can Vet J 2006;47:779–82.
38. Benedict KM, Morley PS, Van Metre DC. Characteristics of biosecurity and infection control programs at veterinary teaching hospitals. J Am Vet Med Assoc 2008;233:767–73.
39. Murphy CP, Reid-Smith RJ, Weese JS, et al. Evaluation of specific infection control practices used by companion animal veterinarians in community veterinary practices in southern Ontario. Zoonoses Public Health 2010;57:429–38.
40. Morgan DJ, Day HR, Harris AD, et al. The impact of contact isolation on the quality of inpatient hospital care. PLoS One 2011;6(7):e22190. http://dx.doi.org/10.1371/journal.pone.0022190.
41. Morgan DJ, Diekema DJ, Sepkowitz K, et al. Adverse outcomes associated with contact precautions: a review of the literature. Am J Infect Control 2009;37:85–93.
42. Ekiri AB, House AM, Krueger TM, et al. Awareness, perceived relevance, and acceptance of large animal hospital surveillance and infection control practices by referring veterinarians and clients. J Am Vet Med Assoc 2014;244:835–43.
43. Amass SF, Arighi M, Kinyon JM, et al. Effectiveness of using a mat filled with a peroxygen disinfectant to minimize shoe sole contamination in a veterinary hospital. J Am Vet Med Assoc 2006;228:1391–6.
44. Dunowska M, Morley PS, Patterson G, et al. Evaluation of the efficacy of a peroxygen disinfectant-filled footmat for reduction of bacterial load on footwear in a large animal hospital setting. J Am Vet Med Assoc 2006;228:1935–9.
45. Hartman FA, Dusick AF, Young KM. Impact of disinfectant-filled foot mats on mechanical transmission of bacteria in a veterinary hospital. J Am Vet Med Assoc 2013;242:682–8.
46. Siegel JD, Rhinehart E, Jackson M, et al. 2007 guideline for isolation precautions: preventing transmission of infectious agents in health care settings. Am J Infect Control 2007;35(10 Suppl 2):S65–164.

ADDITIONAL RESOURCES

Centers for Disease Control and Prevention. Veterinary safety and health: hazard prevention and infection control recommendations for employers. Available at: http://www.cdc.gov/niosh/topics/veterinary/hazard.html. Accessed October 12, 2014; provides a gateway to other tools and guidelines.

Centers for Disease Control and Prevention. Healthcare-associated infections (HAIs): guidelines and recommendations. Available at: http://www.cdc.gov/hai/prevent/prevent_pubs.html. Accessed October 12, 2014; provides a gateway to multiple guidelines for infection control in human health care.

Steneroden K. Stationary veterinary clinic biological risk management, March 2005. Center for Food Security and Public Health. Available at: http://www.cfsph.iastate.edu. Accessed August 29, 2014.

Rocky Mountain Regional Center of Excellence for Biodefense and Emerging Infectious Diseases, Specialized Biodefense Training Group: veterinary guide to personal protective equipment. Available at: http://c.ymcdn.com/sites/www.colovma.org/resource/resmgr/imported/PPE%20Guide.pdf. Accessed August 24, 2014; a comprehensive guide for personal protective equipment use in veterinary medicine.

Environmental Cleaning and Disinfection

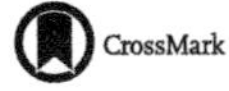

Michelle Traverse, BS, CVT[a], Helen Aceto, PhD, VMD[b,*]

KEYWORDS

- Small animal • Veterinary clinic • Environmental contamination • Infection prevention
- Surveillance

KEY POINTS

- As in human medicine, hospital-associated infections (HAIs) exist in veterinary medicine and must be subject to control measures.
- Environmental contamination with pathogens of concern is widespread in veterinary hospitals and should be an important target of proactive measures to prevent (limit) HAI.
- For environmental cleaning and disinfection (C/D) to be effective, all stakeholders should be educated as to the need for appropriate C/D and the participation of all (at any level) should be encouraged to accomplish this goal.
- Veterinary practices should seriously consider identifying personnel responsible for establishing infection control practices, establishing monitoring/audit procedures, and determining whether their practice situation warrants proactive environmental surveillance.
- More research is required to identify the precise relationship between environmental contamination and HAI and to establish control and surveillance/monitoring procedures of direct relevance to veterinary medicine.

BACKGROUND

The concept of infection control and prevention in veterinary medicine outside the surgical suite or epidemic disease control/eradication in livestock populations was more or less unheard of until the last 1 or 2 decades. During that time, there has been a paradigm shift, such that veterinary infection control is a growing discipline that is becoming part of the customary way in which veterinarians practice medicine. This shift is seen primarily in large academic teaching hospitals associated with specific veterinary schools and in specialty clinics dedicated to advanced diagnostics and care for animals. However, the nature of medicine and mission of veterinary hospitals

---

The authors have nothing to disclose.

[a] Department of Clinical Studies, Matthew J. Ryan Veterinary Hospital, University of Pennsylvania, 3900 Delancey Street, Philadelphia, PA 19104, USA; [b] Department of Clinical Studies, New Bolton Center, University of Pennsylvania, 382 West Street Road, Kennett Square, PA 19348, USA

* Corresponding author.

E-mail address: helenwa@vet.upenn.edu

Vet Clin Small Anim 45 (2015) 299–330

http://dx.doi.org/10.1016/j.cvsm.2014.11.011 **vetsmall.theclinics.com**

0195-5616/15/$ – see front matter

are such that animals clinically affected by the agents that have the potential to spread among the hospital population, as well as subclinical carriers that may go unrecognized, are always likely to be present in veterinary medical facilities, regardless of size or specialty. The standard of care at every veterinary hospital should include a high level of hygiene, awareness of the dangers of transfer of infectious agents between both animals and people, and procedures to reduce infection risk wherever possible. Such infection control procedures are intended to prevent (limit) introduction and spread of infectious diseases within a group of patients and their human caregivers, thereby, protecting human, animal, and environmental health against biological threats. This article provides an overview of environmental considerations in infection control rather than an exhaustive review. There are numerous excellent resources that cover various aspects in greater detail, many of which are referenced in the following sections.

HEALTH CARE–ASSOCIATED INFECTIONS IN HUMAN MEDICINE

Nosocomial infection, otherwise known as hospital-acquired or more recently health care–associated infections (HAIs), are the subject of high-profile press coverage and government or internal regulation in human medicine. The latest published figures from human medicine in the United States suggest that in 2011, 722,000 patients contracted HAI in acute-care hospitals, more than half of which were acquired outside the intensive care unit (ICU).[1] These infections resulted in 75,000 deaths and constitute the seventh leading cause of death in the United States.[2] Although they may be artificial constructs, when these numbers are averaged out over time, they indicate that on any given day in the United States, 1 in 25 patients has at least 1 HAI, and every day of the year, 205 people die from HAIs. As shocking as these figures are, stringent control efforts instituted over the last 2 to 3 decades in human medicine, which were formalized in 2008,[3,4] seem responsible for an apparent decline in rates of HAI compared with the 1970s to 1990s, during which approximately 2 million HAIs were estimated to occur each year and were, in turn, associated with 100,000 annual deaths.[2–4] In 2011, the most common HAIs included central line–associated bloodstream infections (54,500), catheter-associated urinary tract infections (30,100), surgical site infections (53,700), and *Clostridium difficile* infections (107,700).[1,2] The pathogens principally associated with these infections include methicillin-resistant *Staphylococcus aureus* (MRSA), vancomycin-resistant enterococci (VRE), *Clostridium difficile*, *Acinetobacter*, norovirus, and most recently, carbapenemase producing enterobactericeae.[2] HAIs are estimated to account for $40 billion in excess health care costs each year.[5]

ENVIRONMENTAL CONTAMINATION IN HUMAN HOSPITALS

In the early 1990s, initial estimates of the sources of HAI among adult ICU patients suggested that endogenous microbiota accounted for 40% to 60% of infections, cross-infection from the hands of health care personnel for 20% to 40%, changes in the microbiota driven by antimicrobial drug use for 20% to 25%, and other factors, such as environmental contamination, for 20%.[6] In the interim, much compelling evidence has accumulated to confirm an important role for the environment in pathogen transmission.[7] Surfaces in the room of a patient colonized/infected with a hospital pathogen are frequently contaminated, pathogens can remain viable on hospital surfaces and equipment for extended periods, the hands, gloves, and other apparel of health care personnel are readily contaminated after being in contact with a contaminated environment, a person admitted to a room previously occupied by a patient colonized/infected with a hospital pathogen has an increased likelihood of being colonized/infected themselves, and improvements in terminal cleaning and disinfection (C/D) lead to decreased rates of infection.[7–9] The organisms for which data implicating a role for environmental contamination are strongest include norovirus, *Clostridium difficile*, VRE, *Acinetobacter* spp, MRSA, and *Pseudomonas aeruginosa*.[7,9] It should be obvious that the list of organisms with the strongest links to environmental contamination is essentially the same as that for pathogens most closely related to HAI.

HEALTH CARE–ASSOCIATED INFECTIONS IN VETERINARY MEDICINE

In veterinary medicine, specific numbers and incidence of HAI are not so well documented, but 2 recently published studies[10,11] sought to estimate the occurrence of HAI using a standardized syndromic surveillance system in 2 clinical settings over a 12-week period at 5 veterinary teaching hospitals (VTHs); first, in hospitalized horses admitted for gastrointestinal disorders and second, in small animals in the critical care unit. Although there was variability between hospitals, when these differences were controlled for, of the 297 horses in the study population, 19.7% (95% confidence interval [CI], 14.5–26.7) were reported to have had at least 1 nosocomial event during hospitalization. Equivalent proportions for 1535 dogs were 16.3% (95% CI, 14.3–18.5), and of 416 cats, 12% (95% CI, 9.3–15.5) had at least 1 nosocomial event. In both horses and small animals, the most commonly reported syndrome was surgical site inflammation, with intravenous catheter site inflammation and urinary tract inflammation being the second most common in horses and small animals, respectively. In addition, in a published survey of biosecurity experts at 38 VTHs,[12] 31 (82%) hospitals reported the occurrence of a nosocomial disease outbreak in the 5 years before the survey interview. Although most of these outbreaks were associated with large animal facilities, there are also published reports of HAIs and outbreaks in small animal clinics.[13–18] There is more than enough evidence to indicate that, as in human medicine, HAIs in veterinary hospitals are a part of the world in which we live. Although certain issues, the principal pathogens, and thus the control measures may differ, it is nonsensical to imagine that reality for veterinary medicine is any different from human medicine, in that HAIs exist and must be subject to control measures.

ENVIRONMENTAL CONTAMINATION IN VETERINARY HOSPITALS

Many of the pathogens associated with HAI in humans are found in VTHs and can cause infections in animals. However, just as data on veterinary HAI are not readily available, the relationship of environmental contamination with most of these pathogens to HAI is not well defined. Nevertheless, as with human medicine, the link between HAIs and the environment of veterinary clinics is becoming more clear. There are numerous descriptions of environmental contamination associated with HAI in large animal hospitals,[19–23] and at the University of Pennsylvania's George D. Widener Hospital for Large Animals, where we conduct routine environmental surveillance for *Salmonella*, we have many examples directly correlating infection in animals (both community associated and HAI) with environmental contamination (Dr H. Aceto, unpublished observations, 2004). In addition, recently documented MRSA events in veterinary settings showed that environmental contamination ranged from 1% to 12%,[24–27] and there are reports of contamination of the environment and equipment in small animal hospitals with enterococci many of which were multidrug resistant (MDR).[28,29] One of these studies[28] investigated the hypothesis that cage doors, stethoscopes, thermometers, and mouth gags used in participating hospitals would have bacterial contamination that could contribute to HAI. This investigation was accomplished by determining the prevalence of surface contamination with enterococci at 10 different veterinary hospitals. Because the locations within the hospitals that were sampled had direct patient contact, it is perhaps not surprising that they all yielded enterococci at 1 or more hospitals. To compare cleaning protocols with bacterial contamination, a veterinarian at each hospital was asked to complete a questionnaire. Results showed that only half of the hospitals had written standard operating procedures for hospital cleaning, and the wide variety of disinfectants used precluded examination of any relationship between cleaning and contamination. Moreover, 5 of 10 veterinarians surveyed reported almost never or never cleaning their stethoscopes, and there were also deficiencies in the cleaning of cage doors, thermometers, and mouth gags at some hospitals.

Despite the relative paucity of data, it should be apparent that veterinary hospitals are inherently contaminated and that any number of bacterial, viral, or fungal organisms may be harbored in the hospital environs. The nature of animals and the challenges they pose in terms of hygiene and containment almost guarantee contamination of a space. The range of species that may require hospitalization is large and varied, and each species may have distinct flora and different susceptibility risks.

As our understanding of HAI in veterinary medicine increases, medical staff and administrators alike are coming to realize the acute threat that HAIs pose to hospitalized veterinary patients and are looking toward proactive preventive measures rather than reactive damage control. The additional financial burden (eg, increased length of hospital stay, increased treatment costs, possible indemnification and legal costs, loss of future business) that HAI in general and outbreaks in particular can impose on a hospital is undoubtedly another motivating factor.[19,23,30] The fact that many of the pathogens of importance to the health of hospitalized animals are also zoonotic is an equally important consideration, and all infection control programs should include measures to protect human health.[31] In common with human medicine, it is becoming clear that the hospital environment is an important target of these proactive measures.

IMPORTANCE OF FACILITY DESIGN

The physical environment can affect many facets of veterinary care, including patient comfort, patient stress, patient and staff safety, staff effectiveness, quality of care, and patient susceptibility to disease. Effective C/D are critical in preventing transmission of infectious agents between patients or from contaminated environments. To aid in this process, it is desirable that surfaces in animal housing and clinical spaces are cleanable and nonporous. This strategy can be as simple as ensuring that wood surfaces are properly sealed and painted or more complex by eliminating furniture and finishes that are not easily disinfected or, in the worst case, those that are essentially not cleanable by standard C/D methods. Furniture and finishes may include carpeting, upholstery, and unfinished or damaged wood surfaces. In a veterinary hospital, in which fecal material and respiratory or other secretions are abundant, frequently defy containment, are more likely to harbor pathogens, and may represent an HAI risk, cleanliness of treatment/procedures spaces, animal housing, and operating rooms is crucial. This necessity is particularly true in critical care and isolation units, where exacting evaluation of all surfaces, construction materials, and equipment is essential to maximize cleanability, environmental safety, and efficient operation of the area. Such considerations should influence the choice of materials and finishes for all kinds of surfaces (eg, floors, walls, benches and work surfaces, doors and frames); solid, nonporous surface materials that are highly durable and with as few seams as possible are best. For example, in personnel areas, such as nursing stations, seamless, highly cleanable and exceptionally durable poured epoxy floors, although more expensive, are preferable to materials such as vinyl tile. Wherever seams are present, regular maintenance to ensure their integrity or that of other interfaces between surfaces is essential. Block walls should be sealed, with urethane-based paints, for example. Although metal doors and frames are nonporous and may be the ideal, some composites are also suitable. Any wood surfaces must be properly sealed and painted. For all materials, regular inspection and maintenance are a must. To facilitate cleaning, there should be adequate provision of drains. Drains should be connected to the sanitary system, and, to limit future disruption for the conduct of work to replace corroded drains, use of stainless steel drain hubs should be considered to prolong the life of the drain in the face of water, cleaners, disinfectants, and animal urine. The choice of heating and ventilation systems and the location of heaters and air vents are all critical components in facility design. Although this factor may be most obvious for the control of pathogens classically considered to be transmitted via the airborne route, it may be less obvious that organisms normally thought of as fecal-oral can be greatly impacted by heating, ventilation, and air conditioning (HVAC) systems. Impacts can be both in terms of contaminating the system and in terms of the system facilitating pathogen spread via, for example, forced hot air systems that circulate contaminated particulates widely throughout a given space. It is imperative that engineers with knowledge about airborne transmission be involved in the design of HVAC systems for veterinary facilities, particularly isolation units.

Frequently unconsidered surfaces, such as in the vicinity of nursing stations, doorknobs and hardware, light switches, telephones, computers and their keyboards, are also becoming recognized hot spots of contamination.[19,22,32,33] When a hospital environment is not easy to both clean and disinfect, the potential for HAI increases, so critical evaluation of the hospital environment is essential.

Intentionally planning a space for improved safety and hygiene is an important concept in human medicine and an easy, although not necessarily inexpensive, idea to adapt to veterinary hospitals. Infection control and ease of disinfection should be essential considerations in newly designed veterinary facilities or those undergoing renovation. Hospital improvements must always consider the role that design plays in infection prevention. The architects and designers hired to plan a new health care facility or renovate current facilities are crucial in establishing design features that improve hospital safety and in identifying and using appropriate surfaces and substrates.[34] The Center for Health Design's internationally recognized Evidence-based Design Accreditation and Certification[35] program awards credentials to individuals who show a thorough understanding of how to apply an evidence-based process to the design and development of health care settings. Evidence-based design is the process of basing decisions about the built environment on credible research to achieve the best possible outcomes; to this end, it also includes measuring and reporting results.

GENERAL CONCEPTS IN ENVIRONMENTAL CLEANING AND DISINFECTION

The goal of environmental C/D is not to completely sterilize the environment but rather to significantly decrease the pathogen load to a point at which disease transmission does not occur. Definitions of C/D terminology are given in **Box 1**. At a minimum, C/D protocols should include the following steps:

1. Detergent to remove organic debris (critical to the efficacy of most disinfectants)
2. Rinsing

Box 1
Basic definitions

Cleaning: removal of foreign material (eg, contaminants, including dust, soil, chemical residues, pyrogens, large numbers of microorganisms) and the organic matter protecting them. Normally accomplished using water with detergents or enzymatic products. Thorough cleaning is required before high-level disinfection and sterilization, because inorganic and organic materials remaining on surfaces interfere with the effectiveness of these processes

Disinfection: the process that destroys most pathogenic microorganisms, especially the vegetative forms, but not necessarily bacterial spores, usually accomplished by use of liquid chemicals

Antisepsis: a special category of disinfection, referring to the inhibition or destruction of pathogenic microbes on the skin and mucous membranes

Biocides: distinct from disinfectants in that they are intended to destroy all forms of life, not just microorganisms

Sanitation: reduction of the number of bacterial contaminants to a safe level. Sanitizers are not concentrated enough or in contact with organisms long enough to effect disinfection

Terminal cleaning: the process carried out after a patient under isolation has been discharged, end of the day cleaning in areas such as operating rooms, or end of procedure cleaning in areas in which a patient known to be infected with a contagious disease has been handled

Sterilization: the process used to render an object free of all microorganisms, excluding prions

Data from Refs.[36,37,48–51]

3. Drying (optimum; or at a minimum water removal, because application of disinfectant to a water-logged area may result in dilution to the point of inefficacy)
4. Disinfectant application at appropriate concentration, ensuring that the disinfectant remains wet on the surface for the required contact time.

Veterinarians and staff should pay strict attention to the role that appropriate environmental C/D plays in the reduction and elimination of veterinary HAI.[36–38] C/D processes are of utmost importance in ensuring patient, client, and staff safety and an uneventful hospital stay in terms of HAI. The steps in a typical practical C/D procedure of broad environmental application are shown in more detail in **Box 2**, with an emphasis on critical concepts such as dilution rates and contact times for disinfectants. The steps provided are suitable for high-level C/D but are readily adaptable to more low-level C/D needs. Some, but not all, disinfectants have good cleaning in addition to disinfecting properties, so the basic number of steps can be reduced in noncritical areas (to determine whether a particular disinfectant product has adequate cleaning properties inspect the manufacturer's label). However, where areas are grossly dirty, a separate detergent step is always required. In addition, some disinfectants require rinsing, because of the potential for toxicity or surface damage, but others may have residual activity, which might be negated by rinsing. The need for rinsing and claims for residual activity are also stated on the product label. Drying after C/D is always beneficial to pathogen control. Characteristics of each disinfectant product, including their compatibility with detergents and other chemicals, can be determined by careful inspection of the label, so it is important that individuals responsible for both choosing and using these products understand how to read the manufacturer's label.[36] More information on characteristics of disinfectants is covered in the section on choosing a disinfectant.

Box 2
Example of an effective, broad-application, environmental C/D protocol

Have all material safety data sheet or product safety data sheets for C/D materials available and follow instructions for proper mixing, disposal, and personal protective equipment (eg, gloves, eye protection).

In the case of animal cages, remove all bedding (if intended for reuse, place in receptacle and send for laundering) and any organic material before cleaning. In other areas, remove any loose organic material (eg, feces, feed, hair, linens, bandage or other materials) before cleaning.

Clean surfaces with an anionic detergent. Scrubbing of surfaces is often necessary to remove biofilms and stubborn organic debris, especially in animal housing areas.

Rinse with clean water. For all rinsing and product application procedures, care must be exercised to avoid overspray. Unless equipment is moved to a dedicated cleaning area, high-pressure washing should generally be avoided. Higher pressures can help remove stubborn organic debris, but may also force debris and organisms into crevices or porous materials, from which they can later emerge, and they cause more aerosolization and overspray, which may spread organisms widely, even into previously uncontaminated areas. For methods not involving hoses see **Box 3**.

Allow to dry or at least ensure that the bulk of surface water is removed. If excess water remains, subsequently applied disinfectants may be diluted to the point of inefficacy

Apply disinfectant solution and allow the appropriate contact time. A dilute solution (1:25–1:50) of household (4%–5.25%) bleach with at least 15 minutes contact time is readily available and inexpensive but may not be the most effective choice. Many other options are available. Alternatives include accelerated hydrogen peroxide (eg, Accel TB [Virox Technologies Inc, Oakville Ontario, Canada]), quaternary ammonium disinfectants (eg, Roccal-D [Zoetis, Florham Park, NJ], Parvosol [Hess and Clark Inc, Randolph, WI]), peroxygen-based disinfectants (eg, Virkon-S [Sudbury, Suffolk, UK]/Trifectant [Vetoquinol, Fort Worth, TX]), or phenolics (eg, 1-Stroke Environ [Steris Corp, Mentor, OH], Tek-Trol [Bio-Tek Industries Inc, Atlanta GA]). Dilution rates and recommended contact times vary by product and are critical to efficacy; be sure to read the product label carefully and follow manufacturer's instructions. Although not suitable for use in all areas, metered hose-end sprayers or foamers (eg, HydroFoamer/Sprayer [Hydro Systems Co, Cincinnati, OH]) are efficient delivery methods and generally ensure accurate dilution. Foamers might enhance surface contact.

Rinse thoroughly with clean water (although some disinfectants indicate that rinsing is unnecessary, it can prevent residue build-up over time).

Allow the treated area to dry as much as possible. Drying is important to achieve maximum effect; allow area to dry as much as possible (completely is preferred), before reintroducing animals or reusing the area. If postcleaning environmental samples are being collected, the area must be completely dry.

In known contaminated or high-risk areas, a second application of disinfectant with, for example, an accelerated hydrogen peroxide product should be considered as a final decontamination step. Ensure appropriate contact time, rinse with clean water, and allow the treated area to dry as much as possible, as stated above.

Several studies in human medicine have shown that less than 50% of hospital rooms are adequately cleaned and disinfected.[39,40] Less obvious environmental sites can be frequently overlooked. "Housekeeping, nurses, and aides will universally clean obviously soiled surfaces; many germ-infected sites go unnoticed."[41] Several methods are being used to improve C/D, including staff education, use of checklists, and hygiene assessment tools. Although there are few examples, hygiene assessments using luminometer readings[33] and fluorescent tagging[42] have been described in veterinary medicine. The Association for Professionals in Infection Control and Epidemiology and the Association for the Healthcare Environment are 2 human-based professional infection control societies that are using all of these approaches and are striving to improve the cooperation between medical staff and environmental services (housekeeping), with the singular goal of improved patient outcomes. Their educational campaign *Clean Spaces, Healthy Patients* incorporates educational resources and training materials. The initiative represents both an evolution and a revolution in infection prevention. Although for many years, the field focused on clean hands, there is now growing recognition that preventing HAIs is about clean hands touching clean equipment in clean environments. It also serves to bridge the gap and remove barriers to success between medical staff and environmental services.[43] Although not all private veterinary practices have dedicated housekeeping personnel and C/D tasks are likely to be carried out by staff members who also have other duties, this training initiative in human medicine and the simple tools that it uses are equally applicable to veterinary medicine.

Depending on size, caseload, and case type, veterinary hospitals should consider appointing a willing individual or a group that represents all relevant constituencies to oversee infection control issues. A preliminary step in establishing an infection control program should be an evaluation of the level of HAI risk and how risk averse you want to be in your practice. The risk evaluation process helps guide the nature and stringency of the infection control procedures to be adopted. Because infection control measures are generally associated with some cost, consideration should also be given to how the risk/benefit ratio of these procedures is assessed (the latter might require evaluation over time). Disinfection protocols, for example, should be frequently reviewed and if necessary altered based on evidence gathered through patient and, potentially, environmental surveillance. In addition, there is ample evidence that, in addition to antimicrobial resistance, microorganisms can be resistant to disinfectants, antiseptics, and sterilants, either constitutively, through acquired means, or by formation of biofilms.[44] Keeping abreast of developments in antimicrobial resistance helps in determining the need for change.

When designing a C/D protocol, consideration should also be given to the effect of disinfectants (some of which are powerful oxidizers) on equipment, personnel, and materials in the environment. A particular disinfectant may be more costly at the outset but overall might be a prudent choice, because of minimal destruction of equipment or damage inflicted to surfaces over time. If prolonged use of a disinfectant is found to damage surfaces, an alternative should be sought, because loss of surface integrity defeats the object of maintaining sealed, cleanable surfaces in critical areas. The use of prepackaged wipes containing disinfectants such as accelerated hydrogen peroxide or quaternary ammonium compounds is a convenient means of disinfecting hand surfaces and certain types of delicate equipment. Clippers, clipper blades, bandage or suture scissors, thermometers, mouth gags, laryngoscopes, endoscopes, and all other equipment used on patients should be subject to appropriate C/D. There are differences between cleaning, disinfection, antisepsis, and terminal cleaning, as defined in **Box 1**. Many valuable resources cover all aspects of cleaning protocols, and the properties and use of disinfectants in significant detail.[32–38,45–55]

AREAS TO ADDRESS

When establishing cleaning protocols, it is important to appreciate that appropriate veterinary hospital C/D is not random. There are certain factors, such as risk, traffic flow, and the critical nature of a given space or item, that must be considered and other decisions that must be made; every aspect of the process, from what type of products and materials should be used, to the order of events, and frequency of cleaning, needs to be scrutinized and researched. In addition to the typical C/D protocol outlined in **Box 2**, steps in the 3 basic methods for performing environmental C/D are shown in **Box 3**.

Box 3
Outline of basic cleaning methods

1. Dry method
   - Use of dust-retaining materials (ie, microfiber cloths; microfiber cloths and mops have shown superior microbe removal to other materials like cotton, particularly when used with a detergent cleaner) rather than traditional brooms or rags, to minimize the dispersion of contaminated dust in the environment
   - When cloths are used for damp cleaning, only clean water should be used; no additional detergents are needed
   - All cloths should be washed after every use
2. Wet method
   - Double bucket technique: first bucket is for clean water and either detergent or disinfectant; second bucket is for clean rinse water
   - Single bucket technique: solution must be changed as soon as it becomes dirty and before moving to any new area
   - All mop buckets should be emptied, cleaned, and left to dry when not in use. Mop heads should be changed a minimum of once a day or sooner when visibly soiled
3. Terminal method
   - Personnel conducting the process must use appropriate personal protective equipment (eg, gloves, disposable apron, eye protection) when indicated
   - Discard all disposable items according to proper waste disposal regulations
   - Remove portable equipment to dirty utility area for C/D or sterilization as needed
   - Place all laundry into an appropriate bag, seal before removal from the space, and send for processing
   - Dry dust patient area, beginning at the top and working toward the bottom (although walls are not considered particularly critical surfaces in human medicine, the fact that veterinary patients may regularly lick those surfaces as well as floors increases their importance in veterinary infection control)
   - Wet dust patient area, beginning at top and working toward the bottom
   - Wash mats, caging or animal housing areas, surgical and examination tables, and other static equipment with detergent and water, rinse, and dry
   - If disinfection is required (mandatory for infectious patients), apply appropriate disinfectant solution to any/all areas, allow contact time, rinse, and dry
   - Use special procedures for static equipment that cannot withstand treatment with water and detergents
   - As needed, repeat washing and disinfection of floors

Data from Refs.[36,49,50,52,53]

As part of the process of developing the most efficient cleaning protocols that are likely to be most effective in mitigating HAI, it is useful to consider the hospital environment divided into 2 principal groups:

1. Surfaces that come into frequent contact with hands
2. Surfaces that have minimal contact with hands

As a rule, hand-touch surfaces are of a larger concern than surfaces having minimal contact.[43,50] At the University of Pennsylvania's large animal hospital, *Salmonella* has been used as an environmental biosensor for more than 10 years. When hand and floor surface samples are compared, of samples identified as positive for *Salmonella* over that period, approximately 60% were collected from hand areas (eg, stall door bolts, light switches, telephones, door knobs, drawer pulls, bench tops in records and preparation areas, refrigerator door handles, computer keyboards).

Picking and choosing which hospital surfaces and areas are of most concern and in most need of high-level C/D must also take other factors into consideration. In particular, the frequency of C/D necessary for an area should take into account:

- Type of hospital unit (eg, high-risk units such as critical care, neonatal, and isolation units and surgical suites require frequent high-level C/D)
- Potential for contamination with bodily fluids
- Potential for contamination with dust, soil, or water

The National Specifications of Cleanliness for the UK National Health Service (NHS)[54] suggest identifying hospital risk categories and the required level of service for each category, as outlined later. Veterinary hospitals should consider this approach and, as mentioned earlier, establish an infection control individual/group, which in the context of C/D ideally includes individuals responsible for C/D of the facilities, clinical representatives, and other relevant stakeholders. In addition to instituting C/D protocols, this group should be prepared to educate other staff to ensure buy-in at all levels and promote compliance. Although not widely adopted in veterinary medicine, auditing of C/D is a means of checking practice against a standard or desired outcome and it has been used to improve health service in human medicine.[54,56] The infection control team should be encouraged to develop and conduct audits of C/D. The NHS materials include some sample cleaning standards and audit score sheets that are eminently adaptable to veterinary use. Cleaning standards for a few selected items are shown in **Table 1**. Elements for consideration of cleaning standards can be divided into 3 overlapping major groups: environment, direct contact, and patient equipment. In terms of the environment, there are several subgroups: floors; fixed assets; electrical appliances; toilets, sinks, and other washing facilities; and furnishings and fixtures; examples of which are indicated in **Table 1**. Issues to be considered when designing and implementing an audit process include frequency, personnel, methodology, sampling, scoring, and action. For human hospitals, personnel involvement and scoring systems can be complex. However, for most veterinary applications, audits could be conducted by an individual or, better yet, a small group, which comprises medical personnel and individuals responsible for C/D. Whoever conducts the audit should be able to competently judge what is acceptable in terms of cleanliness and infection prevention and control. Once the elements and standards criteria to be included in the audit have been identified, the scoring system could be as simple as acceptable (score 1) or unacceptable (score 0) for each element in a given space of a functional area (see later discussion), leading to an overall score for that area. Based on the number of elements scored, the area score can be converted into a percent

Table 1
Examples of cleaning standards for selected elements found in the clinical environment

Element	Standard
Floor: nonslip (environment/floors)	The complete floor, including all edges, corners, and main floor space, should have a uniform finish or shine and be visibly clean, with no blood and body substances, dust, dirt, debris, or spillages
Walls (environment/ fixed assets)	All wall surfaces, including skirting, should be visibly clean, with no blood and body substances, dust, dirt, debris, adhesive tape, or spillages
All doors (environment/ fixed assets)	All parts of the door structure should be visibly clean so that all door surfaces, vents, frames, and jambs have no blood or body substances, dust, dirt, debris, adhesive tape, or spillages
Switches, sockets, and data points (environment/ fixed assets)	All wall fixtures (eg, switches, sockets, data points) should be visibly clean, with no blood and body substances, dust, dirt, debris, adhesive tape, or spillages
Sinks (environment/toilets sinks and other washing facilities)	The sink and wall-attached dispensers should be visibly clean, with no blood and body substances, dust, dirt, debris, lime scale, stains, or spillages. Plugholes and overflow should be free from build-up
Hand hygiene alcohol rub dispensers (environment/ furnishings and fixtures)	All parts of the surfaces of hand hygiene alcohol rub dispensers should be visibly clean, with no blood and body substances, dust, dirt, debris, adhesive tape, or spillages. Dispensers should be kept stocked
Animal cages (environment/ fixtures/direct contact)	All parts of the cage (including bars, interior walls, floor, and corners) should be visibly clean, with no blood and body substances, dust, dirt, debris, adhesive tape, or spillages
Tables (environment/ furnishings and fixtures)	All parts of the table (including wheels, castors, and underneath) should be visibly clean, with no blood and body substances, dust, dirt, debris, adhesive tape, stains, or spillages
Waste receptacles (environment/furnishings and fixtures)	The waste receptacle should be visibly clean, including lid and pedal, with no blood and body substances, dust, dirt, debris, stains, or spillages. Receptacles should be emptied frequently and not allowed to overflow
Fridges and freezers (environment/ furnishings and fixtures)	Fridges and freezers should be visibly clean, with no blood and body substances, dust, dirt, debris, spillages, food debris, or build-up of ice
Medical equipment connected to a patient (eg, intravenous infusion pumps, drip stand) (patient equipment/direct contact)	All parts, including underneath, should be visibly clean, with no blood and body substances, dust, dirt, debris, or spillages
Cleaning equipment (environment/fixtures, maybe electrical)	Cleaning equipment should be visibly clean, with no blood and body substances, dust, dirt, debris, or moisture

acceptable. As a guideline, the NHS system uses the following percentages as targets for the 4 functional risk areas described later: very high, 98%; high, 95%; significant, 85%; low, 75%; areas with scores lower than this are considered for predetermined remedial action.

Ideally, regular audits should form part of the quality assurance program of your clinic. Issues raised should be followed up according to their magnitude and location. Lead times should be identified for remediation. For example, a problem in the surgical area needs to be resolved immediately, whereas one in a storeroom for noncritical items may require checking within some reasonable time, such as during the next scheduled audit. Although it is important that deficiencies be identified and corrected, efforts should be made to avoid the perception that audits will be punitive in nature. Functional areas for evaluation can be categorized as follows:

1. Very high-risk functional areas
    - Operating rooms, critical care units, departments in which invasive procedures are performed or in which immunocompromised patients are receiving care, isolation units
    - Desired outcomes are achieved only through intensive and frequent cleaning
    - Initially audit at least once a week, until the lead cleaning manager and infection control team are satisfied that consistently high standards are being achieved, after which the audit frequency may be reduced to no less than twice monthly
2. High-risk functional areas
    - Include examination rooms, general wards, sterile supplies, public thoroughfares, and public toilets
    - Desired outcomes maintained by regular and frequent cleaning, with spot cleaning in between
    - Initially audited at least once a month, until it is clear that consistently high standards are being achieved, after which the audit frequency may be reduced to no less than monthly
3. Significant-risk functional areas
    - Pathology, outpatient areas, and laboratories
    - Desired outcomes maintained by regular and frequent cleaning with spot cleaning in between
    - Audited at least once every 3 months
4. Low-risk functional areas
    - Administrative areas, nonsterile supply areas, record storage, and archives
    - Desired outcomes maintained by regular and frequent cleaning with spot cleaning in between
    - Audit at least twice a year

CHOOSING A DISINFECTANT

There are numerous chemical agents available to disinfect health care facilities. These agents are mostly liquid based and fall into 9 broad categories: acids, alcohols, aldehydes, alkalis, biguanides, halogens (hypochlorites and iodine-based iodophors), oxidizing agents, phenolics, and quaternary ammonium compounds. Accelerated hydrogen peroxide products (eg, Accel, Virox Technologies, Oakville, ON, Canada), which claim virucidal, bactericidal, fungicidal, and tuberculocidal activity, have been introduced recently for disinfection of noncritical environmental surfaces and equipment. In addition, there are some newer disinfectant combinations that have synergistic actions (eg, Siloxycide, Preserve International, Reno, NV), a combination of hydrogen peroxide plus silver nitrate; the latter provides extended peroxide stability, and the combination claims increased efficacy compared with products containing only hydrogen peroxide; this combination is approved for use in health care settings. Quaternary ammonium/glutaraldehyde combinations (eg, Synergize, Preserve International; Reno, NV) were developed for use in livestock facilities and have been successful, but they are not approved for use in veterinary hospitals. There are also newer technologies, such as no-touch methods of surface disinfection.[7,48,49] These methods include ultraviolet (UV) light and hydrogen peroxide dry-mist or vapor (HPV) fogging procedures.[49] Both can be used for whole room decontamination and are more suited to occasional use either in response to a specific problem or as part of a program of thorough disinfection of specific spaces scheduled to occur at predetermined intervals. HPV is capable of killing a wide range of pathogens, including *Cryptosporidium* and ~6 logs spores, whereas UV is reliably biocidal at 3 to 4 logs against vegetative bacteria. No animals or people can be present during the decontamination process. The use parameters for both are sensitive and require specialized equipment, representing a considerable capital investment, but unlike HPV, UV systems need no additional consumable products. Room decontamination is rapid with UV (~15 minutes) compared with 3 to 5 hours for HPV. In addition, for HPV, the HVAC system must be disabled and the rooms sealed to prevent unwanted dilution of the vapor, which requires considerable staff time. HPV is uniformly distributed throughout the room via an automated dispersal system and is particularly useful for disinfecting temperature-sensitive or complex equipment and furniture. It has been speculated that over time HPV might cause damage to sensitive electronics as a result of microcondensation, but this should not be an issue with the dry-mist form. HPV leaves no toxic residues (aeration units convert HPV into oxygen and water), and it requires no rinsing. Similarly, UV systems generate no residues and are not associated with health and safety concerns, but the environmental penetration of these systems is probably less than HPV. Neither procedure removes dust or stains, so the area must be clean before decontamination. Although these systems have been used widely in human medicine, there are no data to show whether or not the incidence of HAI decreases.[49] Other no-touch methods increasingly being used include self-disinfecting surfaces impregnated with heavy metals (eg, copper and silver) or germicides (eg, the bisphenolic compound triclosan). At our large animal hospital, we have successfully used silver-impregnated sticky mats (Dycem, Warwick, RI) in place of footbaths in main entry areas to our high-risk isolation and colic facilities as well as the entry way to the necropsy facility. Although we have not encountered specific problems with these mats, which are sampled weekly for the presence of *Salmonella*, it is well known that bacteria (particularly gram-negative organisms, including *Escherichia coli*) can be resistant to heavy metals by both intrinsic and, in some cases, acquired mechanisms. Five mechanisms of intrinsic resistance have been described that allow bacteria to survive in the presence of inhibitory or microbicidal concentrations of toxic metals[44] Bacterial resistance to biocides such as triclosan can be intrinsic or acquired by mutation or plasmid or transposon acquisition and can be via several mechanisms: exclusion; efflux mechanisms; mutation to decrease target sensitivity; or target overproduction.[44] The likelihood of resistance development should always be considered when choosing products, particularly because some items, such as the mats mentioned earlier, are expensive. Antimicrobial surface coatings based on nanoparticles are under development for both biomedical devices and environmental surfaces[57,58] and may have the advantage over microbicidal coatings based on metals or agents, such as triclosan, because they have prolonged activity, and some seem unlikely to be associated with the development of microbial resistance.[57] Steam disinfection systems offer an alternative to liquid chemical disinfectants and can kill a diverse group of pathogenic organisms in seconds, but they are not suitable for all surfaces and introduce additional safety considerations.

Characteristics of the ideal disinfectant are shown in **Box 4**. The possibility of achieving all of these qualities for all scenarios is unrealistic. Therefore, individuals

Box 4
Characteristics of an ideal disinfectant

1. Broad spectrum: wide antimicrobial spectrum (including sporicidal), should have kill claims for the pathogens that are the common causes of HAIs and outbreaks
2. Fast acting: high germicidal activity, rapid kill and short kill/contact time listed on the label
3. Remains wet: surfaces stay wet long enough to meet listed kill/contact times with a single application or meet wet times recommended by evidence-based guidelines
4. Not affected by environmental factors: stable and effective in the presence of organic matter (eg, blood, feces)
5. Chemical compatibility: should be compatible with soaps, detergents, and other chemicals encountered in use, such that the effectiveness of neither chemical is affected, and that mixing does not result in toxicity, increased corrosiveness, or other reactivity
6. Nontoxic: not irritating to user, other staff, clients, or patients. No induction of allergies (especially asthma and dermatitis). Disinfectant toxicity ratings are danger, warning, caution, and none. Ideally, choose products with the lowest toxicity rating
7. Surface compatibility: be capable of penetration without destruction, proven compatible with common surfaces and equipment found in veterinary settings
8. Persistence: sustained antimicrobial activity or residual postapplication antimicrobial effect
9. Easy to use: ideally available in multiple forms (eg, wipes, sprays, concentrates); simple directions for use with information about PPE as required
10. Acceptable odor: odor and aesthetics should be acceptable to users and others
11. Economical: costs should not be prohibitively high but when considering the costs of a disinfectant product capabilities, cost per compliant use, and so on should also be considered
12. Solubility: soluble in water
13. Stability: stable in concentrate and use dilution
14. Cleaner: good cleaning properties
15. Nonflammable: flash point higher than 65.5°C (150°F)

Data from Refs.[37,45–50]

responsible for developing C/D protocols must learn to discretionarily pick and choose disinfectants based on the properties of the disinfectant, the perceived challenges of the task, and desired results of the disinfection procedure. For example, the disinfectant that might be chosen for a footbath or foot mat is likely different from the agent picked for general purpose C/D, because the footbath must be quick kill and preferably stable in the face of organic debris. Quick kill and lack of surface damage tend to be mutually exclusive characteristics. Even in the case of routine surface disinfection, procedures should not make for slippery floor surfaces, cause films to build up over time, or damage surfaces (film build-up and surface damage preclude effective cleaning). Although footbaths are not used as commonly in small animal compared with large animal clinics, they may be effective in preventing the transmission of infectious agents.[59–63] While opinions about the degree of efficacy vary, in the absence of other control methods, their use should certainly be considered in isolation areas, particularly if it is short-term, without attendant management problems.

There are numerous excellent resources[36,37,45–51] that provide more information on chemical disinfectants, their classes, characteristics, and modes of activity.

Iowa State's Center for Food Safety and Public Health Web site[46,47] is a valuable and trusted resource in the veterinary community; it gives the spectrum of activity of the major disinfectant groups against various microorganisms and the characteristics of selected disinfectants in accessible readily understood tables.[47] The susceptibility of various microorganisms and the level of disinfection required to kill them are summarized in **Table 2**, and the characteristics of the most common disinfectants are shown in **Table 3**. As mentioned earlier, for each chemical disinfectant, the manufacturer's label[36,37] provides important information, including about

Table 2
Decreasing order of resistance of microorganisms to disinfection and sterilization and the required level of disinfection

	Microorganism	Examples	Disinfection Level Required[a]
More resistant	Prions	Scrapie, chronic wasting disease, bovine spongiform encephalopathy	Prion reprocessing
↓	Bacterial spores	*Bacillus, Clostridium*	Sterilization
	Protozoal oocysts	*Cryptosporidium*	High: can be classified as chemical sterilants, kill spores with prolonged contact times, shorter exposure periods kill all microorganisms except large numbers of bacterial spores
	Helminth eggs	*Ancylostoma, Strongyloides, Trichuris*	
	Mycobacteria/ acid fast bacteria	*Mycobacterium tuberculosis, Nocardia*	
	Small nonenveloped (nonlipid) viruses	Calicivirus, circovirus, paramyxovirus, parvovirus	Intermediate: may be cidal for mycobacteria, vegetative bacteria, most viruses, and most fungi but do not necessarily kill bacterial spores
	Protozoal cysts	*Giardia*	
	Fungal spores	*Aspergillus, Coccidioides, Microsporum canis, Trichophyton*	
	Gram-negative bacteria	*Acinetobacter, Escherichia, Pseudomonas, Salmonella*	
	Vegetative fungi and algae	*Aspergillus, Trichophyton, Candida, Malassezia*	
	Vegetative helminths and protozoa	*Ancylostoma, Strongyloides, Trichuris, Cryptosporidium, Giardia*	
	Large, nonenveloped (nonlipid) viruses	Adenovirus, rhabdovirus, rotavirus	
	Gram-positive bacteria	*Staphylococcus, Streptococcus, Enterococcus*, MRSA, VRE	Low: may kill most vegetative bacteria, some fungi, and some viruses in a practical period $\leq$10 min
	Enveloped (lipid) viruses	Coronavirus, herpesvirus, influenza viruses	
Less resistant	Mycoplasmas	*Mycoplasma canis, M felis*	

[a] The designated disinfection levels were developed for medical and surgical materials and equipment, not the environment. They are included here because, for the most part, the concepts they convey are still valid considerations for environmental surfaces.

Table 3
Characteristics of commonly used disinfectants

Category	Acids	Alcohols	Aldehydes	Alkalis	Biguanides	Chlorine-Releasing Agents	Iodine Iodophors	Oxidizing Agents	Phenolic Compounds	Quaternary Ammonium Compounds
Examples	Acetic acid, citric acid, lactic acid	Ethanol, isopropanol, methanol	G, F, OPA	Sodium hydroxide (lye, caustic soda), calcium hydroxide (slaked lime), sodium carbonate (washing soda, soda ash), ammonium hydroxide	Chlorhexidine diacetate and gluconate (Nolvasan, Chlorhex, Virosan)	Sodium hypochlorite (bleach, Clorox), calcium hypochlorite, chlorine dioxide	Iodine solutions (tinctures) or iodophors (complex of iodine with neutral polymers, most commonly povidone-iodine, Betadine)	HP, AHP (Accel), PAA (Oxy-Sept 333), PMS (Virkon, Trifectant)	Various phenols (2-phenylphenol, benzylphenol, 4-chloro-3,5-dimethy-lphenol; One-Stroke Environ, Tek-Trol, Osyl, Lysol, Pine-Sol)	Various ammonium salts (benzalkonium chloride, benzethonium chloride, cetalkonium chloride, cetyl pyridinium chloride, tetraethy-lammonium bromide, cetyl trimethy-lammonium bromide, and domiphen bromide; Roccal-D, Parvosol, DiQuat, D-256)
Mechanism of action	Precipitate proteins, disrupt nucleic acids	Precipitate proteins, denature lipids, cell lysis	Denature proteins, alkylate nucleic acids	React with membrane lipids	Alter membrane permeability	Denature proteins	Denature proteins, disrupt nucleic acids	Denature proteins and lipids	Alter cell wall permeability, denature proteins	Disrupt cell membrane, denature proteins, inactivate enzymes

Suitable applications	Specialist applications mainly large animal, not recommended for general use	Limited surface disinfection, topical antiseptic, hand sanitizers (Purel)	Surface disinfection, fumigant (F), sterilization (G), high-level disinfectant (OPA)	Have been used for environmental disinfection but not recommended for general use	Surface disinfection, topical antiseptic	Surface disinfection, chlorine dioxide also fumigation and gas sterilization	Surface disinfection (Environmental Protection Agency–registered hard surface iodophors only), topical antiseptic (skin antiseptic iodophors)	Surface disinfection all, HP and AHP topical antiseptic, HP vapor sterilization, PAA fumigation, PMS aerosol fumigation	Surface disinfection	Surface disinfection
Efficacy with organic material	Poor, reduced	Poor, reduced	Moderate, reduced	Sodium hydroxide high, others low to moderate	Very poor, rapidly inactivated	Very poor, rapidly inactivated, except chlorine dioxide moderate	Slightly better than chlorine-releasing agents but still very poor, rapidly inactivated	Variable, HP low, AHP moderate, PMS and PAA high	High, effective	Poor to moderate, reduced
Efficacy with detergents/soap	?	?	Reduced	?	Inactivated	Inactivated	Effective	?	Effective	Inactivated
Efficacy with hard water	?	?	Reduced	?	?	Effective	?	?	Effective	Inactivated, but for some agents higher concentrations work, check label

(*continued on next page*)

Table 3
(continued)

Category	Acids	Alcohols	Aldehydes	Alkalis	Biguanides	Chlorine-Releasing Agents	Iodine Iodophors	Oxidizing Agents	Phenolic Compounds	Quaternary Ammonium Compounds
Residual activity	Some	No	?	?	Yes (skin)	No	Some	Claimed for AHP	Yes	Some, brief
Advantages	Nontoxic, nonirritating at typical concentrations	Fast acting, no residues, overall low toxicity	Broad spectrum, relatively noncorrosive, relatively inexpensive, sporicidal in alkali solution	Ammonium hydroxide effective against coccidial oocysts, sodium hydroxide assists in prion destruction	Broad spectrum against bacteria, activity in aqueous alcohol solutions superior to aqueous only, relatively low toxicity	Broad spectrum, short contact time, inexpensive, sporicidal at higher concentration	Broad spectrum, stable in storage, relatively safe	Fast acting, broad spectrum, considered environmentally friendly, sporicidal	Broad spectrum, stable in storage, noncorrosive, effective over large pH range	Relatively broad spectrum (although variable between products), stable in storage, generally nonirritating to skin, effective at high temperatures and high pH (9–10)

Disadvantages	Change environmental pH, hazardous at high concentrations, corrosive, toxic	Rapid evaporation, flammable, irritation to injured skin	Toxic (F carcinogenic risk), irritating to mucous membranes and tissues, use in well-ventilated areas, toxic to fish	Very caustic, corrosive to metals, ammonium hydroxide intense pungent fumes, toxic to aquatic life	Limited activity against viruses, functions only in narrow pH range (5–7), toxic to fish (environmental concern), keratitis	Inactivated by sunlight and some metals, reduced activity at high pH and low temperatures, frequent application needed, surface to be disinfected must be clean and dry, corrosive to metals (not stainless steel) and some other materials, discolors fabrics, irritating to mucous membranes and skin, mixing with acids release toxic chlorine gas	Stains clothes, some surfaces and plastics, frequent application needed, corrosive, inactivated by quaternary ammonium compounds, contact sensitivity	Some (notably PMS, PAA) are damaging to plain metals, concrete, and some other surfaces, discolor fabrics, eye irritation	Toxic to animals, particularly cats and pigs, can cause skin and eye irritation, unpleasant odor, some have disposal restrictions, not recommended for food surfaces	Toxic to fish, lose activity at pH<3.5 and low temperatures

(*continued on next page*)

Table 3
(continued)

Category	Acids	Alcohols	Aldehydes	Alkalis	Biguanides	Chlorine-Releasing Agents	Iodine Iodophors	Oxidizing Agents	Phenolic Compounds	Quaternary Ammonium Compounds
Gram-positive bacteria	+	+	+	+	+	+	+	+	+	+
Gram-negative bacteria	+	+	+	+	+	+	+	+	+	+
Myco-bacteria	—	+	—	+	—	+	+	+	+	±
Enveloped viruses	+	+	+	+	±	+	+	+	±	±
Large nonen-veloped viruses	—	±	+	+	±	+	±	+	±	—
Small nonen-veloped viruses	±	±	+	±	±	+	±	+	±	—
Fungi	±	±	+	+	±	+	+	±	+	±
Spores	±	±	+	±	—	±	±	±	—	—

Abbreviations: AHP, accelerated hydrogen peroxide; F, formaldehyde; G, glutaraldehyde; HP, hydrogen peroxide; OPA, orthophthalaldehyde; PAA, peroxyacetic acid; PMS, peroxymonosulfate.
Data from Refs.[18,36,37,45–53]

microorganisms against which it has been shown to be effective, appropriate contact time, correct dilutions for the desired outcome (may be higher for bactericidal activity and lower for bacteriostatic claims, and different for parvicidal activity vs routine use), as well as other factors that may alter effectiveness of the agent. These other factors can include the length of time that a product remains effective when diluted; shelf-life of the concentrate; temperature range in which it is maximally effective; water hardness (because dilution rates of some disinfectants [eg, quaternary ammonium compounds] may vary depending on hardness of the water); interaction with detergents (which can alter the pH of a disinfectant and reduce its effectiveness); features of the surface to be disinfected (as previously mentioned, integrity of the surface, or lack thereof, can greatly affect disinfectant effectiveness); and organic load (**Box 5**).

LAUNDRY

Soiled hospital laundry and animal bedding may be considered a potential source of infection to both staff and patients and may cause cross-contamination of the environment. All reusable linens and bedding that have been contaminated with blood, urine, feces, or any other bodily fluids or exudates must be subjected to a decontamination process.[64,65] The following list of suggestions regarding laundry applies to all situations:

1. All workers involved in the collection, transport, sorting, or washing of soiled bedding must:
   - Be appropriately trained
   - Wear required personal protective equipment (PPE), including gloves of a sufficient thickness to minimize sharps injuries, face mask and eye protection

Box 5
Additional considerations in choosing cleaners and disinfectants

A surface cannot be properly disinfected if it is not clean. A plain, anionic detergent should be chosen as a basic cleaner for animal housing and handling areas, including surgical suites.

Cost is important but should not be the only consideration; efficacy, ease of use, and potential deleterious effects must be part of the equation.

Make sure that the properties of all of the cleaners and disinfectants that you chose are compatible (eg, avoid combinations that lead to generation of chlorine gas).

Potential negative effects of disinfectants on equipment, personnel, and the environment. For example, prolonged use of some disinfectants, particularly powerful oxidizers such as the peroxygens, can damage surfaces (notably metals other than stainless steel, concrete, and tile). Loss of surface integrity defeats the object of maintaining sealed cleanable surfaces and makes cleaning more difficult.

Some disinfectants cause a surface film build-up over time, particularly around footbaths/mats but even with general use. Films can be slippery, can impede proper cleaning, and may promote biofilm formation. Although not widely used in small animal practice, footbaths/mats may be necessary in isolation units. Careful siting of footbaths/mats or changing disinfectant may avoid potential problems.

Prepackaged disinfectant wipes can be useful in C/D of delicate equipment and hard surfaces in sensitive areas. In general, accelerated hydrogen peroxide–based wipes are preferred over those containing quaternary ammonium compounds.

Data from Refs.[37,45–50]

when appropriate (eg, when there is a zoonotic risk in the handling of urine-soaked bedding from known or suspected cases of canine leptospirosis)
  - Cover any exposed broken skin or lesions
  - Have access to hand washing facilities
2. Every effort should be made to eliminate the inadvertent disposal of harmful objects, such as sharps or instruments
3. Animal bedding must be carefully shaken free of all loose debris and fecal matter before processing; such matter should be disposed of appropriately
4. All soiled laundry must be held and transported in bins or bags impervious to liquids
5. Clean and dirty laundry must have separate transport receptacles and storage facilities

In addition, it is worthwhile to sort and label used laundry into categories for processing. This practice is adopted to protect both workers, patients, and the environment from potentially infectious agents.

1. General: bedding from patients not considered infectious or contagious
2. Infectious: bedding contaminated with microorganisms that pose a hazard to workers who may have contact with it, the environment, or other animals; laundry associated with infected animals should be bagged and sealed before being removed to the laundry area
3. Heat labile: bedding likely to be damaged by the normal laundering process

The average laundry process in a hospital setting is adequate to render bedding hygienically clean[66] This level of cleaning is achieved through a combination of dilution with water, loosening with detergent, agitation, and heat (both in the washing and, just as importantly, drying processes). In regard to appropriate temperatures for the laundry cycle, it is suggested[64–66] that the process should

- Maintain 65°C for no less than 10 minutes or
- Maintain 71°C for no less than 3 minutes or
- Contain the addition of chemicals (ie, bleach) for heat-labile materials or lower temperatures[1]

WASTE MANAGEMENT

The handling of the waste generated by the veterinary industry is both complex and regulated. Waste is everything that no longer serves a purpose and needs a form of disposal. In professional settings such as veterinary clinics, there are specific guidelines in place regarding waste disposal. Most waste in the world is considered solid waste, regardless if it is in solid form. In a veterinary clinic, this waste may include but is not limited to animal tissues, bodily fluids and waste, carcasses, cleaning and laboratory chemicals, general medical waste, radiographic by-products, medications, chemotherapeutic agents, batteries, and solvents. The American Veterinary Medical Association (AVMA) has excellent resources available to guide the appropriate disposal of solid wastes generated by the veterinary industry and has developed categories for them (**Fig. 1**).[67] Complete definitions of each of the categories are available at the AVMA Web site. Other

---

[1] Low temperature (used to mitigate the cost of using high heat) laundry cycles rely heavily on bleach to reduce levels of microbial contamination. Regardless of the temperatures used for washing, the temperatures achieved in drying provide additional significant microbicidal action.[66]

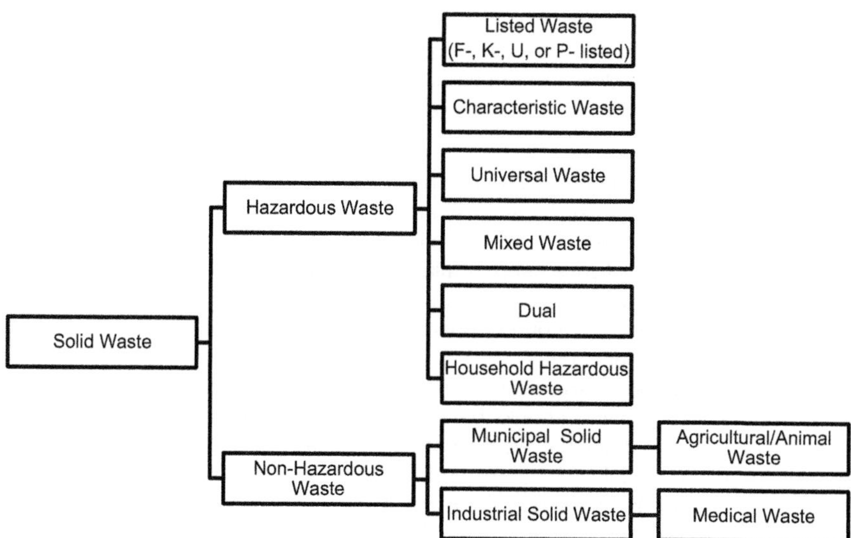

Fig. 1. Categories of solid waste. (*Data from* AVMA. Available at: https://www.avma.org/PracticeManagement/Administration/Pages/Definitions-What-is-Waste.aspx. Accessed September 17, 2014. For full descriptions of the above categories visit the AVMA Web site.)

jurisdictions may, of course, categorize wastes and the means of handling them differently, so veterinary hospitals should always check the regulations in their local jurisdiction.

More complete information on appropriate waste management is available at the AVMA Web site.[67] Bearing in mind the breadth of differences in both type of waste and regulatory body responsible for the different types (**Table 4**), it is important that there is a methodology associated with how a veterinary facility disposes of its waste. Decisions about waste disposal must include and may not be limited to:

- Awareness of the options available for waste disposal in the physical area
- Knowing which authorities have oversight so questions may be directed appropriately

Table 4
Federal agencies that regulate veterinary waste disposal in the United States

United States Federal Agency	Waste Regulated
Environmental Protection Agency	All waste with an environmental impact
Occupational Health and Safety Administration	Waste associated with potential employee exposure to hazardous substances
National Institute of Occupational Safety and Health	Workplace products that affect both human and public health
Drug Enforcement Agency	Disposal of controlled substances
Department of Transportation	Shipping of chemicals and specimens
Nuclear Regulatory Commission	Chemotherapeutic agents

Data from AVMA. Available at: https://www.avma.org/PracticeManagement/Administration/Pages/Federal-Regulation-of-Waste-Disposal.aspx. Accessed September 17, 2014.

- Following specific material safety data sheet (MSDS) or product safety data sheet (PSDS) instructions for disposal
- Specific practice policy and procedures regarding waste disposal
- The need for training of individuals to ensure both safe handling and organizational compliance

Although VTHs in academic institutions generally have their own offices of environmental health and safety, which can answer questions and assist in ensuring compliance with federal, state, local, and institutional policies, veterinary facilities without such resources should always keep in mind that overall, when in doubt, the default agency for questions and concerns regarding waste management is the Environmental Protection Agency (or country-specific equivalent) and direct enquires to their state office or the federal agency.

For the average veterinary clinic, a few specific guidelines for waste disposal and adequate staff training should be sufficient for compliance. The first step is categorizing waste. Traditional waste categories may include clinical, sharps, laboratory, pharmaceutical, infectious, and hazardous. What defines a category is both how the waste is handled at its point of collection and how it must be disposed of.[53,66,68] Responsible medical waste producers should consider it their obligation to:

- Describe the waste categories
- Provide for safe collection and handling of waste by workers
- Provide employee training to ensure safety
- Establish a contract with a reputable waste disposal contractor
- Investigate the waste disposal contractor for compliance
- Pack the waste in accordance with regulations
- Store waste properly on site before disposal

The adoption of a color-coded waste disposal system is another useful tool that could be implemented in the veterinary industry. Potential suggestions for waste color codes could be:

- Red: biohazardous/infectious
- Yellow: for incineration
- Orange: biological/carcass/body parts
- Purple: for incineration at a facility regulated to handle cytotoxic or chemotherapeutic agents
- Green: recyclable
- Black: general disposal/landfill

ENVIRONMENTAL SURVEILLANCE

Hospital surveillance exists in many forms, each with a precise goal.[68] Some methods are culture based, meaning that a sample is taken and processed for results. Other methods are non–culture based, meaning that the activity relies on the observation of situations and their various outcomes. Either way, surveillance, when conducted properly, can be a useful and meaningful aspect of a complete hospital infection control program.[10–12,19,22,23] However, random surveillance of a hospital environment is not recommended. This advice is because random surveillance activities, either culture based or non–culture based, produce results, but they are results with no viable context.[12] Therefore, when considering surveillance, always proceed methodically, with the intention of carrying out an associated and appropriate action. See the article elsewhere in this issue entitled "Veterinary hospital surveillance systems" by Burgess and Colleagues for more information.

Veterinary hospitals are inherently contaminated; any number of microorganisms might be harbored in its environs. Monitoring and surveillance are essentially the sensory mechanisms to any infection control program. Microbiological surveillance of the hospital environment can be a critical component of a successful infection control program.[13–16,19,22] Data to support this contention include findings indicating that many organisms of concern can survive for prolonged periods on surfaces and equipment.[69] For example, *Acinetobacter* persists for 3 days to 5 months, *Bordetella* 3 to 5 days, *Campylobacter jejuni* up to 6 days, *Chlamydophila psittaci* 15 days, *Clostridium difficile* spores for 5 months, *Enterococcus* (including VRE) 5 days to 4 months, *E coli* as little as 1.5 hours to 16 months, *Klebsiella* 2 hours to 30+ months, canine parvovirus greater than 1 year, influenza viruses 1 to 2 days, norovirus up to 28 days, *Pseudomonas aeruginosa* 6 hours to 16 months, *Staphylococcus aureus* (including MRSA) 7 days to 7 months, and *Salmonella enterica* 1 day to years![69] Clearly, then, surveillance of the environment for pathogens associated with HAI is feasible and could be considered as part of an infection control program.

As mentioned earlier, environmental surveillance does not always imply microbiological evaluation, but it should certainly encompass monitoring/auditing to ensure proper hygiene and control of clutter that might impede effective cleaning. If undertaken, environmental sampling can be useful in determining which patient populations, traffic patterns, and protocols present a risk for hospital contamination, and in assessing how well containment efforts are performing.[12,19,22,33] Thus, if active environmental surveillance is undertaken, high traffic areas, critical spaces or equipment, treatment areas, and areas that house high-risk patients should be evaluated as the focus of that surveillance. Even in the absence of active surveillance of the environment, monitoring of the clinical status of patients can be a helpful indicator of when both patients and the environment require closer scrutiny.[12] It should be the responsibility of designated infection control personnel to adjust the intensity or focus of surveillance (active or passive), based on developments in the hospital, the picture of disease prevalence in the referral area, literature, and so forth. In concert with these considerations, individual hospitals need to determine characteristics of their case population (size and type, critical care vs elective, both of which have been associated with increased risk),[12] level of risk aversion, cost-benefit analysis, and so forth, either before initiating a surveillance program or, just as importantly, evaluating an ongoing infection control program. In either case, an end-all determination makes little sense, and periodic review is warranted.

A major difficulty with environmental surveillance is one of context if it is not conducted in a repeatable, methodical manner. For instance, with culture-based surveillance, at any point in time when surfaces are sampled[19,22] and cultured, bacteria may be found, but without a baseline point of reference, what does that positive finding mean? Establishment of a useful, active environmental sampling strategy might require collection of environmental and HAI baseline data, without which it is often not possible to assess the likelihood that particular infections are HAI, determine whether there has been an increase in such infections, or evaluate the efficacy of any interventions. However, in deciding whether or not to pursue a targeted surveillance program, even with good baseline data, it can be difficult to make such assessments on every occasion.

If the goal of hospital surveillance is to eliminate HAI, collecting data is futile if the process does not lead to an immediate action. Some of the potential actions associated with surveillance may be:

- Establishment of baseline rates of infection or contamination
- Provision of proof needed to convince practitioners to adopt best practices
- Identification and control of outbreaks
- Evaluation of the success of the infection control program
- Drive potential changes to current policy and procedure

For the desired effect to be positively achieved, the collected information must be disseminated to individuals who can interpret and effect the desired change. In the case of HAIs and outbreak scenarios, surveillance can even be the foundation for a facility organizing and instituting or modifying an infection control program. If a facility is experiencing a suspected outbreak or is interested in introducing an infection control program, it is important for individuals to understand both the object of surveillance activities and various surveillances types (**Box 6**). However, in general, available reports suggest that most veterinary hospitals, including academic institutions, do not practice methodical collection and analysis of either patient or environmental data.[12]

If a decision is taken to initiate active surveillance for a particular organism(s), it might be useful to consider factors that went into the choice of *Salmonella* as the general biosensor most commonly used in large animal hospitals. *Salmonella* is among the most important cause of HAIs in large animal hospitals, it is a significant zoonotic threat, and it has been associated with numerous outbreaks at VTHs. In addition, the following characteristics favor *Salmonella* as an effective biosensor:

- Survives well in the environment
- Can spread readily on fomites
- Relatively difficult to kill
- Relatively easy to detect
- Good indicator of effectiveness of infection control programs
- Increase in environmental prevalence widely regarded as an early warning of problems

Box 6
Potential surveillance types

1. Laboratory based: focused on the various types and numbers of concerning or alert (ie, likely to cause outbreaks or infection) organisms being isolated from the patient population
2. Targeted: focused on high-risk areas, specific types of infections, procedures or a single organism
3. Patient: focused on the potential for pre/post screenings at the times of entry and exit to the hospital to determine/prevent incidences of HAI
4. Outbreak: focused on locating the source of a cluster of infection in various patients with the same organism
5. Procedural: focused on determining the effectiveness of current C/D policies and procedures
6. Clinical/ward liaison: focused on the activity of a medical health care worker visiting various hospital departments to evaluate patients, review records, attend rounds, or advise individuals about the most appropriate care and housing of patients to prevent HAI

All of the same considerations should be part of the decision in choosing an environmental biosensor(s) for a small animal veterinary hospital, but this is easier said than done. Although evidence-based choices for large animal hospitals are straightforward, the options for small animal clinics are less clear. In this context, although still useful in evaluating the effectiveness of C/D, the value of measuring organisms like generic *E coli* to assess HAI and overall effectiveness of infection control programs is increasingly questioned. Potential targets include MDR pathogens of concern, microorganisms causing the most significant problem in your facility, or evidence from multi-institutional surveys, but further research is necessary to provide veterinarians with better guidance. For these same reasons, some advocate using non–culture-based techniques, such as fluorescent tagging, because they are not tied to specific pathogens.[42] If specific pathogens are identified as targets, in addition to classic epidemiologic measures for the sensitivity, specificity, and predictive values of detection methods, another critical characteristic of testing that should be considered is speed to return of results. In terms of the environment, if it takes days to get results, there could be wide dissemination to patients and other parts of the hospital before corrective measures are initiated. These considerations explain the move away from traditional culture methods to more rapid techniques such as polymerase chain reaction, which often offer enhanced sensitivity and specificity, as well as greater speed.

Environmental surveillance can also be a useful tool for determining the effectiveness of C/D (**Box 6**).[28,33,42,68,70] In this case, the methods and goals differ slightly from those associated with investigating HAIs or a potential disease cluster or outbreak. Basically, methods that evaluate the presence or absence of generic bacteria preferably with quantitation could suffice for C/D evaluation,[33,42] but the incorporation of specific indicator organisms increases the value of any such surveillance.[68,70] There are almost no studies of this type in veterinary medicine, but those that are available clearly indicate that environmental contamination exists and that like human medicine, although the cleaning of some surfaces (eg, examination tables, countertops) may just about be adequate, others are seriously deficient (eg, computer keyboards and other hand contact equipment).[42] More research is needed to fully evaluate selected deficiencies, define such deficiencies in the context of C/D policies and practices, and further determine their relationship, if any, to HAIs.

SUMMARY

Hospitalized animals are not the same as the general animal population; they are more likely to shed or acquire an infectious agent for a variety of reasons, including stress; immunosuppression; altered nutrition or disturbances to normal microbiota; administration of antimicrobials; being subject to procedures that are known risk factors for infection of various types; concentration close to other animals with similar risk factors. The standard of care at every veterinary hospital should therefore include a high standard of hygiene, awareness of the dangers of transfer of infectious agents between both animals and people, and procedures to reduce infection risk wherever possible. It is becoming increasingly clear that the environment of health care facilities is subject to contamination with pathogens and plays a role in at least some HAIs. Consequently, environmental management, with or without active surveillance, should be a component of risk reduction designed to limit HAIs. Effective C/D procedures are critical in preventing transmission of infectious agents between patients or from contaminated environments. Development of well-understood protocols and schedules for C/D, waste disposal, and environmental maintenance to ensure that surfaces remain sealed and cleanable is important. Education of veterinarians and all staff as to the need for thoroughness and vigilance when it comes to C/D is critical to successful mitigation of HAI risks.

REFERENCES

1. Magill SS, Edwards JR, Bamberg W, et al. Multistate point-prevalence survey of health care-associated infections. N Engl J Med 2014;370:1198–208.
2. US Centers for Disease Control and Prevention. Healthcare-associated infections. Atlanta (GA). Available at: http://www.cdc.gov/hai/. Accessed September 17, 2014.
3. US Department of Health and Human Services. National action plan to prevent health care–associated infections: road map to elimination. Available at: http://www.hhs.gov/ash/initiatives/hai/actionplan/. Accessed September 17, 2014.
4. Yokoe DS, Anderson DJ, Berenholtz SM, et al. A compendium of strategies to prevent healthcare-associated infections in acute care hospitals: 2014 updates. Infect Control Hosp Epidemiol 2014;35(8):967–77.
5. Scott RD. The direct medical costs of healthcare-associated infections in US hospitals and the benefits of prevention. Atlanta (GA): Division of Healthcare Quality Promotion; Centers for Disease Control and Prevention; 2009. Available at: http://www.cdc.gov/HAI/pdfs/hai/Scott_CostPaper.pdf. Accessed September 17, 2014.
6. Weinstein RA. Epidemiology and control of nosocomial infections in adult intensive care units. Am J Med 1991;91(Suppl 3B):179S–84S.
7. Weber DJ, Anderson D, Rutala WA. The role of the surface environment in healthcare-associated infections. Curr Opin Infect Dis 2013;26:338–44.
8. Morgan DJ, Rogawski E, Thom KA, et al. Transfer of multidrug-resistant bacteria to healthcare workers' gloves and gowns after patient contact increases with environmental contamination. Crit Care Med 2012;40(4):1045–51.
9. Weinstein RA. Intensive care unit environments and the fecal patina: a simple problem? Crit Care Med 2012;40(4):1333–4.
10. Ruple-Czerniak AA, Aceto H, Bender JB, et al. Nosocomial infection rates in small animal referral hospitals: using syndromic surveillance to establish baseline rates. J Vet Intern Med 2013;27(6):1392–9.
11. Ruple-Czerniak AA, Aceto H, Bender JB, et al. Syndromic surveillance for evaluating the occurrence of healthcare-associated infections in equine hospitals. Equine Vet J 2014;46(4):435–40.
12. Benedict KM, Morley PS, Van Metre DC. Characteristics of biosecurity and infection control programs at veterinary teaching hospitals. J Am Vet Med Assoc 2008; 233:767–73.
13. Weese JS, Stull J. Respiratory disease outbreak in a veterinary hospital associated with canine parainfluenza virus infection. Can Vet J 2013;54(1):79–82.
14. Weese JS, Armstrong J. Outbreak of *Clostridium difficile*-associated disease in a small animal veterinary teaching hospital. J Vet Intern Med 2003;17(6):813–6.
15. Wright JG, Tengelsen LA, Smith KE, et al. Multidrug-resistant *Salmonella typhimurium* in four animal facilities. Emerg Infect Dis 2005;11(8):1235–41.
16. Ogeer-Gyles JS, Mathews KA, Boerlin P. Nosocomial infections and antimicrobial resistance in critical care medicine. J Vet Emerg Crit Care 2006;16:1–18.
17. Sanchez S, McCrakin MA, Stevenson CR, et al. Characterization of multidrug resistant *Escherichia coli* isolates associated with nosocomial infections in dogs. J Clin Microbiol 2002;40(10):2586–95.

18. Greene CE. Environmental factors in infectious disease. In: Greene CE, editor. Infectious diseases of the dog and cat. 3rd edition. St Louis (MO): Saunders Elsevier; 2006. p. 991–1013. Chapter 94.
19. Dallap Schaer BL, Aceto H, Rankin SC. Outbreak of salmonellosis caused by *Salmonella enterica* serovar Newport MDR-ampC in a large animal veterinary teaching hospital. J Vet Intern Med 2010;24:1138–46.
20. Dunowska M, Morley PS, Traub-Dargatz JL, et al. Comparison of *Salmonella enterica* serotype Infantis isolates from a veterinary teaching hospital. J Appl Microbiol 2007;102:1527–36.
21. Ewart SL, Schott HC II, Robison RL, et al. Identification of sources of *Salmonella* organisms in a veterinary teaching hospital and evaluation of the effects of disinfectants on detection of *Salmonella* organisms on surface materials. J Am Vet Med Assoc 2001;218:1145–51.
22. Burgess BA, Morley PS, Hyatt DR. Environmental surveillance for *Salmonella enterica* in a veterinary teaching hospital. J Am Vet Med Assoc 2004;225(9):1344–8.
23. Ekiri AB, Morton AJ, Long MT, et al. Review of the epidemiology of and infection control aspects of nosocomial *Salmonella* infections in hospitalized horses. Equine Vet Educ 2010;22(12):631–41.
24. Weese JS, DaCosta T, Button L, et al. Isolation of methicillin-resistant *Staphylococcus aureus* from the environment in a veterinary teaching hospital. J Vet Intern Med 2004;18:468–70.
25. Hoet AE, Johnson A, Nava-Hoet RC, et al. Environmental methicillin-resistant *Staphylococcus aureus* in a veterinary teaching hospital during a nonoutbreak period. Vector Borne Zoonotic Dis 2011;11(6):609–15.
26. Heller J, Armstrong SK, Girvan EK, et al. Prevalence and distribution of methicillin-resistant *Staphylococcus aureus* within the environment and staff of a university veterinary clinic. J Small Anim Pract 2009;50(4):168–73.
27. Loeffler A, Boag AK, Sung J, et al. Prevalence of methicillin-resistant *Staphylococcus aureus* among staff and pets in a small animal referral hospital in the UK. J Antimicrob Chemother 2005;56(4):692–7.
28. KuKanich KS, Ghosh A, Skarbek JV, et al. Surveillance of bacterial contamination in small animal veterinary hospitals with special focus on antimicrobial resistance and virulence traits of enterococci. J Am Vet Med Assoc 2012;240(4):437–45.
29. Ghosh A, KuKanich KS, Brown CE, et al. Resident cats in small animal veterinary hospitals carry multidrug resistant enterococci and are likely involved in cross-contamination of the hospital environment. Frontiers in Microbiol 2012;3:1–14.
30. Kim LM, Morley PS, Traub-Dargatz JL, et al. Factors associated with *Salmonella* shedding among equine colic patients at a veterinary teaching hospital. J Am Vet Med Assoc 2001;218(5):740–8.
31. Scheftel JM, Elchos BL, Cherry B, et al. Compendium of veterinary standard precautions for zoonotic disease prevention in veterinary personnel: National Association of State Public Health Veterinarians Veterinary Infection Control Committee 2010. J Am Vet Med Assoc 2010;237:1403–22. Available at: http://nasphv.org/Documents/VeterinaryPrecautions.pdf. Accessed September 17, 2014.
32. Girling SJ, Fraser MA. Bacterial carriage of computer keyboards in veterinary practices in Scotland. Vet Record 2009;165(1):26–7.
33. Bender JB, Schiffman E, Hiber L, et al. Recovery of staphylococci from computer keyboards in a veterinary medical centre and the effect of routine cleaning. Vet Record 2012;170(16):414–6.

34. Lee D. Controlling infection through design. Long Term Living Magazine 2012. Available at: http://www.ltlmagazine.com/article/controlling-infection-through-design. Accessed September 17, 2014.
35. The Center for Health Design, Evidence-based design accreditation and certification (EDAC). Available at: http://www.healthdesign.org/edac. Accessed September 17, 2014.
36. Caveney L. Guidelines for effective cleaning and disinfection. In: Caveney L, Jones B, editors. Veterinary infection prevention and control. 1st edition. Chichester (United Kingdom): Wiley-Blackwell John Wiley and Sons; 2012. p. 107–27. Chapter 6.
37. Dvorak G, Petersen CA. Sanitation and disinfection. In: Miller L, Hurley K, editors. Infectious disease management in animal shelters. 1st edition. Ames (IA): Wiley-Blackwell John Wiley and Sons; 2009. p. 49–60. Chapter 4.
38. Center for Food Security and Public Health, Iowa State University. Infection control for veterinarians. Available at: http://www.cfsph.iastate.edu/Infection_Control/overview-of-infection-control-for-veterinarians.php. Accessed September 17, 2014.
39. Carling PC, Parry F, von Beheren M. Identifying opportunities to enhance environmental cleaning in 23 acute care hospitals. Infect Control Hosp Epidemiol 2008;29:1–7.
40. Goodman ER, Platt R, Bass R, et al. Impact of environmental cleaning intervention on the presence of methicillin-resistant *Staphylococcus aureus* and vancomycin-resistant enterococci on surfaces in intensive care unit rooms. Infect Control Hosp Epidemiol 2008;29:593–9.
41. LaVecchia-Ragone G. Where are the germs? Long Term Living Magazine 2013. Available at: http://www.ltlmagazine.com/article/where-are-germs. Accessed September 17, 2014.
42. Weese JS, Lowe T, Walker M. Use of fluorescent tagging for assessment of environmental cleaning and disinfection in a veterinary hospital. Vet Rec 2012;171(9):217–9.
43. Association for Professionals in Infection Control and Epidemiology (APIC) and the Association for the Healthcare Environment (AHE). Clean spaces healthy patients project. Available at: http://cleanspaces.site.apic.org/. Accessed September 17, 2014.
44. McDonnell GE. Mechanisms of antimicrobial resistance. In: Antisepsis, disinfection, and sterilization: types, action, and resistance. Washington, DC: ASM Press; 2007. p. 253–334. Chapter 8.
45. Perry K, Caveney L. Chemical disinfectants. In: Caveney L, Jones B, editors. Veterinary infection prevention and control. 1st edition. Chichester (United Kingdom): Wiley-Blackwell John Wiley and Sons; 2012. p. 129–43. Chapter 7.
46. Dvorak G. Disinfection 101. Center for Food Security and Public Health, Ames, IA: Iowa State University; 2005. Available at: http://www.cfsph.iastate.edu/BRM/resources/Disinfectants/Disinfection101Feb2005.pdf. Accessed September 17, 2014.
47. Center for Food Security and Public Health, Iowa State University. Disinfection. Available at: http://www.cfsph.iastate.edu/Disinfection/index.php. Accessed September 17, 2014.
48. Rutala WA, Weber DJ. Selection of the ideal disinfectant. Infect Control Hosp Epidemiol 2014;35(7):855–65.
49. Rutala WA, Weber DJ. Selection and use of disinfectants in healthcare. In: Mayhall CG, editor. Hospital epidemiology and infection control. 4th edition. Philadelphia: Lippincott Williams & Wilkins; 2012. p. 1180–212. Chapter 80.

50. Damani N. Disinfection and sterilization. In: Manual of infection prevention and control. 3rd edition. Oxford (United Kingdom): Oxford University Press; 2012. p. 59–95. Chapter 6.
51. McDonnell GE. Antisepsis, disinfection, and sterilization: types, action, and resistance. Washington, DC: ASM Press; 2007.
52. Fraise AP. Decontamination of the environment and medical equipment in hospitals. In: Fraise AP, Maillard JY, editors. Russell, Hugo and Ayliffe's principles and practice of disinfection, preservation and sterilization. 4th edition. Oxford (United Kingdom): Blackwell Publishing; 2004. p. 563–85 Part 2, Practice. Chapter 18.
53. Fraise AP, Bradley C. Decontamination of equipment, the environment and the skin. In: Fraise AP, Bradley C, editors. Ayliffe's control of healthcare-associated infection: a practical handbook. 5th edition. London: Hodder Arnold Publishing; 2009. p. 107–49. Chapter 6.
54. The national specifications for cleanliness in the NHS: a framework for setting and measuring performance outcomes. 2007. p. 25–7. Available at: http://www.nrls.npsa.nhs.uk/resources/?entryid45=59818. Accessed September 17, 2014.
55. McLay C. Preventing/controlling the transmission of infectious agents. In: McLay C, editor. Infection prevention competency review guide. 4th edition. Washington, DC: Association for Professionals in Infection Control and Epidemiology (APIC); 2010. p. 163–241. Chapter 3.
56. Khamis N, van Knippenberg-Gordebeke G. Audits in infection prevention and control. In: Friedman C, Newsom W, editors. Basic concepts of infection control. 2nd edition. Northern Ireland (United Kingdom): International Federation of Infection Control (APIC); 2011. p. 71–80. Chapter 6.
57. Park D, Larson AM, Klibanov AM, et al. Antiviral and antibacterial polyurethanes of various modalities. Appl Biochem Biotechnol 2013;169(4):1134–46.
58. Varghese S, Elfakhri S, Sheel DW, et al. Novel antibacterial silver-silica surface coatings prepared by chemical vapour deposition for infection control. J Appl Microbiol 2013;115(5):1107–16.
59. Morley PS, Morris SN, Hyatt DR, et al. Evaluation of the efficacy of disinfectant footbaths as used in veterinary hospitals. J Am Vet Med Assoc 2005;226: 2053–8.
60. Amass SF, Arighi M, Kinyon JM, et al. Effectiveness of using a mat filled with peroxygen disinfectant to minimize shoe sole contamination in a veterinary hospital. J Am Vet Med Assoc 2006;228:1391–6.
61. Dunowska M, Morley PS, Patterson G, et al. Evaluation of the efficacy of a peroxygen disinfectant-filled footmat for reduction of bacterial load on footwear in a large animal hospital setting. J Am Vet Med Assoc 2006;228:1935–9.
62. Stockton KA, Morley PS, Hyatt DR, et al. Evaluation of the effects of footwear hygiene protocols on nonspecific bacterial contamination of floor surfaces in an equine hospital. J Am Vet Med Assoc 2006;228:1068–73.
63. Hartmann FA, Dusick AF, Young KM. Impact of disinfectant-filled foot mats on mechanical transmission of bacteria in a veterinary teaching hospital. J Am Vet Med Assoc 2013;242(5):682–8.
64. McDonald LL, Pugliese G. Textile processing service. In: Mayhall CG, editor. Hospital epidemiology and infection control. 2nd edition. Philadelphia: Lippincott Williams & Wilkins; 1999. p. 1031–4.
65. Hoffman P. Laundry, kitchens and healthcare waste. In: Fraise AP, Bradley C, editors. Ayliffe's control of healthcare-associated infection: a practical handbook. 5th edition. London: Hodder Arnold Publishing; 2009. p. 107–49. Chapter 6.

66. Damani N. Support services. In: Manual of infection prevention and control. 3rd edition. Oxford (United Kingdom): Oxford University Press; 2012. p. 327–47. Chapter 18.
67. American Veterinary Medical Association, Veterinary practice waste disposal decision maker. Available at: https://www.avma.org/PracticeManagement/Administration/Pages/Veterinary-Practice-Waste-Disposal-Decision-Maker.aspx. Accessed September 17, 2014.
68. Sehulster LM, Rose LJ, Noble-Wang J. Microbiologic sampling of the environment in healthcare facilities. In: Mayhall CG, editor. Hospital epidemiology and infection control. 4th edition. Philadelphia: Lippincott Williams & Wilkins; 2012. p. 1059–75. Chapter 72.
69. Kramer A, Schwebke I, Kampf G. How long do nosocomial pathogens persist on inanimate surfaces? A systematic review. BMC Infect Dis 2006;6:130–7.
70. Dancer SJ. How do we assess hospital cleaning? A proposal for microbiological standards for surface hygiene in hospitals. J Hosp Infect 2004;56:10–5.

Cleaning and Disinfection of Patient Care Items, in Relation to Small Animals

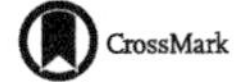

J. Scott Weese, DVM, DVSc

KEYWORDS

• Cleaning • Disinfection • Equipment • Sterilization

KEY POINTS

- Many items pose a potential risk for pathogen transmission because they have contact with high-risk patients or high-risk patient sites or are used on multiple patients.
- The incidence of infection associated with patient care items in veterinary medicine is unknown and likely low, but the consequences can be devastating.
- Different approaches to cleaning, disinfection, and sterilization are required for different items; this may range from basic cleaning to sterilization, and the required level of processing and specific practices must be determined for all items.
- Reprocessing of items that are marketed for single use is often justifiable and routinely done in veterinary clinics, but care must be taken to ensure proper cleaning, disinfection, or sterilization and that processing does not compromise function of the item.

INTRODUCTION

Myriad items come into contact with patients on a regular basis, ranging from commonly used items like stethoscopes to specialized diagnostic and surgical tools. Any item that comes into contact with a patient, person or the environment carries with it some risk of pathogen contamination and transmission, yet the risk of contamination, risk of transmission, and clinical implications vary greatly. For example, *Staphylococcus pseudintermedius* on the bell of a stethoscope pose limited risk, whereas the same bacterium on a surgical implant would pose tremendous risk. Because of the potential risk associated with such a wide range of patient care items, protocols must be established to reduce the risk of hospital-associated infection (HAI) from contaminated items.

There has been intensive study of the role of medical and surgical items in HAIs in human medicine and measures to reduce the risk. Despite this evidence and the

The author has nothing to disclose.
Ontario Veterinary College, University of Guelph, Guelph, Ontario N1G2W1, Canada
E-mail address: jsweese@uoguelph.ca

Vet Clin Small Anim 45 (2015) 331–342
http://dx.doi.org/10.1016/j.cvsm.2014.11.004 vetsmall.theclinics.com
0195-5616/15/$ – see front matter

presence of comprehensive infection control measures, a wide range of HAIs continues to be associated with contaminated items (**Table 1**). Often, investigations implicate failure to adhere to established practices or compromised item surfaces as leading causes, demonstrating the importance of protocol compliance on this (like virtually every) aspect of infection control.

The incidence of HAIs from contaminated patient care items in veterinary medicine is unknown. Whether this is because of limited risk, lack of investigation, or lack of reporting is unclear, and all probably play some role. However, although reports are limited, contaminated patient care items can result in hospital-associated infections and also likely pose some risk for zoonotic pathogen transmission.

Principles of Cleaning, Disinfection, and Sterilization

While "cleaning and disinfection" is often referred to as a single entity, they are separate steps, each with different objectives. Further, disinfection can be subdivided into different categories, depending on the degree of microbial elimination that is required (**Table 2**). Regardless of the level of disinfection that is chosen, it is important to remember that disinfection is not designed to eliminate all microbes; sterilization is a separate approach, designed to eliminate all microbes, required for certain items.

The level of processing that is needed should be determined for every patient item as a guide to identify the appropriate level of cleaning, disinfection, or sterilization that is required. A classification developed by Earle H. Spaulding almost 50 years ago[1] still forms the foundation of this approach. Spaulding's classification system is a straightforward approach to identification of the risk associated with an item and its management (**Table 3**). Although useful and still the basis of risk assessments today, this classification is not absolute, as some contradictions are apparent even in human medicine. For example, forks and spoons come into contact with mucosal surfaces and technically would be classified as semicritical devices, yet they are not routinely disinfected in hospital kitchens. Thus, these classifications should be used as general guidance, and the level of desired and achievable disinfection or sterilization should be

Table 1
Examples of reported human hospital-associated outbreaks linked to contaminated patient care items

Item	Pathogen	Comment
Multidose vials	*Serratia marcescens*	Heparin saline flush
Multidose vial	*S marcescens*	Bevacizumab injection
Endoscope	*Pseudomonas aeruginosa*	
Cystoscope	*P aeruginosa*	Multiple breaches of processing guidelines
Arthroscope	*P aeruginosa*	Contamination during processing
Endoscopes	*Mycobacterium chelonae*	Contamination from automated bronchoscope washer
Endoscope	*Klebsiella pneumonia*	Inadequate cleaning and drying before storage
Thermometers	*Enterobacter cloacae*	Inadequate disinfection between patients
Thermometers	*Salmonella* Eimselbuettel	Inadequate disinfection between patients
Endoscopic biopsy forceps	*P aeruginosa*	Defective instruments that compromised cleaning and disinfection

Data from Refs.[16,18,23–30]

Table 2
Categories of cleaning and disinfection

Category	Description
Cleaning	Reduction of bioburden and foreign material
Low-level disinfection	Destruction of vegetative bacteria, some fungi and viruses (mainly enveloped viruses) but no mycobacteria or bacterial spores
Intermediate-level disinfection	Destruction of vegetative bacteria, mycobacteria, most viruses (except some nonenveloped viruses), most fungi
High-level disinfection	Destruction of all microorganisms except high numbers of bacterial spores
Sterilization	Elimination of all microbial life

considered for individual items. Regardless, this simple approach should be considered when evaluating the need for disinfection or sterilization of patient care items.

APPROACH/GOALS

Steam Sterilization (Autoclave)

Both dry heat and steam under pressure are effective for sterilization; however, steam sterilization is more widely used in veterinary clinics because it is easy, cost effective, nontoxic, and dependable.[2,3] Typically, steam sterilization is used for all items that can tolerate the process. The efficacy of steam sterilization is through a combination of steam, pressure, temperature, and time. Higher pressures facilitate generation of higher temperatures and more rapid microbial killing, and 121°C for 30 minutes in a gravity displacement autoclave is most commonly used.[2,3]

Proper autoclaves should be used for steam sterilization. Pressure cookers, although occasionally used in veterinary clinics, are inappropriate because they are not designed to provide the desired conditions and do so consistently.

Flash sterilization is a process in which an item is sterilized in an autoclave in a more rapid manner for immediate use. Items that are flash sterilized are typically unwrapped, so this process must occur close to where the item will be used. Typical conditions are 132°C for 3 minutes and 27 to 28 pounds of pressure in a gravity

Table 3
Spaulding's classification system for patient care items

Classification	Use	Examples	Required Decontamination
Noncritical	Touches intact skin	Thermometers, stethoscopes	Cleaning, then low- or intermediate-level disinfection
Semicritical	Touches mucous membranes and nonintact skin	Upper respiratory and gastrointestinal endoscopes, endotracheal tubes, laryngoscopes	Cleaning, then high-level disinfection
Critical	Enters sterile tissue, vascular system, or body space	Surgical instruments, implants, needles	Cleaning, then sterilization

From Spaulding EH. Chemical disinfection of medical and surgical materials. In: Lawrence C, Block SS, editors. Disinfection, sterilization and preservation. Philadelphia: Lea & Febiger; 1968.

displacement autoclave.[3] Ineffective flash sterilization has been implicated as a cause of surgical site infections[4] and patient burns from hot instruments,[5] and this approach must only be used as an emergency measure. Typically, this method is indicated when an item is dropped (or otherwise contaminated) during surgery and no sterilized replacements are available. It is also acceptable for items that cannot be packaged, sterilized, and stored before use,[3] a rare situation in veterinary clinics. Flash sterilization should never be used for surgical implants,[3,6] as a replacement for purchasing adequate numbers of routine surgical instruments, to save time, or because of poor operating room and central supply organization.[3,7] The need to flash sterilize an item should be considered an adverse event and the reasons investigated to minimize use of this emergency measure.

Dry Heat Sterilization

Dry heat sterilization is an effective method but is uncommonly used. The combination of temperature and time determines the efficacy, with 170°C for 60 minutes, 160°C for 120 minutes or 150°C for 150 minutes being recommended approaches.[2] This method is reserved for materials that might be damaged by moisture or that are impenetrable to moist heat.

Ethylene Oxide

Ethylene oxide gas is a highly effective sterilant that can be used on many items that cannot tolerate steam (eg, endoscopes). Ethylene oxide is a true sterilant, as it can kill effectively and reliably kill organisms like mycobacteria, enveloped viruses, and bacterial spores. Gas concentration, temperature, humidity, and time impact efficacy,[2] and commercial systems are used to ensure proper and safe use of this toxic substance. Typical recommended ranges for concentration, temperature, humidity, and time are 450 to 1200 mg/mL, 29°C to 65°C, 45% to 85% and 2 to 5 hours, respectively.[2] Processing time (eg, 2–5 hours plus 8–12 hours of aeration at 50°–60°C) and system costs limit the use of this approach, which is largely restricted to facilities that require frequent sterilization of steam-intolerant items. Ethylene oxide is also flammable, explosive, and toxic[2] but quite safe to use with properly installed and maintained commercial systems.

Hydrogen Peroxide Vapor Sterilization

Hydrogen peroxide vapor is another option of sterilization of heat-intolerant items. Hydrogen peroxide has advantages over ethylene oxide; it is a much safer chemical that requires shorter processing times. Hydrogen peroxide vapor is compatible with a wide range of materials and can effectively penetrate lumens with small internal diameters or long lengths (eg, 1 mm or greater diameter and 125 mm or shorter length),[8] making it suitable for most endoscopes and similar items. Commercial systems are available but rarely used outside of large facilities because of equipment costs.

Liquid Immersion (Cold) Sterilization

A variety of chemical sterilants can be used for heat-intolerant items. When used properly, true sterilization can be achieved; however, in practice, this method is fraught with issues that render it an unreliable sterilization method. Improper dilution, inadequate contact time, improper pH, inadequate changing of solutions, failure to ensure no air pockets are present, and poor choice of a product are common problems. Immersion sterilization typically requires 3 to 12 hours,[3] and the time is reset any time a new item is added to the container, regardless of how long other items have been present.

Efficacy of cold sterilization has not been evaluated in veterinary facilities, but a high rate of bacterial contamination of cold sterile solutions was identified in one study,[9] likely a result of inadequate precleaning of instruments, inadequate contact time, adding dirty instruments to solutions containing sterile instruments, inadequate pH, inadequate changing of solutions, and inadequate dilution. This method is not appropriate for surgical instruments or other items that come into contact with sterile sites, regardless of the minor nature of the procedure being performed. Therefore, this method is strongly discouraged.

Chemical Disinfection

Disinfection can be achieved using various chemical disinfectants (**Table 4**). Choices must be made based on the level of disinfection that is required, the physical characteristics of the item, equipment manufacturer recommendations, surface compatibility, and potential toxicity concerns from residual disinfectant exposure. Rarely are evidence-based guidelines available, and much of what is done in veterinary clinics is based on anecdotal experiences and trial and error.

Problems that may be encountered include use of a disinfectant that does not adequately cover the spectrum of pathogens that might be present, inadequate contact time, use of improper disinfectant concentrations, failure to properly clean the item, surface characteristics that limit penetration of the disinfectant, damage to materials from the disinfectant, and toxicity or other adverse reactions to residual chemicals. These problems can be reduced by using a disinfectant with a broad spectrum (one that is commonly used on similar items), having clear guidelines for disinfectant use (concentration, contact time), using good cleaning practices before disinfection, rinsing items with water after the required contact time to remove residual disinfectant, and monitoring items for disinfection-related damage.

Little specific guidance can be provided for disinfection of most items that are used in veterinary facilities because of a lack of research and limited information

Table 4
Examples of chemical disinfectants for equipment

Process	Chemical
Low-level disinfection	70%–90% ethanol Quaternary ammonium products Phenolics Iodophors Some chlorine-based products (eg, 1:100 household bleach, 500 ppm hypochlorite) Chlorhexidine
Intermediate-level disinfection	Some chlorine-based products (eg, 1:10 household bleach/5000 ppm hypochlorite) Some phenolics
High-level disinfection	>2% glutaraldehyde (20–45 min) 0.55% orthophthaldehyde (12 min) 1.12% glutaraldehyde + 1.93% phenol (12 h) 7.35% hydrogen peroxide + 0.23% peracetic acid (3 h) 7.5% hydrogen peroxide (6 h) 1% hydrogen peroxide + 0.08% peracetic acid (25 min)

Adapted from Rutala WA, Weber DJ. Cleaning, disinfection and sterilization. In: Association for Professionals in Infection Control, editor. APIC text of infection control and epidemiology. Washington, DC: APIC; 2009. p. 21–7.

that can be obtained from manufacturers. Equipment manufacturers are often reluctant to provide disinfection guidelines for items that are marketed as single use, when they have not performed surface compatibility studies, or when they have not performed efficacy studies. A recent study evaluated the elimination on experimentally inoculated *Streptococcus zooepidemicus* and *Bordetella bronchiseptica* on endotracheal tubes and found that soaking tubes in accelerated hydrogen peroxide or 2% chlorhexidine for 5 minutes effectively reduced or eliminated bacterial growth (JS Weese, unpublished data, 2014). Beyond that, data are extremely limited.

Cleaning

Although last in this list, cleaning must not be ignored, as it can be the most important part of the cleaning and disinfection process. Cleaning must precede any disinfection or sterilization method to remove debris and substances that might inhibit the efficacy of disinfection or sterilization. Careful physical cleaning and the use of appropriate detergents, enzymatic cleaners, and proteolytic products (or combinations thereof) for the type and degree of contamination are important, with inadequate effort or attention to detail being the main problems that are encountered. Typically, cleaning agents should be rinsed off of items before reuse or subsequent disinfection. Compatibility between the cleaner and disinfectant must also be considered, as disinfectants may be inactivated by some cleaning agents (eg, inactivation of quaternary ammonium disinfectants by anionic disinfectants).

QUALITY CONTROL/QUALITY ASSURANCE

Assessment of Sterilization

Because of the potentially disastrous consequences of inadequate sterilization, a structured quality control program is required for all sterilization practices. Assessment of sterilization is, in general, easier to perform than assessment of cleaning and disinfection because there is a clear objective (elimination of viable microorganisms) and that objective can be tested. A variety of methods are available to assess sterilization (**Table 5**), and these vary in their accuracy, ease of use, cost, and time requirements.

Autoclave

Assessment of autoclave function is an important quality control and quality assurance practice that must be performed by all facilities that use an autoclave. However, an overly simplistic approach that only partially assesses autoclave efficacy is often used in veterinary facilities. Autoclave assessment can involve methods that assess temperature, temperature/time/pressure combinations, and actual bactericidal activity.

Chemical indicators (eg, indicator tape, indicator strips) monitor temperature or combinations of temperature, time, and pressure and should be included outside and inside every pack that is put in the autoclave.[3] External indicator tape is used as an initial assessment of the autoclave run, as it is directly visible. This tape should be examined by the person removing items from the autoclave. The internal indicator provides a more accurate assessment of conditions to which items inside the pack were exposed. Internal indicator strips are not useful if they are not evaluated, and the job of checking the strip should be preassigned (eg, technician opening the pack, surgeon making the incision, assistant surgeon).

Table 5
Common sterilization testing methods

Testing Method	Sterilization Method	Assesses	Comments
External indicator tape	Autoclave	Temperature and time	Only indicates conditions on the outside of the package. Not a sole quality assurance tool. Should be used on every autoclaved pack.
Steam indicator strips	Autoclave	Temperature and time	Should be included *in* every autoclaved pack. Do not directly indicate microbial killing.
Dry heat indicator strips	Dry heat sterilization	Temperature and time	Should be included *in* every dry heat sterilized pack. Do not directly indicate microbial killing.
Biological indicators	Any	Successful killing of hardy bacterial spores	Should be used regularly and any time a problem is suspected.

Biological indicators provide an actual assessment of microbicidal activity by demonstrating killing of hardy bacterial spores. Most autoclave biological indicators consist of *Geobacillus stearothermophilus* spores,[3] which are in vials that are processed in an autoclave run. After completion of the autoclave cycle, the spore container is incubated to confirm that no bacterial growth is present. Easy-to-use commercial systems allow for this to be done in the veterinary facility, with results available within 24 hours. There are no standards regarding the frequency of biological indicator use, and factors such as the amount of autoclave use, the items that are being placed in the autoclave (eg, higher concern would be present with surgical implants), the autoclave type, and autoclave service history need to be considered. Weekly testing is probably appropriate for most veterinary hospitals, but more frequent use may be indicated in busy facilities, particularly those with a caseload involving complex surgical patients, and consideration should be given to including biological indicators with every load containing implantable devices.[3,6]

Dry Heat

Indicator strips are available for dry heat sterilization assessment. These are different from those used with autoclaves because of the differences in temperature, time, and pressure that are used for the different techniques. Biological indicators may also be used, as they are for autoclaves.

Ethylene Oxide and Hydrogen Peroxide Vapor

Biological indicators can (and should) be used to assess ethylene oxide or hydrogen peroxide vapor sterilization. *Bacillus* spores are used to assess ethylene oxide, while *Geobacillus stearothermophilus* spores are recommended for hydrogen peroxide vapor.[6] Biological indicators should be placed in the most challenging location in an autoclave load, typically in the center of the load. Assessment of sterilization of small diameter items (eg, endoscope channels) is not possible; therefore, one must rely on a combination of use of biological indicators in other areas of the load and manufacturer guidelines for minimum diameter and maximum length of channels or tubing.

Immersion Sterilization

No standard methods exist for assessment of sterilization of items processed by immersion sterilization, which is another reason that this method is not acceptable for items that truly need sterilization.

Labeling and Storing of Sterilized Items

All sterilized items should be labeled with the date of sterilization. They should be stored in an area where they will be protected from water and excessive movement. Packs should be stored in a manner that they do not need to be moved, as movement increases the chances for creation of small, undetectable breaks in the packing.

There are no clear criteria for shelf life of sterilized and properly packaged items. Because spontaneous germination of microbial life does not occur, any contamination must work its way into the packaging through surface breaks or seals. Properly sterilized and packaged items that are not subjected to ongoing manipulation likely remain sterile for prolonged periods,[6,8] yet packaging breakdown times have not been studied. A 1-year shelf life is a reasonable recommendation. Packs sterilized in an autoclave should be stored and labeled so that older items are used first, ensuring adequate rotation of supplies and reducing the likelihood of long-term storage.

Recording of Sterilization Quality Control Testing Results

A log of quality control testing should be kept to record results of quality control testing. It is impractical (and unnecessary) to record indicator tape and indicator strip results from each pack. However, any failed indicators must be recorded in a log and acted on as discussed below. Biological indicator data should be recorded, as they represent the definitive assessment of sterilization efficacy. Failure to record results means that one has no way to provide sterilization efficacy if problems arise and no definitive baseline date to return to in the event of ineffective sterilization (ie, if one does not know when the sterilizer definitely worked last, all items processed in the clinic must be considered potentially nonsterile).

Responding to Failure of Sterilization Efficacy Testing

Quality control testing is only effective if results are monitored and actions are taken in response to any problems. Failure of any of the above-described quality assurance methods must be immediately investigated. If internal or external indicators fail, the sterilization cycle should be repeated with different indicator strips from different packages and with biological indicators. In the event of biological indicator failure (with or without external or internal indicator strip failure), all items that were sterilized in that run must be resterilized. Further, consideration must be given to the status of any other items that have been sterilized since the last proven (ie, no growth of biological indicators) sterilization cycle. High-risk items such as surgical implants should be removed immediately and not be used until resterilized (with sterilization confirmed by biological indicators). Recall of other items is prudent but not considered necessary while the investigation ensues if there is reasonable suspicion that the sterilization failure was a single event.[6] Three consecutive runs should be performed with biological indicators, and if any are positive, then all items processed since the last successful biological indicator run must be recalled and reprocessed.[3] The above highlights the importance of maintaining adequate detailed records so that dates can be used to identify particular items that may be at risk when responding to a sterilization failure.

With any possible sterilization failure, the sterilizer should be promptly serviced and postservice biological indicator testing performed. If a reason for failure is not identified and the equipment is not replaced, more frequent use of biological indicators in the following period is indicated.

Assessment of Cleaning and Disinfection

Assessment of cleaning and disinfection practices is a potentially useful quality assurance practice in routine circumstances and may be of additional relevance during outbreaks. Yet, objective assessment can be difficult because of the lack of a clear outcome measure. Visual appearance of an item after cleaning can provide some information, because, if gross debris is visible, cleaning either did not occur or was suboptimal. Direct observation can be used to assess cleaning and disinfection practices, yet the Hawthorne effect (changes in an individual's actions because they know they are being observed) can affect results. Further, direct observation is time consuming. Equipment cultures are of limited use because the goal of cleaning (and disinfection) is not necessarily to eliminate all viable microorganisms. Thus, a properly cleaned surface may still have viable bacteria, including various opportunistic pathogens. Equipment culture is best reserved for targeted surveillance of specific pathogens when there is a clear suspicion that contaminated equipment might be a source of infection and when the results of culture will alter actions (eg, testing and holding equipment until negative cultures are obtained). Equipment cultures are rarely justifiable as a routine practice and are mainly reserved for outbreak investigations. Environmental tagging is a potentially effective, easy, and low-cost approach to assessment of cleaning.[10] This involves contamination of surfaces with fluorescent dye that is not visible to the naked eye. After cleaning (or after a period in which cleaning should have been performed), the area can be investigated with a handheld UV light. If residual dye is evident, cleaning was not performed or was inadequate.

OTHER CONSIDERATIONS

Reprocessing Single Use Items

Many patient care items that are used in veterinary medicine are designed and marketed for human medicine. Often, items are marketed as single-use items that are disposed of in human hospitals but reprocessed and reused in veterinary facilities (eg, endotracheal tubes). This is often justifiable from an economic and environmental standpoint and can be safe if done logically and carefully. However, because these items are not typically designed or tested for multiple uses, and reprocessing practices have not been scrutinized, there may be issues with efficacy of disinfection or material degradation.[11]

Information about optimal disinfection or sterilization methods and the number of times an item can be reused and resterilized is also valuable, although formal data are typically lacking, and anecdotal experiences drive most guidelines. Care must be taken to monitor for reprocessed item degradation, particularly items that are put in the autoclave repeatedly, as this can result in damage to some products, either with a single run or gradually over time.[11] Chemical disinfectants can also damage surfaces or change their physical properties (eg, render them stiff or brittle). Further, proper cleaning and sterilization may be difficult to impossible for some items based on the materials (eg, porous materials) or design (eg, small channels).

Facilities should be cognizant of potential risks associated with reuse of single use items, although properly characterizing these risks is essentially impossible. In human medicine, the US Food and Drug Administration considered hospitals that reprocess single-use items to assume the role of the manufacturer and, therefore, holds them to the same standards and scrutiny as the original manufacturer.[3,8] Whether this applies to veterinary medicine and other countries is unclear, but it bears consideration. Essentially, veterinary facilities must consider the benefits (eg, cost, convenience) and risks (e.g. contamination, malfunction) that could occur, whether there are any data pertaining to processes or risk, and develop a policy that they can justify. If re-processing is performed, written guidelines should be available and items must be carefully inspected before and after processing to detect any potential problems.

Contamination of Multidose Items

Any substance that is injected into the body poses a risk of infection if contaminated. Contamination of substances such as intravenous fluids, parenteral nutrition solutions, vaccines and drugs is therefore of concern. Rarely are these contaminated at the time of processing, and the risks are usually encountered from contamination of items that are used multiple times or on multiple patients.

Contamination of multidose items is not uncommon, and contamination of 18% of multidose drug vials and fluid bottles was reported in a study of one veterinary hospital.[12] This included various concerning bacteria such as *Pseudomonas, Serratia, Acinetobacter, Salmonella, Klebisella, Listeria* and methicillin-resistant *Staphylococcus aureus*. Human studies have reported contamination rates of 0.9%–5.6%,[13,14] with contamination and HAIs leading to changes in product manufacturing to reduce or eliminate the re-use of substances in vials, bags or other containers.

Although contamination rates may be high, the overall risk to patients appears to be limited. Presumably this is because the number of contaminating microorganisms tends to be low and the immune system is able to eliminate them. However, multidose vial-associated infections certainly occur in human medicine, and there is no reason to think that they would not also occur in veterinary medicine. Examples from humans include outbreaks of invasive *Staphylococcus aureus* infection from contaminated analgesic vials,[15] *Serratia marcescens* outbreak from heparin-saline catheter flush solution,[16] sepsis from propofol,[17] *S marcescens* endophthalmitis outbreak from bevacizumab,[18] *Enterobacter cloacae* bloodstream infections from human albumin,[19] hepatitis C infection from anesthetic agents,[20] and *S aureus* joint and soft tissue infections from lidocaine.[21] A large outbreak of fungal meningitis occurred from contamination corticosteroids that were being used for epidural injection.[22]

Contamination of injectable substances should be considered when there are clusters of HAIs, when infections occur at an injection site or when infections caused by organisms often associated with contamination (eg, *Serratia, Pseudomonas*) are identified. If there is any concern about contamination, the potentially contaminated product should not be used, the manufacturer should be contacted and an adverse drug reaction report filed with the appropriate regulatory body.

Multidose vials will inherently pose increased risk because of the potential for contamination with every entry. Accordingly, they should not be used for medications that will be injected into high-risk sites (eg, joints, eye, central nervous system) unless it is the first withdrawal from the bottle. Where available and economically justifiable, single-use vials should be chosen over multidose alternatives. When multidose vials must be used, careful withdrawal practices should be used to reduce the risk of contamination, including use of a sterile needle, wiping the stopper with alcohol,[12] and withdrawing from bottles in a clean area.

SUMMARY

Infections caused by contaminated patient care items are rarely reported in veterinary medicine, and although surveillance is limited, the incidence is probably truly rare. Cases are rare because of standard practices that are used. However, inadequate practices, inadequate equipment, and poor compliance increase the risk of contamination and, correspondingly, the risk to patients. Veterinary facilities should have documented practices for equipment processing and handling to reduce the risk of hospital-associated infections and to facilitate prompt identification of any issues.

REFERENCES

1. Spaulding EH. Chemical disinfection of medical and surgical materials. In: Lawrence C, Block SS, editors. Disinfection, sterilization and preservation. Philadelphia: Lea & Febiger; 1968. p. 517–31.
2. Rutala W, Weber D. Infection control: the role of disinfection and sterilization. J Hosp Infect 1999;(Suppl 43):S43–55.
3. Centers for Disease Control and Prevention. Guideline for disinfection and sterilization in healthcare facilities, 2008. Atlanta, GA: Centers for Disease Control and Prevention; 2008. p. 1–158.
4. Hood E, Stout N, Catto B. Flash sterilization and neurosurgical site infections: guilt by association. Am J Infect Control 1997;25:156.
5. Rutala WA, Weber DJ, Chappell KJ. Patient injury from flash-sterilized instruments. Infect Control Hosp Epidemiol 1999;20:458.
6. Jefferson JA. Central services. In: Association for Professionals in Infection Control, editor. APIC text of infection control and epidemiology. Washington, DC: APIC; 2009. 55/1–18.
7. Mangram AJ, Horan TC, Pearson ML, et al. Guideline for prevention of surgical site infection, 1999. Hospital infection control practices advisory committee. Infect Control Hosp Epidemiol 1999;20:250–78 [quiz: 279–80].
8. Rutala WA, Weber DJ. Cleaning, disinfection and sterilization. In: Association for Professionals in Infection Control, editor. APIC text of infection control and epidemiology. Washington, DC: APIC; 2009. p. 21–7.
9. Murphy CP, Weese JS, Reid-Smith RJ, et al. The prevalence of bacterial contamination of surgical cold sterile solutions from community companion animal veterinary practices in southern Ontario. Can Vet J 2010;51:634–6.
10. Weese JS, Lowe T, Walker M. Use of fluorescent tagging for assessment of environmental cleaning and disinfection in a veterinary hospital. Vet Rec 2012;171:217.
11. Serbetci K, Kulacoglu H, Devay AO, et al. Effects of resterilization on mechanical properties of polypropylene meshes. Am J Surg 2007;194:375–9.
12. Sabino C, Weese J. Contamination of multiple-dose vials in a veterinary hospital. Can Vet J 2006;47:779–82.
13. Motamedifar M, Askarian M. The prevalence of multidose vial contamination by aerobic bacteria in a major teaching hospital, Shiraz, Iran, 2006. Am J Infect Control 2009;37:773–7.
14. Mattner F, Gastmeier P. Bacterial contamination of multiple-dose vials: a prevalence study. Am J Infect Control 2004;32:12–6.
15. Radcliffe R, Meites E, Briscoe J, et al. Severe methicillin-susceptible *Staphylococcus aureus* infections associated with epidural injections at an outpatient pain clinic. Am J Infect Control 2012;40:144–9.

16. Liu D, Zhang LP, Huang SF, et al. Outbreak of *Serratia marcescens* infection due to contamination of multiple-dose vial of heparin-saline solution used to flush deep venous catheters or peripheral trocars. J Hosp Infect 2011;77:175–6.
17. Muller AE, Huisman I, Roos PJ, et al. Outbreak of severe sepsis due to contaminated propofol: lessons to learn. J Hosp Infect 2010;76:225–30.
18. Lee SH, Woo SJ, Park KH, et al. *Serratia marcescens* endophthalmitis associated with intravitreal injections of bevacizumab. Eye 2010;24:226–32.
19. Wang SA, Tokars JI, Bianchine PJ, et al. *Enterobacter cloacae* bloodstream infections traced to contaminated human albumin. Clin Infect Dis 2000;30:35–40.
20. Branch-Elliman W, Weiss D, Balter S, et al. Hepatitis C transmission due to contamination of multidose medication vials: summary of an outbreak and a call to action. Am J Infect Control 2013;41:92–4.
21. Kirschke DL, Jones TF, Stratton CW, et al. Outbreak of joint and soft-tissue infections associated with injections from a multiple-dose medication vial. Clin Infect Dis 2003;36:1369–73.
22. Chiller TM, Roy M, Nguyen D, et al. Clinical findings for fungal infections caused by methylprednisolone injections. N Engl J Med 2013;369:1610–9.
23. Diaz Granados CA, Jones MY, Kongphet-Tran T, et al. Outbreak of *Pseudomonas aeruginosa* infection associated with contamination of a flexible bronchoscope. Infect Control Hosp Epidemiol 2009;30:550–5.
24. Wendelboe AM, Baumbach J, Blossom DB, et al. Outbreak of cystoscopy related infections with *Pseudomonas aeruginosa*: New Mexico, 2007. J Urol 2008;180: 588–92 [discussion: 592].
25. Tosh PK, Disbot M, Duffy JM, et al. Outbreak of *Pseudomonas aeruginosa* surgical site infections after arthroscopic procedures: Texas, 2009. Infect Control Hosp Epidemiol 2011;32:1179–86.
26. Chroneou A, Zimmerman SK, Cook S, et al. Molecular typing of *Mycobacterium chelonae* isolates from a pseudo-outbreak involving an automated bronchoscope washer. Infect Control Hosp Epidemiol 2008;29:1088–90.
27. Aumeran C, Poincloux L, Souweine B, et al. Multidrug-resistant *Klebsiella pneumoniae* outbreak after endoscopic retrograde cholangiopancreatography. Endoscopy 2010;42:895–9.
28. van den Berg RW, Claahsen HL, Niessen M, et al. *Enterobacter cloacae* outbreak in the NICU related to disinfected thermometers. J Hosp Infect 2000;45:29–34.
29. McAllister TA, Roud JA, Marshall A, et al. Outbreak of *Salmonella* Eimsbuettel in newborn infants spread by rectal thermometers. Lancet 1986;1:1262–4.
30. Corne P, Godreuil S, Jean-Pierre H, et al. Unusual implication of biopsy forceps in outbreaks of *Pseudomonas aeruginosa* infections and pseudo-infections related to bronchoscopy. J Hosp Infect 2005;61:20–6.

Contact Precautions and Hand Hygiene in Veterinary Clinics

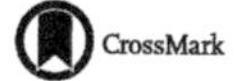

Maureen E.C. Anderson, DVM, DVSc, PhD

KEYWORDS

• Hand hygiene • Barrier nursing • Contact precautions • Infection control culture • Interventions • Hospital-associated infections • Zoonoses

KEY POINTS

- Contact precautions and hand hygiene prevent the physical translocation of microbes between patients, staff, and the environment, thus decreasing potential host exposure and preventing infection.
- Hand hygiene is considered the single most important measure for infection control in hospitals and other health care facilities. The same is likely true in veterinary clinics.
- Compliance with contact precautions and hand hygiene protocols is the most challenging component of ensuring efficacy. Available evidence suggests compliance in veterinary clinics is low.
- Monitoring these practices through means, such as direct observation or video surveillance, is feasible and provides data for evaluating interventions and providing feedback to staff.
- Development of a clinic infection control culture is the ultimate means of improving compliance with infection control measures, including hand hygiene and contact precautions.

THE IMPORTANCE OF HAND HYGIENE AND CONTACT PRECAUTIONS

There are 3 main categories of infection prevention and control measures: those that decrease host susceptibility, those that increase host resistance, and those that decrease host exposure to infectious agents. Of these, decreasing exposure is the most effective (and often the most practical) approach. If a host does not encounter a particular pathogen, or if exposure can be limited to a level below the infectious dose, then disease simply cannot occur. For some organisms, however, in particular

The author has nothing to disclose.
Animal Health and Welfare Branch, Ontario Ministry of Agriculture, Food and Rural Affairs (OMAFRA), 1 Stone Road West, Guelph, Ontario N1G 4Y2, Canada
E-mail address: maureen.e.c.anderson@ontario.ca

Vet Clin Small Anim 45 (2015) 343–360
http://dx.doi.org/10.1016/j.cvsm.2014.11.003 vetsmall.theclinics.com
0195-5616/15/$ – see front matter

those that may cause short- or long-term colonization, avoiding exposure may be difficult or impossible.

Contact precautions are measures used in health care settings specifically to help prevent the physical translocation of microbes between patients, staff, and the environment, particularly via direct or indirect contact or droplet transmission (as opposed to airborne transmission). In most cases, these include hand hygiene and glove use as well as use of disposable gowns or other designated overwear (eg, laboratory coats). Additional measures may include specific patient placement or cohorting and use of masks, eye protection, and shoe covers (also called personal protective equipment [PPE]) (**Table 1**).[1] There are several different sets of contact precautions that have been proposed or recommended in human health care, referred to as standard precautions, universal precautions, body substance precautions, isolation precautions, or barrier nursing protocols, depending on the setting, goals, and criteria for use (eg, some patients vs all patients or preventing transmission of microbes in general vs specific pathogens).[1] There is still considerable variation in how and what contact precautions are applied in human hospitals,[2] but it is nonetheless standard for each facility to have its own set of protocols for PPE and associated practices.

There is limited published research regarding the use of contact precautions and other infection control measures in veterinary facilities.[3–5] Guidelines for these practices can be found in textbooks and other publications,[6–10] but their implementation has seldom been assessed. Many of these infection control measures are simple to perform, but they all require varying amounts of time and effort, which can make achieving adequate compliance difficult, particularly in a busy clinic setting. Protocols for use of PPE, including what, when, and how, should be established and documented by each veterinary clinic and included as part of a tailored infection control program (see **Table 1**).

Of all the contact precautions, hand hygiene is considered the single most important measure for infection control in hospitals and other health care facilities.[11] It is universally applicable in all patient (and patient environment) contact scenarios. In veterinary medicine, hand hygiene is a key measure in preventing the spread of common zoonotic pathogens, such as enteropathogens and multidrug-resistant bacteria, including methicillin-resistant staphylococci. Hand hygiene also has the potential to help decrease the risk of nonzoonotic pathogen transmission between animals in veterinary clinics via the hands of clinic personnel. Recommendations regarding hand hygiene, including when, how, and how often it should be performed, appear in guidelines from several health care–associated organizations[11–13] as well as veterinary infectious disease control guidelines,[6,9,10] but achieving uptake and compliance with these recommendations remains challenging, particularly in veterinary facilities where a strong infection control culture is often lacking.

Hand Hygiene Basics

The goal of hand hygiene in the context of modern health care is to reduce or eliminate the transient (superficial) microbiota of the hands as atraumatically as possible and ideally to prevent rebound growth to decrease the likelihood of transfer of pathogenic or opportunistic microbes from the hands to other surfaces or individuals/tissues.[14,15] This may be accomplished by physical removal of the microbes from the skin or use of antimicrobial compounds that kill or neutralize the microbes. The resident microbiota of the skin is more difficult to remove but is also less likely to include pathogens and is important to maintain because it can play a role in competitively excluding other pathogens.[11,13] Maintaining the integrity of the skin even after repeated hand hygiene attempts is crucial, because skin damage provides niches for opportunistic pathogens to cause infection, resulting in pain and discomfort as well as increased risk of transmission due to the larger number of pathogenic bacteria present on the skin.[13,14] Reported total bacterial counts on the hands of health care workers range from 2.0×10^4 to 4.6×10^6 colony-forming units, including a wide range of bacterial groups, such as staphylococci (eg, *Staphylococcus aureus* and coagulase-negative staphylococci), streptococci, enterococci, corynebacteria, *Pseudomonas* spp, *Klebsiella* spp, *Acinetobacter* spp, *Serratia* spp, and fungal organisms, such as *Candida* spp.[11,16,17]

Although simply rinsing hands with water can mechanically remove some superficial skin cells and loosely adherent bacteria,[14] in the clinical setting the use of soap (either antimicrobial or nonantimicrobial, depending on the specific situation) and water is recommended.[1,10,11] All soaps must be used in combination with water to be effective. Soaps or detergents are primarily emulsifying agents that break up oils to help remove contamination from the hands via the flushing action of the water.[11,13] Plain soap has no residual activity against microorganisms but is suitable for use in lower-risk situations (eg, homes and general public restrooms). In some cases, washing with plain soap has been shown inadequate for removal of pathogens from the hands of health care workers and may even result in increased bacterial counts on hands.[18,19] Use of antibacterial soap is, therefore, typically recommended in health care settings, and this could be reasonably extended to include veterinary clinics. Innate or acquired resistance to the biocides used in many antibacterial soaps has been reported, however, including increased chorhexidine resistance among human clinical isolates associated with higher chlorhexidine use,[20] and there is concern that some of the resistance mechanisms involved may either coselect for antimicrobial-resistance or offer cross-protection against certain antimicrobials.[21,22] For this reason, antimicrobial soap should not be used in lower-risk situations where it is likely unnecessary. Bar soap should not be used in health care settings, because bars can become contaminated with dirt and debris and ultimately increase transmission of microbes from person to person with sequential use.[23] Liquid soap in a convenient dispenser should be used instead.

Alcohol-based hand sanitizers (ABHSs) rely on the action of the alcohol component to rapidly kill microorganisms by denaturing and coagulating proteins and disrupting the cellular membrane, leading to lysis.[14] These products are generally most effective at an alcohol concentration of 65% to 90%, depending on the specific alcohol they contain (typically ethanol or isopropanol).[11,14] The alcohol evaporates quickly, but some ABHSs also contain other active ingredients (eg, chlorhexidine, quaternary ammonium compounds, octenidine, and triclosan) that remain on the skin and provide some residual disinfectant action.[11] Alcohol-based hand sanitizers are convenient because they do not require water (and therefore sinks/plumbing and a drying mechanism), so dispensers are easily placed and used in any point-of-care area. These products have been shown equally effective as hand washing with soap and water in the presence of minimal gross contamination,[24,25] and they are less damaging to the skin with repeated use than soap and water.[14] Despite their many benefits and availability in many veterinary clinics, in a study of 1353 hand hygiene attempts associated with routine outpatient appointments, ABHS was used in only 7% of attempts,[26] and another veterinary ICU-based study reported ABHS use in 18% to 30% of attempts.[27] The main disadvantage of ABHSs is that they do not physically remove microorganisms from the skin. There are some microorganisms that are inherently resistant to even the nonspecific killing action of alcohol (eg, clostridial spores, *Cryptosporidium* oocysts, and certain nonenveloped viruses, such as canine parvovirus); therefore, ABHSs are (theoretically) ineffective in terms of controlling contamination with these types of pathogens. Significant (ie, visible) amounts of dirt/debris/discharge are not removed by using

Table 1
Contact precautions applicable to veterinary clinics

Contact Precaution	Description	Applicable Conditions/Scenarios	Notes
Sterile gloves	Impermeable, sterile single-use latex, nitrile, or vinyl gloves of appropriate size for individuals	Sterile gloves should be used when the primary risk is transmission of microbes to (rather than from) a particular body site or item (eg, surgery, examination of "clean" wounds [surgical incisions], handling sterile equipment).	Not a substitute for hand hygiene. Due to the risk of preexisting defects, puncture, or tears during use and potential contamination of the hands when doffing (and of sterile gloves when donning), hand hygiene before and after glove use remains as important as before-and-after patient contact when gloves are not used.
Nonsterile gloves	Impermeable, nonsterile single-use latex, nitrile, or vinyl gloves of appropriate size for the individual.	Any scenario in which there is increased risk of hand or clothing contamination with a larger number of microbes or any number of highly virulent, resistant or transmissible microbes, for example • Any animal with potential respiratory tract infection, diarrhea, skin infection, fever of unknown origin • Oral manipulation or procedures (eg, dentistry) • Exposure to potentially infectious fluids or discharge (eg, obstetric procedures, necropsy, handling of clinical samples or soiled linens and other items).	
Gowns or dedicated laboratory coats	Single-use disposable gowns or reusable cloth gowns or laboratory coats that are laundered after each applicable patient contact or procedure. Clothing worn underneath must be completely covered from the wrists and waist to the collar at a minimum, depending on the size and type of patient. Use of coveralls is also an option for animals requiring extensive handling, especially on the floor.		Disposable gowns and laboratory coats are typically permeable to liquids, especially with prolonged or heavy contact; therefore, additional precautions may be required to prevent microbial strike-through.

Face mask	Single-use disposable surgical mask or reusable full-face shield consisting of a stiff clear plastic sheet that covers the face from forehead to chin. Each face shield should be dedicated to a single person but should be discarded or fully reprocessed (ie, cleaned and disinfected) if it becomes visibly contaminated or comes in contact with a contaminated surface (including used glove), and between patients.	Any scenario in which there is a significant splash risk or risk of droplet transmission, for instance • Dental procedures • Wound lavage • Potentially zoonotic respiratory disease with productive coughing or sneezing • Necropsy (especially if any potential risk of rabies)	A face shield may be more appropriate for individuals with heavy facial hair that is not adequately covered by a mask. Does not protect against airborne pathogens—this requires a properly fitted respirator (N95 or higher).
Eye protection	Typically reusable plastic goggles that wrap around the sides of the face or include side-protectors or a full-face shield (described previously)		Poorly fitted eye protection can cause visibility issues due to fogging or slipping. Regular eyeglasses are not a substitute, because they do not fully protect the eyes, particularly from the lateral aspect.
Shoe covers or dedicated footwear	Single-use disposable cloth or plastic boots that fit over regular footwear or reusable slip-on footwear that is easily cleaned and disinfected (eg, rubber boots)	Any scenario in which there is suspected to be significant contamination of the floor with a high-risk substance, for instance • Dog with leptospirosis housed on the floor • Infectious vomiting or diarrhea, particularly in large dogs housed on the floor • Management of large open wounds if floor could become contaminated with discharge or lavage fluid	Disposable plastic shoe covers can create a slipping hazard if they do not have treads. Not commonly needed in small animal clinics; however, contamination of the floor must always be carefully considered due to the high degree of contact of patients and staff with the floor.

ABHSs and may protect microorganisms from the action of the active ingredients. If hands are visibly soiled, or if there is suspected contamination with an alcohol-resistant pathogen, it is recommended that soap and water be used instead of ABHSs, but otherwise use of ABHSs are considered the standard of care in human health care.[11,12] In veterinary practice, hand washing has been recommended over use of ABHSs whenever running water is available.[6] Nonetheless, it has been shown that ABHSs may still be more effective than soap and water at reducing bacterial counts when small amounts of contamination (eg, blood) are present on the hands.[25] Another disadvantage of ABHSs is that the liquid is flammable due to its high alcohol content, which has been an issue in terms of placing ABHS dispensers in some public places and requires precautions for storage of large volumes and clean-up of large-volume spills.[28] See **Table 2** for a summary of the advantages and disadvantages of soap and water washing versus ABHS use.

Some non-ABHSs (NABHSs) are also available containing a variety of biocides with various mechanisms of action intended to have the same rapid-kill effect as alcohol. Objective studies demonstrating the efficacy of NABHSs in vitro or in vivo, as well as studies comparing NABHSs and ABHSs, are few, which is why NABHSs were not considered in the most recent hand hygiene guidelines produced by the US Centers for Disease Control and Prevention.[11,14] More recently, novel guanidine-based disinfectants have been investigated for potential use in topical prophylaxis and treatment

Table 2
Comparison of the advantages and disadvantages of the use of soap and water versus alcohol-based hand sanitizer for hand hygiene in veterinary clinics

	Soap and Water	Alcohol-Based Hand Sanitizer
Pros	• Physical removal of pathogens from hands (resistance not an issue) • Can be used even if hands are grossly contaminated • Very familiar and currently most commonly used method of hand hygiene	• Bottles/dispensers can be carried/placed anywhere, greatly facilitating access at point of care • Tends to cause less skin damage with repeated use (products contain emollients) • Takes less time (no additional rinsing or drying steps) • Additional biocides in products may provide some residual antibacterial action after use • Use associated with improved hand hygiene compliance
Cons	• Requires clean running water (access limited by availability of sinks in different rooms/areas) • Requires a drying method (disposable towels create additional waste, reusable towels can lead to cross-contamination) • Potential recontamination of hands when turning off faucet • Takes longer due to additional steps (ie, going to sink, rinsing, or drying) • Causes more skin damage with repeated use (eg, drying, cracking, or chapping) if proper skin care is not practiced	• Does not remove contaminants from hands (relies on bactericidal action of alcohol); therefore, ineffective against alcohol-resistant pathogens (eg, clostridial spores, *Cryptosporidium*, parvovirus) • Discomfort if applied to damaged skin • Some products may feel like they leave a residue on the hands, which some individuals dislike. • Flammable • Toxic if ingested

of skin infections[29,30] and as NABHSs.[31] The NABHS investigated by Agthe and colleagues[31] showed equal microbiological efficacy to ABHS in vitro, was well tolerated by hospital personnel, and was not significantly irritating to the skin. The clinical efficacy and cost of this product has yet to be directly compared with ABHS, but it has the potential to become an alternative in situations where waterless hand sanitizer is desirable but there is a need or desire to avoid alcohol-based products. Emergence of resistance to the active ingredient, however, as has been detected for other biocides, will need to be monitored carefully.

Hand Hygiene Technique and Timing

How well hand hygiene is performed when it is attempted is equally important to timing and frequency for hand hygiene to be effective. To effectively reduce or kill the transient microflora of the hands, it is generally recommended that soap be applied for a minimum of 10 to 20 s before rinsing or for ABHS that enough product be applied to cover all surfaces of the hands and then rubbed until dry (which should take at least 10–20 s as well).[6,11,13] The World Health Organization Guidelines on Hand Hygiene in Health Care, which are currently the definitive guidelines in human health care, recommend, however, 40 to 60 s for complete hand washing (from wetting hands to completion of drying) and 20 to 30 s for complete application of ABHS.[28] Recommended hand hygiene techniques are well described (**Table 3**).[6,11–13] Anderson and colleagues[26] reported that contact times with products during routine hand hygiene in primary care veterinary clinics are most often far shorter than recommended. Areas of the hand most often missed during washing are under the nails, back of fingers, back of the hands, and parts of the thumbs.[13]

Table 3
Comparison of the steps involved in a complete hand hygiene attempt using soap and water versus alcohol-based hand sanitizer

Hand Wash (Soap and Water)	Hand Rub (Alcohol-Based Hand Sanitizer)
Turn on water	—
Wet hands	—
Dispense appropriate amount of product directly onto hands (eg, 1–2 pumps from dispenser)	Dispense appropriate amount of product directly onto hands (eg, 1–2 pumps from dispenser)
Apply product to all surfaces of hands—minimum 15 s contact time	Apply product to all surfaces of hands—minimum 15 s contact time
Palms	Palms
Back of hands	Back of hands
Between fingers	Between fingers
Finger tips	Finger tips
Thumb and thumb web	Thumb and thumb web
± Wrists	± Wrists
Rinse all surfaces of hands with water	—
Dry hands thoroughly with single-use towel	Rub hands until dry
Turn water off, using drying towel to avoid direct contact with faucet handles (unless automatic faucet present)	—
Discard towel	—
TOTAL TIME: approximately 30–60 s	TOTAL TIME: approximately 20–30 s

Drying of hands is also an important step in the hand washing process, because bacteria are more easily transferred from hands when the skin is wet.[32] Disposable towels are the preferred means of hand drying, because they ensure there is no transmission of bacteria from hand to hand through sequential use of reusable towels by different people and are more efficient in terms of drying time than warm air dryers.[13] The results of studies comparing use of towels and warm air driers for reducing bacterial counts on hands are equivocal.[33–35] Disposable towels are also important to help prevent immediate recontamination of hands after washing through contact with faucet controls (if not automatic) and in some cases door handles. This is done by using the used towel to protect the hands when turning off the water faucet and/or opening the door to exit the room.[12,13] If reusable towels are used for hand drying instead due to cost or environmental concerns, the towels should be changed and laundered as frequently as possible and disposable towels should always be used in higher-risk areas, such as isolation. Another advantage of ABHSs is that the risk of recontamination of the hands immediately after use is decreased by the lack of a need to touch any object or surface once the product has been dispensed.

Hand hygiene should be used after activities that may result in contamination of the hands as well as before activities that may result in transmission of the transient flora of the hands to a common surface or another person or animal. Individuals have an easy time remembering to wash their hands when they are visibly soiled, with the possible exception of veterinary personnel working in a situation when their hands are expected to be (or accepted as) dirty, such as in a barn environment. Unfortunately, microbial contaminants on the hands are frequently not accompanied by visible dirt. In health care, human or veterinary, hand hygiene should ideally be performed[6,11–13]

- Before patient contact
- Before invasive procedures
- After potential exposure to bodily fluids, discharge, and so forth (eg, dirty procedures or specimen handling)
- After glove removal
- After patient contact

As much as possible, hand hygiene should be performed immediately before and after patient contact to minimize the opportunity for contamination of the hands or by the hands of the person in question. This requires hand hygiene stations to be readily available in all patient contact areas, but this has not been a consideration in the design of many veterinary clinics (ie, clinics that do not have a sink in all examination rooms and wards).

Gowning and Gloving Technique and Timing

As for hand hygiene, technique and timing for donning and doffing PPE have a great impact on the effectiveness of gloves, gowns, and similar items as barrier precautions. Misuse of PPE has significant potential to actually increase the risk of pathogen transmission and environmental contamination. There are 2 critical principles to bear in mind:

1. Particularly when dealing with high-risk infectious patients, most PPE must be single-use only, even for interactions with the same patient. It is essentially impossible to remove used gloves, gowns, or shoe covers and store them for any length of time in a manner that allows them to be redonned without contaminating the “clean” (typically inside) surface of the item, other clothing or hands, or environmental

surfaces. This is not to say that it is always necessary to use disposable items; reusable items, such as laboratory coats are acceptable if they can be adequately cleaned (eg, laundered) after each use (eg, a fresh laboratory coat could be used for each contact with a patient, collected in a laundry bag after each use, and then washed for reuse on a subsequent day). The exceptions to the single-use rule are items, such as facemasks or eye protection, which typically do not come in direct contact with patients or the environment. These items can potentially be reused if necessary by the same individual if care is taken to follow the appropriate doffing procedure and sequence (**Table 4**), assuming droplet/splash/direct contamination of the equipment does not occur during patient care.

2. When doffing PPE, contact between surfaces/sides must always be ensured as either clean to clean or dirty to dirty. This typically involves rolling off items, such as gowns and gloves, so that the dirty surface is contained on the inside of the ball, and then all items are dropped directly into an appropriate receptacle (garbage or laundry bag). Doffing of PPE should always be followed by hand hygiene (see **Table 4**).

For patients in isolation, PPE (gowns, gloves, with or without shoe covers, with or without masks) should be donned immediately before entering the isolated environment and doffed as the individual exits, leaving all potentially contaminated items within the isolated (contaminated) environment. Use of anterooms for isolation areas can be problematic, because it is often unclear to staff whether the anteroom is considered "clean" or "dirty." Although the anteroom should be less heavily contaminated than the adjacent isolation room, to err on the side of caution it nonetheless should be considered contaminated and treated appropriately in terms of timing and location for donning and doffing PPE. (See article entitled "Patient Management" by L. Guptill elsewhere in this issue for details on isolation protocols).

The impression that use of gloves negates the need for hand hygiene is problematic and has been reported as a barrier to hand hygiene compliance in human health care studies.[15,36,37] Although gloves provide an additional barrier between the skin of the wearer and the patient and/or objects the wearer may touch, preexisting defects, damage/punctures that may occur during use, and contamination of the hands during glove removal make gloves an imperfect barrier.[11,38] Because gloves are most often

Table 4
Sequence for donning and doffing of personal protective equipment

Donning Personal Protective Equipment	Doffing Personal Protective Equipment
1. *Perform hand hygiene*	1. Remove shoe covers (if applicable)
2. Put on shoe covers (if applicable)	2. Remove gown and gloves together[a]
3. Put on gown	3. *Perform hand hygiene*
4. Put on mask/respirator (if applicable)	4. Remove eye protection (if applicable)
5. Put on eye protection (if applicable)	5. Remove mask/respirator (if applicable)
6. Put on gloves	6. *Perform hand hygiene*

[a] If gloves are removed first, hands must only touch uncontaminated surfaces of the gown, typically behind the neck (ties) and at the back of the shoulders. The gown is then peeled down off the body and arms, balling or rolling in the contaminated surfaces (front and sleeves). This is difficult to do, however, without contaminating the hands. The preferred method for doffing a disposable gown and gloves is, therefore, to break the ties at the neck by pulling on the upper front portion of the gown with the hands still gloved, balling or rolling in the contaminated surfaces, and pulling the gloves off inside-out as the hands are withdrawn from the gown's sleeves. The gown and gloves can then be placed in a disposal receptacle together.

used in situations when there is a need to take additional precautions to prevent contamination of a site with bacteria from the hands or when heavy contamination of the hands or contamination with a serious infectious pathogen is expected to occur, hand hygiene before and after glove use remains necessary for infection control, although one recent randomized controlled trial has suggested that hand hygiene prior to donning nonsterile gloves may not be beneficial.[39] Gloved hands should not touch surfaces or items that are touched by nongloved personnel.

Compliance with Hand Hygiene and Contact Precautions in General

As with many infection control measures, compliance with contact precautions and hand hygiene protocols is the most challenging component of ensuring efficacy. Numerous studies have investigated hand hygiene compliance in human hospitals.[11,40] In general, compliance is poor (<50%) among health care workers, with physicians tending to have lower compliance with hand hygiene protocols than nurses.[15,41] Major barriers to compliance in many situations include skin irritation (irritant contact dermatitis), lack of accessibility of hand hygiene stations, time constraints (ie, too busy), and lack of perceived importance (ie, that it is generally unimportant or more likely that it is less important than other tasks/procedures, which, therefore, take precedence over hand hygiene).[11,36] Another barrier to hand hygiene compliance is that in some cases people may simply forget to perform hand hygiene[11]; to prevent this, hand hygiene needs to become an automatic habit for health care and veterinary personnel, like covering a sneeze or a cough. Some studies include evaluation of compliance with other contact precautions as well as hand hygiene, which is typically also suboptimal and in some cases inversely proportional to the number of patients requiring barrier nursing.[1,2,42] Use of contact precautions can also inadvertently lead to decreased patient contact, delays in procedures that may lead to noninfectious adverse events, negative psychological impact on patients, and decreased patient satisfaction.[43]

Compliance with Hand Hygiene and Contact Precautions in Veterinary Medicine

Literature regarding hand hygiene in veterinary health care specifically is limited. A household-based study by Hanselman and colleagues[44] showed that some dogs and cats share indistinguishable strains of *S aureus* and *S pseudintermedius* with humans living in the same household, and self-reported regular hand washing was protective for *S pseudintermedius* colonization in humans. Traub-Dargatz and colleagues[24] examined the effectiveness of traditional hand washing versus ABHS after basic physical examination of a horse and found the ABHS more effective at reducing bacterial counts on the hands. Anderson and colleagues[45] found that hand washing after contact with infectious cases and between farms had a protective effect against colonization with methicillin-resistant *S aureus* in veterinary personnel who work with horses.

There are only a few studies regarding compliance with hand hygiene recommendations in veterinary practices.

- In the survey conducted by Wright and colleagues,[4] 48% (516/1066) of small animal practitioners and only 18% (57/314) of large animal and 18% (83/456) of equine practitioners reported always sanitizing or washing their hands before patient contact. Only 55% (590/1069) of small animal practitioners in the same study reported always washing their hands before eating, drinking, or smoking while at work, and the same was true for less than a third of large animal and equine practitioners.[4]

- Self-reported compliance among veterinary support staff in another survey-based study was 42% (76/182).[46] The same study found that although 86% (154/182) of respondents believed they should perform hand hygiene more often, only 53% (96/182) had been given information on the importance of hand hygiene from their employers. The most commonly reported barrier to hand hygiene compliance was being too busy (72%).[46]
- In one study using direct observation of personnel in a companion animal teaching hospital, baseline hand hygiene compliance was 21% (117/568 opportunities), which increased to 42% (78/187) 2 weeks after the end of a multimodal educational campaign emphasizing use of a foaming ABHS product.[47] It was not possible, however, to separate the effect of the campaign from the potential effect of the presence of observers (ie, Hawthorne effect), and, unfortunately, there was no additional follow-up performed to determine if there was any longer-term effect.
- Hand hygiene compliance was 27% to 29% in a similar study using direct observation in a small animal ICU at another hospital, with compliance among technicians and assistants specifically ranging from 42% to 48%.[27]
- Anderson and colleagues[26] conducted the first hand hygiene compliance study in primary care veterinary hospitals using video observation. Overall compliance during outpatient appointments was 14%, ranging from 1% to 28% at individual clinics. Similar to patterns seen in human health care, compliance was highest after "dirty" procedures (39%) and lowest prior to patient contact (2%).

There is even less information on compliance with recommended use of PPE in veterinary clinics.

- In the study using direct observation practices in a small animal ICU, compliance with a mandatory glove use policy was reported to be 51% to 56% overall, ranging from 20% in veterinary assistants to 70% in veterinary students.[27]
- In Wright and colleagues'[4] survey of 1070 small animal practitioners in the United States, less than 30% of those who were concerned about zoonotic transmission of rabies, gastrointestinal bacterial or parasitic infections, or dermatophytosis reported using appropriate PPE when handling animals with compatible clinical signs of neurologic, gastrointestinal, or dermatologic disease.[4] Use of face or eye protection in clinical scenarios was reported by 5% or less of veterinarians, other than during surgical procedures (75%) and necropsies (37%).
- Murphy and colleagues[3] reported that 66 of 101 small animal clinics surveyed did not have an isolation area, and, of these, 61% did not use any specific infection control measures for potentially infectious cases in the clinic, including contact precautions.
- In a survey of 344 veterinarians in Australia, only 34% of respondents indicated that complete PPE kits were available for use in their clinics, and training on proper use of PPE was only provided to staff in 25% of clinics. Use of adequate PPE was reported by more than 75% of respondents for dental, surgical, and necropsy procedures but by less than a third of respondents for handling animals with neurologic, gastrointestinal, or respiratory disease. Factors positively correlated with use of PPE included postgraduate education, perceived likely risk of zoonotic disease exposure, concern regarding liability issues, and awareness of industry guidelines.[48]
- Appropriate use of routine personal protective clothing (eg, designated clinic clothing, such as scrubs and laboratory coats used in place of or to cover street clothes) during outpatient appointments was reported for 72% of staff-animal

contacts in a video observation study. In a majority of cases of inappropriate use, designated clothing was worn but in a manner that rendered it ineffective for protecting clothing worn underneath.[49]

Monitoring Infection Control Practices

The ability to monitor and evaluate infection control practices, in particular hand hygiene, is important from both a research and a routine infection control perspective. Accurate monitoring can be challenging, however, in the clinical setting, including human health care facilities and veterinary clinics. The gold standard for measuring hand hygiene compliance in human health care is direct observation, typically performed by an observer on the clinic floor,[11,12] although this has been challenged as the optimal means of monitoring hand hygiene.[50] Direct observation is labor intensive and also prone to bias on the part of the observer and due to Hawthorne effect (ie, behavioral changes in the subject that occur due to knowledge of the presence of the observer), so it may produce a falsely elevated estimate of compliance.[51,52]

Other less time-consuming approaches exist, but each has its own advantages and disadvantages as well. Total volume of hand hygiene product used based on supply orders can be used as a surrogate measure of hand hygiene compliance, or electronic counters can be installed in wall dispensers to record how often soap or ABHS is used, providing slightly more information.[53,54] These counting systems do not provide information on timing or adequacy of hand hygiene attempts nor an estimate of hand hygiene compliance as a percentage of hand hygiene opportunities but may be useful for inferring improvement in hand hygiene compliance after an intervention if there is evidence of increased use in the same clinical setting. Recently, more-advanced remote computer-based monitoring systems have been designed and marketed for use in health care facilities.[55,56] Unfortunately, there are few published reports describing the implementation and accuracy of many of the automated hand hygiene monitoring systems that are currently available.[55]

Video surveillance has not been frequently used for monitoring hand hygiene compliance or infection control practices in hospitals[52,57]; however, use of such a system in a small animal veterinary clinic is more feasible, because many clinics are designed around a central treatment room or area where a majority of nonsurgical procedures are performed, and many have small numbers of staff working at any given time. Video observation has several potential advantages over direct observation by a live observer.[26,58] Use of strategically placed or hidden cameras may also be less intrusive and less readily apparent than a live observer. Cameras can also be put in place in advance of the observation period to desensitize study subjects to their presence, which may help decrease Hawthorne effects and provide a more accurate measure of the practices of interest.[57] Like direct observation, video review is time-consuming, but observational specificity may also be improved by the ability to watch and rewatch video segments in real time or slow motion as needed.[26] Verification of observations by a second reviewer is also possible.[58] Video observation of hand hygiene practices has been used successfully in food handling studies[58,59] and can also be used to monitor infection control practices other than hand hygiene.

Improving Compliance

Education is often the first intervention considered to improve compliance with infection control protocols, but, although important or even essential, improving knowledge alone is often insufficient to change behavior. Behavioral achievement depends on both individual ability to perform the behavior and intention (motivation). Intention is determined by 3 factors: attitude toward the action (ie, what an individual thinks about the practice), subjective norms (ie, what an individual thinks others think about the practice), and perceived behavior control (ie, whether an individual believes he/she can effectively perform the required action).[60] Multimodal interventions that address more than one of these areas and in more than one way are likely to be more effective.

Providing better access to hand hygiene stations and supplies helps improve the ability of staff to perform the desired behavior, because it aids in minimizing the time required to comply with protocols and acts as a visual reminder to perform hand hygiene. Because renovating facilities to improve the location of sinks for hand washing is often not feasible, improving access typically involves introducing or changing the location or number of ABHS dispensers.[11] From an infection control standpoint, sink placement is a critical consideration in the design of new clinics to facilitate hand hygiene as much as possible, particularly in the most common patient contact areas (ie, examination rooms, treatment rooms, and wards). In a study of 38 veterinary clinics in Ontario, Canada, only 66% of clinics had a sink in the examination room, and 11% had neither a sink nor available ABHS in the examination room.[26]

Monitoring and feedback systems themselves can have a significant impact on compliance, in part by affecting subjective norms. Feedback may be from fellow staff, patient owners (in the case of veterinary clinics), researchers, or infection control personnel. Making people aware of how often they neglect to perform hand hygiene and/or giving them positive feedback when their compliance improves (the stick and carrot approach) seems to provide additional incentive to further improve compliance. Particularly when first implementing a monitoring and feedback system, it is important to strike a balance between positive feedback and constructive criticism, and the use of any kind of penalty system must be done with great caution so as not to create a negative attitude toward the infection control program and personnel. Just as hand hygiene compliance among physicians is often lower than among nurses,[15,41] the same may be true of veterinarians and technicians in some cases.[27] Empowering technicians to remind veterinarians to perform hand hygiene and observe other infection control protocols may help improve overall compliance.

Convincing staff of the importance and utility of hand hygiene and other contact precautions to curbing the spread of infectious agents is crucial to achieving compliance.[11] The perception that hand hygiene is unimportant is likely more problematic in veterinary medicine compared with human medicine. Because there are many common nonzoonotic diseases that affect veterinary patients, and fewer known diseases that can be transmitted from animal to person compared with person to person, some veterinary personnel have a cavalier attitude toward contamination of hands/clothing/equipment with animal blood, body fluids, and excreta. Hand hygiene, however, is also a critical means of preventing potential indirect transmission of nonzoonotic pathogens from animal to animal, thus protecting veterinary patients. The potential of a pathogen, brought into a clinic by a single person or animal, to spread first through the clinic and then into the community is significant. Examples of this kind of event have been described,[61,62] and many more likely are unreported or simply unrecognized.

Ideally hand hygiene and other basic contact measures should be things that everyone wants to do rather than things everyone must be asked to do. To be effective, infection control measures need to be practiced by every member of a clinic team, from veterinarians and technicians to kennel staff and volunteers. Several studies have suggested that involvement and support of upper-level management and administration are necessary for effective implementation of hand hygiene protocols in human health care facilities,[63,64] and it is likely that the same is true in veterinary

Table 5
Six easy things to help improve hand hygiene compliance and infection control in veterinary clinics

Put hand sanitizer where it is needed	• Provides access at point of care to reduce risk of cross-contamination of other surfaces • Saves time and facilitates compliance
Use the sink in the examination room	• Reduces risk of cross-contamination by negating need to leave room before performing hand hygiene • Demonstrates best practices and commitment to infection control in front of clients
Do "dirty" tasks last	• Facilitates opportunity to perform hand hygiene immediately after highest-risk tasks • Often allows a single hand hygiene attempt to fulfill 2 hand hygiene indications (after potential exposure and after patient contact)
Empower all staff	• Infection control is a team effort, and the chain is only as strong as its weakest link • Promotes clinic infection control culture • Encourages feedback to help improve and adapt infection control practices to clinics needs
Make the time and take the time	• Infection control practices such as hand hygiene do take extra time • The more they are practiced, the more they become routine/habitual, which also improves efficiency
Be a good example	• Never underestimate the power of your own example (good or bad) • Leadership and buy-in to sound infection control practices from senior staff/owners/hospital administration is particularly important

clinics. Nonetheless, the power of an individual's own good (or bad) example when it comes to promoting infection control and other behaviors must not be underestimated. Development of a clinic infection control culture, whereby infection control practices and principles become integrated into the group mentality through ongoing communication, conversation, training, and strong support from team leaders/management, is the ultimate means of improving compliance with hand hygiene and other infection control measures (**Table 5**).[65]

SUMMARY

Hand hygiene, contact precautions, and other basic infection control measures are crucial in veterinary clinics, because these facilities can be community mixing pots of animals and people with a wide range of health and disease-carrier states. Although the issue of hospital-associated infections in veterinary medicine is poorly defined, prevention of these events is becoming increasingly important with continued medical advances, rising antimicrobial resistance, and client expectations. There is limited information on use of contact precautions and hand hygiene practices among veterinary staff, but what there is suggests that compliance is low. Better compliance with these measures has the potential to have a positive impact on the health of patients, staff, and animal owners, but investigation of interventions to improve compliance is needed to determine effective means of achieving this goal. Improving the infection control culture in clinics and in veterinary medicine overall will be critical to these efforts moving forward.

REFERENCES

1. Siegel JD, Rhinehart E, Jackson M, et al. 2007 guideline for isolation precautions: preventing transmission of infectious agents in health care settings. Am J Infect Control 2007;35(10 Suppl 2):S65–164.
2. Dhar S, Marchaim D, Tansek R, et al. Contact precautions: more is not necessarily better. Infect Control Hosp Epidemiol 2014;35(3):213–21.
3. Murphy CP, Reid-Smith RJ, Weese JS, et al. Evaluation of specific infection control practices used by companion animal veterinarians in community veterinary practices in southern Ontario. Zoonoses Public Health 2010;57(6):429–38.
4. Wright JG, Jung S, Holman RC, et al. Infection control practices and zoonotic disease risks among veterinarians in the United States. J Am Vet Med Assoc 2008; 232(12):1863–72.
5. Lipton BA, Hopkins SG, Koehler JE, et al. A survey of veterinarian involvement in zoonotic disease prevention practices. J Am Vet Med Assoc 2008;233(8):1242–9.
6. Scheftel JM, Elchos BL, Cherry B, et al. Compendium of veterinary standard precautions for zoonotic disease prevention in veterinary personnel: national association of state public health veterinarians veterinary infection control committee 2010. J Am Vet Med Assoc 2010;237(12):1403–22.
7. Portner J, Johnson J. Guidelines for reducing pathogens in veterinary hospitals: disinfectant selection, cleaning protocols, and hand hygiene. Compend Contin Educ Vet 2010;32(5):E1–12.
8. Greene CE, editor. Infectious diseases of the dog and cat. 4th edition. St Louis (MO): Elsevier Saunders; 2012.
9. Australian Veterinary Association. Guidelines for veterinary personal biosecurity [Internet]. 1st edition. St. Leonards (Australia): Australian Veterinary Association; 2011. p. 1–59. Available at: http://www.ava.com.au/biosecurity-guidelines.
10. Canadian Committee on Antibiotic Resistance. Infection prevention and control best practices for small animal veterinary clinics. Guelph (Canada): Canadian Commitee on Antibiotic Resistance; 2008. p. 1–71. Available at: http://www.wormsandgermsblog.com/promo/services/.
11. Boyce JM, Pittet D, Healthcare Infection Control Practices Advisory Committee, HICPAC SHEA APIC IDSA Hand Hygiene Task Force. Guideline for hand hygiene in health-care settings. Recommendations of the healthcare infection control practices advisory committee and the HICPAC/SHEA/APIC/IDSA hand hygiene task force. Am J Infect Control 2002;30(8):S1–46.
12. Pittet D, Allegranzi B, Boyce J. The World Health Organization Guidelines on Hand Hygiene in Health Care and their consensus recommendations. Infect Control Hosp Epidemiol 2009;30(7):611–22.
13. Larson EL. APIC guideline for handwashing and hand antisepsis in health care settings. Am J Infect Control 1995;23(4):251–69.
14. Kampf G, Kramer A. Epidemiologic background of hand hygiene and evaluation of the most important agents for scrubs and rubs. Clin Microbiol Rev 2004;17(4): 863–93.
15. Pittet D. Improving adherence to hand hygiene practice: a multidisciplinary approach. Emerg Infect Dis 2001;7(2):234–40.
16. Larson EL, Hughes CA, Pyrek JD, et al. Changes in bacterial flora associated with skin damage on hands of health care personnel. Am J Infect Control 1998;26(5): 513–21.
17. Larson E. Effects of handwashing agent, handwashing frequency, and clinical area on hand flora. Am J Infect Control 1984;12(2):76–82.

18. Larson EL, Leyden JJ, McGinley KJ, et al. Physiologic and microbiologic changes in skin related to frequent handwashing. Infect Control 1986;7(2): 59–63.
19. Winnefeld M, Richard MA, Drancourt M, et al. Skin tolerance and effectiveness of two hand decontamination procedures in everyday hospital use. Br J Dermatol 2000;143(3):546–50.
20. Suwantarat N, Carroll KC, Tekle T, et al. High prevalence of reduced chlorhexidine susceptibility in organisms causing central line-associated bloodstream infections. Infect Control Hosp Epidemiol 2014;35(9):1183–6.
21. Russell AD. Biocide use and antibiotic resistance: the relevance of laboratory findings to clinical and environmental situations. Lancet Infect Dis 2003;3(12): 794–803.
22. Russell AD. Mechanisms of bacterial insusceptibility to biocides. Am J Infect Control 2001;29(4):259–61.
23. Subbannayya K, Bhat GK, Junu VG, et al. Can soaps act as fomites in hospitals? J Hosp Infect 2006;62(2):244–5.
24. Traub-Dargatz JL, Weese JS, Rousseau JD, et al. Pilot study to evaluate 3 hygiene protocols on the reduction of bacterial load on the hands of veterinary staff performing routine equine physical examinations. Can Vet J 2006;47(7): 671–6.
25. Larson EL, Bobo L. Effective hand degerming in the presence of blood. J Emerg Med 1992;10(1):7–11.
26. Anderson ME, Sargeant JM, Weese JS. Video observation of hand hygiene practices during routine companion animal appointments and the effect of a poster intervention on hand hygiene compliance. BMC Vet Res 2014;10(1): 1–16.
27. Smith JR, Packman ZR, Hofmeister EH. Multimodal evaluation of the effectiveness of a hand hygiene educational campaign at a small animal veterinary teaching hospital. J Am Vet Med Assoc 2013;243(7):1042–8.
28. World Health Organization. WHO guidelines on hand hygiene in health care: first global patient safety challenge clean care is safer care. Geneva (Switzerland): World Health Organization Press; 2009.
29. Kratzer C, Tobudic S, Macfelda K, et al. In vivo activity of a novel polymeric guanidine in experimental skin infection with methicillin-resistant Staphylococcus aureus. Antimicrob Agents Chemother 2007;51(9):3437–9.
30. Buxbaum A, Kratzer C, Graninger W, et al. Antimicrobial and toxicological profile of the new biocide Akacid plus. J Antimicrob Chemother 2006;58(1):193–7.
31. Agthe N, Terho K, Kurvinen T, et al. Microbiological efficacy and tolerability of a new, non-alcohol-based hand disinfectant. Infect Control Hosp Epidemiol 2009; 30(7):685–90.
32. Patrick DR, Findon G, Miller TE. Residual moisture determines the level of touch-contact-associated bacterial transfer following hand washing. Epidemiol Infect 1997;119(3):319–25.
33. Ansari SA, Springthorpe VS, Sattar SA, et al. Comparison of cloth, paper, and warm air drying in eliminating viruses and bacteria from washed hands. Am J Infect Control 1991;19(5):243–9.
34. Matthews JA, Newsom SW. Hot air electric hand driers compared with paper towels for potential spread of airborne bacteria. J Hosp Infect 1987;9(1):85–8.
35. Taylor JH, Brown KL, Toivenen J, et al. A microbiological evaluation of warm air hand driers with respect to hand hygiene and the washroom environment. J Appl Microbiol 2000;89(6):910–9.

36. Pittet D. Improving compliance with hand hygiene in hospitals. Infect Control Hosp Epidemiol 2000;21(6):381–6.
37. Ashraf MS, Hussain SW, Agarwal N, et al. Hand hygiene in long-term care facilities: a multicenter study of knowledge, attitudes, practices, and barriers. Infect Control Hosp Epidemiol 2010;31(7):758–62.
38. Olsen RJ, Lynch P, Coyle MB, et al. Examination gloves as barriers to hand contamination in clinical practice. J Am Med Assoc 1993;270(3):350–3.
39. Rock C, Harris AD, Reich NG, et al. Is hand hygiene before putting on nonsterile gloves in the intensive care unit a waste of health care worker time?–a randomized controlled trial. Am J Infect Control 2013;41(11):994–6.
40. Larson EL, Quiros D, Lin SX. Dissemination of the CDC's Hand Hygiene Guideline and impact on infection rates. Am J Infect Control 2007;35(10):666–75.
41. Pittet D, Mourouga P, Perneger TV. Compliance with handwashing in a teaching hospital. Infection Control Program. Ann Intern Med 1999;130(2): 126–30.
42. Clock SA, Cohen B, Behta M, et al. Contact precautions for multidrug-resistant organisms: current recommendations and actual practice. Am J Infect Control 2010;38(2):105–11.
43. Anderson DJ, Weber DJ, Sickbert-Bennett E. On contact precautions: the good, the bad, and the ugly. Infect Control Hosp Epidemiol 2014;35(3):222–4.
44. Hanselman BA, Kruth SA, Rousseau J, et al. Coagulase positive staphylococcal colonization of humans and their household pets. Can Vet J 2009; 50(9):954–8.
45. Anderson ME, Lefebvre SL, Weese JS. Evaluation of prevalence and risk factors for methicillin-resistant Staphylococcus aureus colonization in veterinary personnel attending an international equine veterinary conference. Vet Microbiol 2008;129(3–4):410–7.
46. Nakamura RK, Tompkins E, Braasch EL, et al. Hand hygiene practices of veterinary support staff in small animal private practice. J Small Anim Pract 2012;53(3): 155–60.
47. Shea A, Shaw S. Evaluation of an educational campaign to increase hand hygiene at a small animal veterinary teaching hospital. J Am Vet Med Assoc 2012;240(1):61–4.
48. Dowd K, Taylor M, Toribio JA, et al. Zoonotic disease risk perceptions and infection control practices of Australian veterinarians: call for change in work culture. Prev Vet Med 2013;111(1–2):17–24.
49. Anderson ME. Video observation of infection control practices in veterinary clinics and a petting zoo, with emphasis on hand hygiene and interventions to improve hand hygiene compliance [PhD dissertaion]. Guelph, Ontario: University of Guelph; 2013. Available at: https://atrium.lib.uoguelph.ca/xmlui/handle/10214/6648.
50. Marra AR, Moura DF, Paes AT, et al. Measuring rates of hand hygiene adherence in the intensive care setting: a comparative study of direct observation, product usage, and electronic counting devices. Infect Control Hosp Epidemiol 2010; 31(8):796–801.
51. The Joint Commission. Measuring hand hygiene adherence: overcoming the challenges. Oakbrook Terrace, Illinois: Monograph; 2009.
52. Haas JP, Larson EL. Measurement of compliance with hand hygiene. J Hosp Infect 2007;66(1):6–14.
53. Boyce JM, Cooper T, Dolan MJ. Evaluation of an electronic device for real-time measurement of alcohol-based hand rub use. Infect Control Hosp Epidemiol 2009;30(11):1090–5.

54. Marra AR, Guastelli LR, de Araújo CM, et al. Positive deviance: a new strategy for improving hand hygiene compliance. Infect Control Hosp Epidemiol 2010;31(1): 12–20.
55. Levchenko AI, Boscart VM, Fernie GR. The feasibility of an automated monitoring system to improve nurses' hand hygiene. Int J Med Inform 2011;80(8):596–603.
56. Fries J, Segre AM, Thomas G, et al. Monitoring hand hygiene via human observers: how should we be sampling? Infect Control Hosp Epidemiol 2012; 33(7):689–95.
57. Haidet KK, Tate J, Divirgilio-Thomas D, et al. Methods to improve reliability of video-recorded behavioral data. Res Nurs Health 2009;32(4):465–74.
58. Chapman B, Eversley T, Fillion K, et al. Assessment of food safety practices of food service food handlers (risk assessment data): testing a communication intervention (evaluation of tools). J Food Prot 2010;73(6):1101–7.
59. Redmond EC, Griffith CJ. A comparison and evaluation of research methods used in consumer food safety studies. Int J Consum Stud 2003;27(1):17–33.
60. Ajzen I. The theory of planned behavior. Organ Behav Hum Decis Process 1991; 50(2):179–211.
61. Weese JS, Caldwell F, Willey BM, et al. An outbreak of methicillin-resistant Staphylococcus aureus skin infections resulting from horse to human transmission in a veterinary hospital. Vet Microbiol 2006;114(1–2):160–4.
62. Wright JG, Tengelsen LA, Smith KE, et al. Multidrug-resistant Salmonella Typhimurium in four animal facilities. Emerg Infect Dis 2005;11(8):1235–41.
63. Whitby M, Pessoa-Silva CL, McLaws ML, et al. Behavioural considerations for hand hygiene practices: the basic building blocks. J Hosp Infect 2007;65(1):1–8.
64. Pittet D, Hugonnet S, Harbarth S, et al. Effectiveness of a hospital-wide programme to improve compliance with hand hygiene. Lancet 2000;356(9238): 1307–12.
65. Attard K, Burrows E, Kotiranta-Harris K, et al. Veterinary infection control in Australia: is there control? Aust Vet J 2012;90(11):438–41.

Antimicrobial Stewardship in Small Animal Veterinary Practice: From Theory to Practice

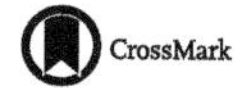

Luca Guardabassi, DVM, PhD[a,*], John F. Prescott, VetMB, DVM, PhD[b]

KEYWORDS

- Antimicrobial resistance • Antimicrobial stewardship • Rational antimicrobial use • Interventions • Infection control • Dogs • Cats

KEY POINTS

- There is increasing recognition of the critical role for antimicrobial stewardship and infection control in preventing the spread of multidrug-resistant bacteria in small animals.
- Establishment of antimicrobial stewardship programs requires (1) coordination ideally by an infectious disease specialist or at least by a clinician with strong interest in and good knowledge of antimicrobial resistance and therapy, (2) commitment by the clinical staff, and (3) collaboration with the microbiology laboratory.
- Even in the absence of specialist help, by accessing the increasingly available resources, veterinary clinics should at least develop, implement, and periodically update local antimicrobial policies indicating first-choice, restricted, and reserve drugs.
- Educational approaches, clinical guidelines, preprescription approval, postprescription review, and computer-based decision support are the most effective strategies to accomplish best practices in antimicrobial stewardship.
- The main barriers to implementation of antimicrobial stewardship programs comprise (1) economic sustainability; (2) lack of formally trained infectious disease specialists; (3) limited use of culture and antimicrobial susceptibility testing; (4) scientific knowledge gaps for assessment of resistance, development of evidence-based guidelines, and optimization of antimicrobial therapy; and (5) absence of standardized methods for evaluating the outcomes of antimicrobial stewardship programs.

INTRODUCTION: NATURE OF THE PROBLEM

Antimicrobial resistance (AMR) is one of the greatest challenges currently facing small animal veterinary medicine. During the past decade, various multidrug-resistant

---

Dr L. Guardabassi has received research funding from Zoetis, ICF, and SSI Diagnostica. Dr J.F. Prescott has nothing to disclose.

[a] Department of Veterinary Disease Biology, Faculty of Health and Medical Sciences, University of Copenhagen, Stigbøjlen 4, 1870 Frederiksberg C, Copenhagen, Denmark; [b] Department of Pathobiology, Ontario Veterinary College, University of Guelph, Guelph, Ontario N1G 2W1, Canada
* Corresponding author.
E-mail address: lg@sund.ku.dk

Vet Clin Small Anim 45 (2015) 361–376
http://dx.doi.org/10.1016/j.cvsm.2014.11.005 vetsmall.theclinics.com
0195-5616/15/$ – see front matter

bacteria (MDR) have emerged and spread among dogs and cats on a worldwide basis. The major current MDR organisms of concern are methicillin-resistant *Staphylococcus pseudintermedius* (MRSP)[1] and *Escherichia coli* producing extended-spectrum β-lactamase (ESBL).[2] However, these bacteria are just the tip of the iceberg because multidrug resistance has diffused in other common bacterial pathogens encountered in general practice, such as *Pseudomonas aeruginosa* and enterococci.[3] Additional MDR bacteria that are more likely to be isolated from animals presenting to referral centers include methicillin-resistant *Staphylococcus aureus* (MRSA),[4] carbapenemase-producing *E coli* and *Klebsiella pneumoniae,*[5] and MDR *Acinetobacter baumannii*.[6] All these MDR bacteria are frequently resistant to all conventional antimicrobials licensed for animal use and therefore pose a serious threat to animal health by increasing the risk of therapeutic failure and the recourse to euthanasia. MRSP/MRSA and MDR gram-negatives are important hospital-associated pathogens that can be transmitted from patient to patient through contact with personnel, with healthy animal carriers, and with contaminated environmental surfaces. Significant public health concerns exist because of the possible risk of animal-to-human transmission and in part also because of the increasing use in small animals of critically important antimicrobials authorized for human use only, such as carbapenems.[5] From the owner's perspective, infections caused by MDR bacteria contribute to increased veterinary expenditures because of additional and more expensive antimicrobial treatments, longer hospitalization, more visits, and more diagnostic tests. Moreover, the negative consequences of MDR infections in household pets include emotional and social effects on the owners and their families. Hospitals and clinics affected by outbreaks of MDR bacterial infections also can be impacted economically by the loss of revenue due to loss of reputation and decreased case load, decontamination procedures, closure, and coverage of patient bills.[7] This situation is worsened by the slow development of new antimicrobial drugs observed over the past decades. The few truly new agents are reserved for human use in hospitals and it is unlikely that these drugs will be authorized for veterinary use in the years to come. Thus, it is of paramount importance to preserve the efficacy of the veterinary antimicrobial products available today.

APPROACH/GOALS

For the reasons described, there is an urgent need to mitigate the escalation of AMR in small animal veterinary practice. Antimicrobial stewardship programs (ASPs) are a cornerstone of the response to the AMR crisis in human medicine but are still largely underdeveloped in veterinary medicine. Because it is a relatively new area of practice, there is poor understanding among practitioners of what constitutes an ASP. The aim of this article is to indicate the necessary steps that should be taken to establish ASPs in small animal veterinary practice, taking into consideration the many and remarkable differences between the human and the veterinary sector, and indeed the remarkable differences within veterinary medicine. Although the article highlights the structural and economic constraints that make implementation of ASPs used in human health care facilities difficult in small animal practice, it provides suggestions and approaches to overcome such constraints and to move toward practical implementation of effective veterinary-specific ASPs in small animal hospitals and clinics. We emphasize the multidimensional and the "mind-set" nature of "good stewardship practice" (GSP), as well the importance of an entire team-based commitment similar to that required for implementation of infection control practices.

THE ANTIMICROBIAL PARADOX IN SMALL ANIMAL PRACTICE

One of the most effective strategies to manage AMR in human hospitals is to reduce the overall consumption of antimicrobial agents and rationalize the use of the most valuable drugs (eg, carbapenems, fourth-generation cephalosporins, glycopeptides), which are generally reserved for empirical treatment of life-threatening infections or infections that cannot be treated otherwise on the basis of susceptibility data. This strategy is almost completely flipped in small animal practice, where the listed drugs are not authorized and the most powerful veterinary antimicrobials, namely β-lactamase–resistant penicillins, cephalosporins, and fluoroquinolones, are widely used as empiric first-line agents in primary care, including treatment of mild or self-limiting infections. Altogether, aminopenicillins combined with β-lactamase inhibitors (mainly amoxicillin/clavulanic acid) and first-generation cephalosporins (mainly cephalexin) account for approximately three-fourths of the total sales of antimicrobial tablets for companion animals in Europe[8]; data on antimicrobial consumption are not readily available in North America, but are likely similar. The sale of tablets containing fluoroquinolones reaches up to 10% of total sales in some European countries[8] and in the United States is enhanced by marketing of generic ciprofloxacin that is cheaper but less effective compared with veterinary-licensed fluoroquinolones.[9] High consumption of these drugs provides a strong selective pressure in favor of MDR bacteria resistant to extended-spectrum β-lactams and fluoroquinolones, including MRSA, MRSP, and ESBL-producing *E coli*. It should be noted that both fluoroquinolones and cephalosporins are known to select for MRSA and ESBL-producing *E coli* in humans and most likely have a similar effect on animals.[10–15] On the other hand, they are indispensable drugs for management of common bacterial infections in small animals, including complicated skin and urinary tract infections and various life-threatening conditions.[16,17] This leads to the paradox that these highly important antimicrobials are the most used and therefore the least preserved.

WHAT IS ANTIMICROBIAL STEWARDSHIP?

The term "antimicrobial stewardship" is used to describe the multifaceted and dynamic approaches required to sustain the clinical efficacy of antimicrobials by optimizing drug use, choice, dosing, duration, and route of administration, while minimizing the emergence of resistance and other adverse effects. The word stewardship implies the obligation to preserve something of enormous value for future generations, and resonates in a way that "prudent use" or "judicious use" does not. GSP is the active, dynamic process of continuous improvement in antimicrobial use, and is an ethic with many steps of different sizes by everyone involved in antimicrobial use. Stewardship thus links, for example, front-line veterinary practitioners with laboratory diagnosticians, owners, drug regulators, and pharmaceutical companies.[18] **Table 1** lists examples of key elements encompassed by the term antimicrobial stewardship.

Antimicrobial stewardship is perceived among veterinarians in a slightly different way compared with physicians. Although antimicrobial stewardship in veterinary medicine encompasses numerous aspects of improved use (see **Table 1**) and is generally associated with country-wide surveillance of AMR and development of national and international guidelines for antimicrobial use, in human medicine, this term generally refers to specific programs or series of interventions to monitor and direct antimicrobial use at the hospital level.[19] Formal ASPs were first established in human hospitals in the late 1970s and 1980s to reduce costs associated with inappropriate use of antimicrobials, and have been shown to reduce total or targeted antimicrobial use, increase appropriate antimicrobial use, reduce resistance, and improve clinical

Table 1
Examples of elements encompassed by the term antimicrobial stewardship that affect the emergence and spread of resistance

Element	Comment
Practice guidelines	Awareness of national or international practice guidelines; development of local practice-specific guidelines; antimicrobial choice and restriction policies; stop orders.
Dosage considerations	Knowledge of pharmacokinetic and pharmacodynamic aspects of effective antimicrobial treatment; knowledge of factors affecting duration of treatment.
Clinical microbiology data	Use of diagnostic microbiology, including susceptibility testing; point-of-care diagnostics; rapid diagnostic approaches.
Resistance and use surveillance	Knowledge of critical resistance problems and benchmarking of antimicrobial use and resistance locally, nationally, or internationally.
Infection control practices	Development of local and national infection control policies and procedures; assessment, review, and certification of practices; identification of specific resistance problems that need to be addressed.
Alternatives to antimicrobials	Use of vaccines and immunostimulants.
National and international regulations	Development and compliance assessment of professional antimicrobial stewardship standards; knowledge and compliance with national regulations.
Owner compliance	Owner education and compliance assessment; educational materials.
Education	Continuing education to ensure antimicrobial use best practices; self-assessment and peer-assessment procedures; ongoing educational reminders.
Responsibility	A 5R approach to stewardship: Acceptance of responsibility for resistance as a potential effect of antimicrobial use, and for reduction, replacement, refinement, and review of antimicrobial use on an ongoing basis. Recognition of potential adverse effects of antimicrobial use in animals on human health. Like safety, antimicrobial stewardship is everyone's responsibility, but specific responsibility can be assigned in a hierarchical manner.

markers (eg, length of hospitalization).[19–21] This practice is largely unknown in small animal clinics and more broadly in the veterinary sector, where the term antimicrobial stewardship is used in a broad sense and includes legal (regulatory) interventions imposed by national authorities to restrict or ban specific drugs, to limit profit derived from antimicrobial dispensation, and taxes or penalties to prevent antimicrobial overuse.[22] This regulatory approach has been used successfully in some countries (eg, Scandinavian countries) for reducing antimicrobial consumption in food-producing animals but its application in small animal practice is rare to date. Implementation of voluntary ASPs at the national and clinic levels appears to be a more appropriate approach to contain AMR in companion animals in view of the strong human-animal bond and the animal welfare and legal issues associated with household pets. Although supporting the use of the term antimicrobial stewardship in veterinary medicine to encompass the broad, multifaceted, approach to sustaining the efficacy of antibiotics for the long term, the authors recognize the need for establishing hospital-based ASPs in small animal practice.

ESTABLISHING AN ANTIMICROBIAL STEWARDSHIP PROGRAM

No guidelines are available for development of ASPs in small animal clinics. The joint guidelines published by the Infectious Diseases Society of America (IDSA) and the Society for Healthcare Epidemiology of America (SHEA) may serve as a source of inspiration for those interested in establishing an ASP in their clinic.[23] The key elements of an ASP are summarized in **Box 1**. Regardless of type and size, every small animal clinic should have some form of ASP in place as part of a formal infection control program coordinated by a designated infection control practitioner (ICP).[24] In human medicine, ASPs, which as noted are hospital-based and practice-based, are initiated and sustained by a dedicated multidisciplinary team composed of an infectious disease physician and a clinical pharmacist, and are supported by a microbiologist, a computer information technologist, and an ICP or hospital epidemiologist.[19] Organization of similar ASP teams is not possible in most veterinary health care facilities. To replace the lack of formally trained infectious disease specialists, a clinician with strong interest in and good knowledge of AMR and antimicrobial therapy may serve as the ASP coordinator. The designated person should lead a multidisciplinary team responsible for deciding the strategies that are needed to improve antimicrobial stewardship, taking into consideration hospital type and size, local patterns in antimicrobial usage, trends in AMR, and available resources. The team should comprise the ICP (if available) and leaders from the clinic services in which most antimicrobials are prescribed (eg, dermatology, internal medicine, surgery, and intensive care). In large facilities, endorsement by the clinic's leadership is necessary to secure the resources needed for program development and to enhance compliance by the clinic staff. In

Box 1
Key elements of a clinic-based antimicrobial stewardship program (ASP)

- Designation of an ASP coordinator with sufficient knowledge in antimicrobial resistance and therapy
- Establishment of an ASP team composed of the infection control practitioner and the leaders from the main clinic services in large facilities, or by the entire staff in small facilities
- Development of a formal-practice ASP, taking into consideration hospital type and size, local patterns in antimicrobial usage, trends in antimicrobial resistance, and available resources
- Participation by the clinic's leadership and staff at early development stages to ensure commitment by all parts
- Liaison with a microbiology laboratory that is able to advise on specimen collection and transportation, interpretation of antimicrobial susceptibility reports, and antimicrobial choice
- Inclusion of basic educational activities and a local antimicrobial policy based on national or international practice guidelines (minimal requirement)
- Inclusion of preprescription approval, postprescription review, and computer-based decision support strategies according to availability of expertise and resources
- Periodic evaluation of the ASP outcome through "benchmarking" of data on antimicrobial prescription at the practice level
- Yearly revision and update of the ASP based on clinicians' experience and cumulative antibiograms provided by the microbiology laboratory

small clinics, the entire staff should be involved. Participation by all parties should be sought early in the process to ensure acceptance and ownership of the program. It is important to understand and address any concerns by highlighting the benefits of the proposed changes. The key steps in the implementation of an ASP are summarized in **Box 2**.

The most basic form of ASP is given by a local antimicrobial policy (LAP) for rational antimicrobial use. An LAP should define distinct categories of antimicrobial prescription/use. Three categories are generally recommended[25]:

1. *First-choice drugs* that can be prescribed without any restrictions.
2. *Restricted drugs* that can be prescribed for specific indications defined by the LAP after consultation of the ASP coordinator.
3. *Reserve drugs* that can be prescribed only after permission from the ASP coordinator and/or the national expert committee.

The ASP team should assign the available antimicrobial drugs to 1 of these 3 categories depending on national and international guidelines, local patterns of antimicrobial usage and antimicrobial resistance, and specific goals of the ASP pursued at the clinic. Ideally the document should be organized into sections dedicated to treatment of different infection types, taking into consideration drug activity, spectrum, pharmacokinetics, pharmacodynamics, risks of resistance development, adverse effects, costs, and special needs of individual patient groups.[25] It should be revised every year based on the clinicians' experience and the susceptibility reports of the microbiology laboratory.

ROLE OF THE MICROBIOLOGY LABORATORY

Liaison with a microbiologist at the diagnostic laboratory, which in contrast to human hospitals is normally placed outside the clinic environment, is an essential aspect for implementation of ASPs in small animal veterinary practice. The microbiology laboratory is not only supposed to provide timely and accurate species identification and antimicrobial susceptibility testing. Its role and responsibilities go beyond correct specimen testing and reporting of results, and include attention to the preanalytical (eg, guidelines for appropriate specimen collection and transportation, and rejection

Box 2
Steps necessary to implement an ASP

1. Frame the problem that needs to be addressed
2. Consider potential solutions to the problem
3. Decide how the solution should be achieved
4. Meet clinic's leadership and administrators
5. Determine the annual cost
6. Determine the costs associated with the target infection of interest
7. Calculate the financial effect
8. Include additional benefits (eg, patient clinical outcomes and owners' satisfaction)
9. Prospectively collect the relevant outcome data

Adapted from Tamma PD, Cosgrove SE. Antimicrobial stewardship. Infect Dis Clin North Am 2011;25:256; with permission.

criteria for specimens inappropriately submitted) and postanalytical (eg, correct interpretation of antimicrobial susceptibility reports and advice on appropriate antimicrobial choice) components of testing. Selective reporting of susceptibility profiles can be used to discourage unnecessary use of broad-spectrum agents that are not licensed for veterinary use (eg, hiding or masking data on carbapenems in strains susceptible to veterinary-licensed drugs). Indiscriminate reporting of positive culture and susceptibility data on likely contaminants or nonpathogenic commensals should be avoided, because this practice may lead to inappropriate antimicrobial use. Last, but not least, the microbiology laboratory should generate annual reports summarizing the trends of AMR at the clinic level or at least at the regional level. These reports, generally referred to as "cumulative antibiograms," potentially allow adjustments of LAPs based on changes in AMR rates over time. It is well recognized that data from susceptibility testing tends to overidentify resistance because samples are more likely to come from treated animals with resistant bacteria rather than from patients who were not previously treated with antimicrobial agents or responded successfully to the treatment. Thus, it is important that veterinary clinicians also submit specimens from the latter categories of patients, allowing generation of antibiograms that reflect the actual levels of AMR in the patient population. Antibiograms are useful to design (eg, identification of the target antimicrobials) and evaluate the outcome of an ASP (eg, assessment of effects on AMR). They should cover common bacterial species that are isolated in sufficient numbers to allow statistical significance of the data (eg, *S pseudintermedius* and *E coli*), exclude multiple isolates from the same patient, and possibly be reported by infection type. Guidelines for collection, analysis, and reporting of cumulative antibiograms have been published by The Clinical and Laboratory Standards Institute.[26]

ANTIMICROBIAL STEWARDSHIP STRATEGIES

Various strategies have been shown to improve appropriateness of antimicrobial use and cure rates, decrease failure rates, and reduce health care–related costs in human hospitals. This topic has been reviewed comprehensively.[19–21] The following provides an overview of the most successful strategies used in human hospitals with focus on their implementation in small animal veterinary practice. It should be noted that one strategy does not exclude the other and that multiple strategies can be successfully used in combination.

Educational Approaches

Teaching of AMR and antimicrobial pharmacology is inadequate in most veterinary university curricula. As a consequence, the prescription habits of young veterinarians are often influenced by the practice of older colleagues and the information acquired from antimicrobial handbooks or from representatives of the pharmaceutical industry. As the information provided by these sources may be in conflict with best practices in antimicrobial stewardship, clinics and national and international veterinary organizations should provide guidelines for antimicrobial use and educate young veterinarians to rational antimicrobial use. Good education reduces inappropriate antimicrobial use and enhances understanding and acceptance of stewardship and of stewardship strategies. Passive educational strategies (eg, posters and leaflets) are easier to implement but less effective compared with active strategies, such as one-on-one educational sessions addressing topics of general interest (eg, discussion of guidelines or local data on antimicrobial use) or patient-specific issues (eg, feedback on prescriptions). These programs should be ideally implemented by an academic educator, usually a physician or pharmacist in human health care.[20]

An outstanding example of a readily and freely accessible Web-based and app-linked resource aimed to support companion animal veterinarians to develop practice policies for antimicrobial stewardship is the PROTECT site of the British Small Animal Veterinary Association (http://www.bsava.com/Resources/PROTECT.aspx). PROTECT stands for Practice policy, Reduce prophylaxis, Other options, Types of bacteria and drugs, Employ narrow spectrum, Culture and sensitivity, and Treat effectively. The advantage of such Web-based resources is the ability to update them regularly and relatively inexpensively. We recommend this as a good place to start the development of LAPs and other clinic-based antimicrobial stewardship practices in the absence of infectious disease specialists. Among other initiatives taken to support education in this field, the Federation of European Companion Animal Veterinary Associations recently released several posters addressing responsible use of antimicrobials, appropriate antimicrobial therapy, and hygiene and infection control in veterinary practice (available at www.fecava.org/content/guidelines-policies). This area is dynamic so that resources of this type are continually being developed.

Development and Implementation of Guidelines

General (generic) guidelines providing statements of principles of prudent antimicrobial use have been developed in recent years by most national veterinary organizations (**Box 3**).[18,27] Although important from a conceptual standpoint, their clinical guidance and impact is likely limited. Standard texts have included investigator recommendations on first-choice, second-choice, and last-resort antimicrobial agents.[28,29] More recently, evidence-based clinical antimicrobial use guidelines have been developed using approaches similar to those for human guidelines. These have typically involved national or international expert panels reviewing and assessing the quality and strength of published literature to produce recommendations for diagnosis and management of specific conditions.[16,17,30,31] The impact of national practice guidelines is likely higher than for international guidelines, because they take into account local factors regarding legislation, drug market availability, and prevalence of resistance. Many veterinary specialty organizations also have developed guidelines, ranging from generic prudent use guidelines to practice-specific or disease-specific guidelines.[32] Veterinary practice guidelines are negatively affected by numerous knowledge gaps regarding dose-effect relationships between antimicrobial use and resistance, antimicrobial consumption, resistance prevalence, drug-to-drug superiority, and optimal duration of treatment. However, although there are limitations, national guidelines are an essential milestone for development of LAPs and more complex ASPs at the clinic level.

Although there has been a marked increase in available guidelines, there has been little assessment of their impact on practice. Data from Sweden indicate that information campaigns on MDR bacteria and local discussions between national experts and veterinarians may have a rapid and significant impact on antimicrobial consumption (**Fig. 1**).[33] The effort spent on introducing guidelines, on educating health care providers, and in monitoring the response to guidelines is often slight compared with the effort of development, but critical to success. Compliance with guidelines may be poor because of inadequate communication, differences in opinion regarding recommended treatments, and resentment of measures to prescribe individual decisions.[18] Thus, it is crucial that national and local veterinary professional and regulatory organizations allocate sufficient time and resources to promote guidelines and facilitate compliance.

Box 3
General principles of rational antimicrobial use

- Antimicrobials should be used only when there is evidence or at least a well-founded clinical suspicion of bacterial infection
- Antimicrobials should not be used for treatment of self-limiting infections
- Antimicrobial, pathogen, infection site, and patient factors should be considered when choosing an appropriate treatment
- Cytology should be used as a point-of-care test to guide antimicrobial choice for relevant disease conditions (eg, otitis and urinary tract infections)
- Antimicrobial susceptibility testing should be performed if
    - There is suspicion of a complicated or life-threatening infection
    - The patient does not respond to initial treatment
    - The patient has a recurring or refractory infection
    - The patient is immunosuppressed
    - There is a need to monitor the outcome of therapy (eg, long treatment period)
    - The patient is at risk of infection with multidrug-resistant bacteria
- As narrow a spectrum therapy as possible should be used
- Topical therapy should be preferred over systemic therapy for treatment of superficial skin infections
- Antimicrobials should be used for as short a time as possible
- Extra-label use should be avoided when on-label options are reasonable
- Use of critically important antimicrobials not authorized for veterinary use should at least be restricted to rare and severe patient conditions (eg, diagnosed, life-threatening bacterial infections that cannot be treated by any other available antimicrobials, provided that treatment has a realistic chance of eliminating infection)
- Antimicrobial therapy should never be used as a substitute for good infection control, and good medical and surgical practices
- Perioperative prophylaxis should be used only when indicated, and follow standard guidelines
- Clients should be educated to ensure compliance

Preprescription Approval

This strategy is based on external control over antimicrobial prescription. It can be accomplished by the use of antimicrobial formularies that limit free prescription/dispensation for certain antimicrobials. Other antimicrobials can be used only if certain criteria are met and/or after approval by an infectious disease specialist or appropriately designated individual. The nature and degree of restriction and specific targeted agents is defined based on the specific goal(s) of the ASP. An initiative based on restriction has been taken in Sweden, where prescription of third-generation cephalosporins and fluoroquinolones is allowed only when susceptibility data show resistance to all the other veterinary-licensed antimicrobials that can be used for the relevant indication. Although based on restriction, this national ASP is implemented on a voluntary basis without specific measures being taken to check for compliance. On a local level, some veterinary facilities restrict the use of certain antimicrobials (eg, carbapenems and vancomycin) and require a formal approval process before those

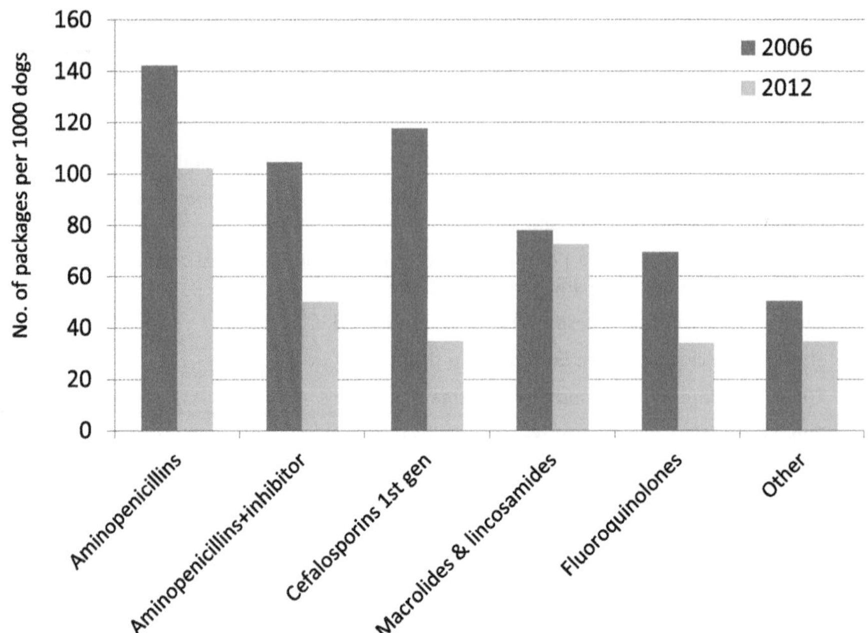

Fig. 1. Sales of antimicrobials for oral use in dogs in Sweden in 2006 and 2012. The marked decrease in antimicrobial sales observed during this period was triggered by the appearance of the first cases of methicillin-resistant staphylococci and the availability of statistics on antimicrobial use. These areas received considerable attention, both among veterinarians and in the media. The consequent debate at the national and the local levels contributed to increase prescribers' awareness and establishment of consensus guidelines, resulting in a downward trend of antimicrobial consumption. (*Adapted from* Greko C. Reductions of sales of antimicrobial for dogs—Swedish experiences. Eur J Comp Anim Pract 2013;23:57.)

drugs can be dispensed. The authors are not aware of any studies investigating the efficacy of restriction strategies in small animal practice. Based on human data, restriction strategies are effective at reducing use of targeted antimicrobials even though they raise issues of prescriber autonomy and require dedicated prescribers to ensure compliance.

Postprescription Review

This strategy involves retrospective (hours to days) review of antimicrobial prescriptions and provision of unsolicited feedback to individual prescribers. It can be used in addition to or as an alternative to restriction strategies. The methods used to provide feedback to the prescriber include one-on-one conversations and written notifications. Specific targets for postprescription review are streamlining (ie, modification of initial empiric therapy based on susceptibility data), discontinuation of empiric therapy when cause of illness does not require antimicrobial treatment (eg, viral upper respiratory tract illness), dose optimization, parenteral-to-oral conversion, identification of organism-antimicrobial mismatch and drug-drug interactions, and therapeutic monitoring. Among the advantages of feedback strategies are that there can be custom applications to small and large health care facilities, the prescriber's autonomy is not affected, and prescription cannot be delayed by their implementation.

The downsides are that recommendations are optional unless specific rules are established to correct unaccepted prescriptions. Although this is a time-consuming effort that requires expert knowledge, periodic review of existing prescribing practices is strongly recommended by the authors, as this has been proven to be one of the most effective ways to rationalize antimicrobial use in hospitals and primary health care facilities.

Computer-Based Decision Support

The increasing computerization of veterinary clinics offers new opportunities for programs to optimize antimicrobial use. Computer-assisted decision support programs have been developed to provide real-time recommendations on antimicrobial choice in human medicine. This strategy consists of linking national or local antimicrobial formularies to computerized order-entry systems. Even though numerous veterinary practice management systems are available in the market, the authors are not aware of any software including specific applications for antimicrobial stewardship. Mobile phone applications, generally referred to as "apps," are another useful IT-based tool to provide clinical decision support. More than 12,000 medical apps have been developed to facilitate rational antimicrobial choice at the point of care.[34] The authors are aware of 2 examples in the veterinary sector: "Antimicrobial Smart/Vet" by the Canadian Veterinary Medical Association (CVMA) and a similar app launched by the Danish Small Animal Veterinary Association for implementation of the national guidelines ("AB Vejledning," in Danish). There is clearly room for further development of IT-based clinical decision support in veterinary medicine.

MEASURING THE OUTCOMES OF ANTIMICROBIAL STEWARDSHIP PROGRAMS

The IDSA/SHEA guidelines recommend measuring the outcomes of ASPs on the basis of data on antimicrobial consumption.[23] Monitoring of antimicrobial prescription patterns can be used to identify irrational antimicrobial use and to evaluate LAPs over time. Data expressed as defined daily dose or antimicrobial days of therapy are used as an internal and external benchmark of antimicrobial consumption in human hospitals.[21] The ASP coordinator responsible for developing and implementing the practice of ASP should play a key role in centralizing, compiling and evaluating data on antimicrobial prescription on a regular basis. IT support may be needed to allow handling of antimicrobial prescription data, especially in large facilities. Baseline data on antimicrobial use should be in place before implementation of the ASP to track the progress of interventions over time.

The effects of ASPs on AMR are difficult to measure, but several studies indicate short-term reductions in the isolation rates of specific MDR bacteria (see **Fig. 1**).[35] The impact of generic or practice-specific guidelines on impairing the development and spread of resistance is especially hard to measure because guidelines are only one part of a multidimensional approach to stewardship, which includes infection control as a complementary approach to prevent the spread of MDR bacteria associated with hospital-associated infections. Some MDR bacteria are mainly controlled by infection control measures whereas others are more affected by stewardship interventions reducing antimicrobial use.

BARRIERS TO IMPLEMENTATION OF ANTIMICROBIAL STEWARDSHIP PROGRAMS

GSP is made up of numerous components and is based on a proactive culture of continuous improvement in identifying factors that impede such practice.[18] Several practical barriers can hinder implementation of ASPs in small animal practice, including allocation of time and resources, lack of perceived value, or lack of confidence in ability to develop an ASP. However, practical barriers can be more easily overcome if structural and organizational barriers are adequately addressed at the political level. Examples of important areas that deserve attention by national and international public health care and veterinary institutions, pharmaceutical companies, and public and private research funding agencies, and that would improve implementation of ASP in small animal practice, are discussed later in this article.

Economic Sustainability of Antimicrobial Stewardship Programs

Veterinary small animal hospitals and clinics are operated as private companies without the support of national health care systems, and the costs for antimicrobial therapy are paid by the animal owners. Thus, there is a lack of economic interest and possibly even a subtle conflict of interest in reducing the costs for antimicrobial therapy. Although veterinary facilities range in size from a few large referral hospitals to a multitude of small or medium-sized clinics, where implementation of large ASPs in the fashion of human hospitals is not economically sustainable, every veterinary clinic can and should implement at least rudimentary but functional ASP. Antimicrobial stewardship should be promoted by generating concrete evidence for veterinarians, clinic leaders, and hospital administrators that ASPs improve patient care without increasing costs. Research is warranted to investigate the sustainability of ASPs in small animal practice and ultimately to show how their implementation correlates with quality of patient care and owners' satisfaction. Taxes on antibiotics[36] might even be used to support the cost of establishing veterinary ASPs, while contributing to reduce overall antimicrobial use.

Lack of Formally Trained Infectious Disease Specialists

Formal training of veterinary infectious disease specialists and clinical microbiologists is not readily available. Thus, implementation of ASPs in small animal practice would be facilitated by the establishment of formal training programs, including continuing education activities organized by national and international veterinary associations and relevant specialty colleges (eg, American College of Veterinary Internal Medicine (ACVIM), European College of Veterinary Internal Medicine (ECVIM), and International Society for Companion Animal Infectious Diseases (ISCAID). University veterinary curricula should contain teaching activities on antimicrobial stewardship and interpretation of susceptibility reports. There is a need to build a new generation of specialists in this area.

Limited Use of Antimicrobial Susceptibility Testing

Antimicrobial susceptibility data are indispensable to establish and evaluate the outcome of any ASP. A recent survey by the Federation of Veterinarians in Europe has indicated a clear need to improve antimicrobial susceptibility tests and services in veterinary medicine, with the availability of rapid, reliable, and cheaper testing being key factors.[37] More reliable laboratory results, accurate in-house sampling kits, and easier methods for collection and shipment of samples were among the factors that veterinarians considered important to increase the use of susceptibility testing. Various technologies could provide valuable alternatives to the existing methodologies in the near future.[38,39] The use of antimicrobial susceptibility tests should be promoted by national clinical guidelines and made compulsory before the use of certain antimicrobial agents. In addition, the frequency of samples submitted to microbiology laboratories could be increased through implementation of national pet health insurance schemes covering the costs for culture and susceptibility testing, which are largely underdeveloped in most countries.

Scientific Knowledge Gaps

Development of evidence-based clinical guidelines is hampered by the lack of adequate scientific knowledge to assess drug superiority and optimize dosage regimens in small animals. For some infections (eg, urinary tract infections), there is great uncertainty with regard to the optimal treatment duration, which is significantly longer than for human patients. There is a lack of data on etiology and pathogen distribution for respiratory infections and other infections for which samples are rarely submitted to the clinical microbiology laboratory. The reliability of clinical breakpoints for assessing resistance to older drugs is limited by the lack of animal species-specific pharmacokinetic (PK), pharmacokinetic/pharmacodynamic (PK/PD), and clinical outcome data. These knowledge gaps are not easy to fill because of the limited funds allocated for research on antimicrobial therapy in companion animals.

Lack of Standard Methods and Data to Assess the Outcomes of Veterinary Antimicrobial Stewardship Programs

Monitoring and analysis of antimicrobial usage is critical to measure the effects of ASPs. There is a broad need to establish metric approaches and reliable baseline data against which to measure the effect of ASPs; this will require local, national, and international efforts to improve surveillance of antimicrobial use in small animal practice. There is an important role for veterinary professional standards bodies in developing ways to assess implementation of antimicrobial stewardship measures at the individual practice and national levels. Metrics could include the following: documentation that the guidelines have been implemented; comparison of international, national, local, or practice use of antimicrobials, linked to rates of resistance in specific pathogens; and the absence of identified local or national problems of nosocomial infections based on comparison with other practices or countries. Development of assessment rubrics that could lead to certification as meeting GSP standards, with periodic recertification, is an area that could be developed by veterinary professional standard bodies to promote antimicrobial stewardship.

CONCLUDING REMARKS

The emergence and spread of resistance is a complex process that demands multiple responses, including a stewardship approach. The cumulative effect of these responses should help preserve existing antimicrobials and should provide time for the development of new antimicrobials and other interventions, such as improvements in diagnostics or alternative treatments.[40] Establishment of sustainable and functional ASPs is a key issue for both better care of patients and combating AMR. The concept of antimicrobial stewardship and of its continuous improvement is in its relative infancy in small animal veterinary practice, but every clinic has the responsibility and access to a wide range of resources to develop an ASP. This can be improved over time by an approach of continuous improvement (see **Table 1**). Various practical, structural, and organizational barriers may hinder full implementation of ASPs at the clinic level, but the time to start is now. Overcoming some of these barriers requires significant investments in research and training by national and international veterinary organizations, funding agencies, and animal health industries. At the national level, development and implementation of ASPs require coordination of the activities of national public health and veterinary authorities, veterinary organizations, clinics, and individual practitioners.

Antimicrobial stewardship should be seen as a collective approach that not only encompasses the potential for numerous interventions, as well as the potential for certification, but also involves everyone responsible in some way or another for antimicrobial use in small animals. Like good infection control, it's everyone's responsibility.

REFERENCES

1. Perreten V, Kadlec K, Schwarz S, et al. Clonal spread of methicillin-resistant *Staphylococcus pseudintermedius* in Europe and North America: an international multicentre study. J Antimicrob Chemother 2010;65:1145–54.
2. Rubin JE, Pitout JD. Extended-spectrum β-lactamase, carbapenemase and AmpC producing Enterobacteriaceae in companion animals. Vet Microbiol 2014;170:10–8.
3. Papich MG. Antibiotic treatment of resistant infections in small animals. Vet Clin North Am Small Anim Pract 2013;43:1091–117.
4. Vincze S, Stamm I, Kopp PA, et al. Alarming proportions of methicillin-resistant *Staphylococcus aureus* (MRSA) in wound samples from companion animals, Germany 2010–2012. PLoS One 2014;9:e85656.
5. Abraham S, Wong HS, Turnidge J, et al. Carbapenemase-producing bacteria in companion animals: a public health concern on the horizon. J Antimicrob Chemother 2014;69:1155–7.
6. Endimiani A, Hujer KM, Hujer AM, et al. *Acinetobacter baumannii* isolates from pets and horses in Switzerland: molecular characterization and clinical data. J Antimicrob Chemother 2011;66:2248–54.
7. Bengtsson B, Greko C. Antibiotic resistance—consequences for animal health, welfare, and food production. Ups J Med Sci 2014;119:96–102.
8. European Medicines Agency (EMA) (2013). Sales of veterinary antimicrobial agents in 25 EU/EEA countries in 2011. Available at: www.ema.europa.eu/docs/en_GB/document_library/Report/2013/10/WC500152311.pdf. Accessed August 10, 2014.
9. Papich MG. Ciprofloxacin pharmacokinetics and oral absorption of generic ciprofloxacin tablets in dogs. Am J Vet Res 2012;73:1085–91.
10. Trott DJ, Filippich LJ, Bensink JC, et al. Canine model for investigating the impact of oral enrofloxacin on commensal coliforms and colonization with multidrug-resistant *Escherichia coli*. J Med Microbiol 2004;53:439–43.
11. Damborg P, Gaustad IB, Olsen JE, et al. Selection of CMY-2 producing *Escherichia coli* in the faecal flora of dogs treated with cephalexin. Vet Microbiol 2011;151:404–8.
12. Gibson JS, Morton JM, Cobbold RN, et al. Risk factors for dogs becoming rectal carriers of multidrug-resistant *Escherichia coli* during hospitalization. Epidemiol Infect 2011;139:1511–21.
13. Gibson JS, Morton JM, Cobbold RN, et al. Risk factors for multidrug-resistant *Escherichia coli* rectal colonization of dogs on admission to a veterinary hospital. Epidemiol Infect 2011;139:197–205.
14. Lawrence M, Kukanich K, Kukanich B, et al. Effect of cefovecin on the fecal flora of healthy dogs. Vet J 2013;198:259–66.
15. Guardabassi L, Larsen J, Weese JS, et al. Public health impact and antimicrobial selection of methicillin-resistant staphylococci in animals. J Glob Antimicrob Resist 2012;1:55–62.
16. Weese JS, Blondeau JM, Boothe D, et al. Antimicrobial use guidelines for treatment of urinary tract disease in dogs and cats: Antimicrobial Guidelines Working

Group of the International Society for Companion Animal Infectious Diseases. Vet Med Int 2011;2011:263768 Article 263768.

17. Hillier A, Lloyd DH, Weese SJ, et al. Guidelines for the diagnosis and antimicrobial therapy of canine superficial bacterial folliculitis (Antimicrobial Guidelines Working Group of the International Society for Companion Animal Infectious Diseases). Vet Dermatol 2014;25:163.e43.
18. Weese JS, Page SW, Prescott JF. Antimicrobial stewardship in animals. In: Giguère S, Prescott JF, Dowling PM, editors. Antimicrobial therapy in veterinary medicine. 5th edition. Ames, Iowa: Wiley Blackwell; 2013. p. 117–32.
19. Tamma PD, Cosgrove SE. Antimicrobial stewardship. Infect Dis Clin North Am 2011;25:245–60.
20. MacDougall C, Polk RE. Antimicrobial stewardship programs in health care systems. Clin Microbiol Rev 2005;18:638–56.
21. Owens RC Jr. Antimicrobial stewardship: concepts and strategies in the 21st century. Diagn Microbiol Infect Dis 2008;61:110–28.
22. Wegener H. Antibiotic resistance—linking human and animal health. In: Choffnes ER, Relman DA, Olsen LA, et al, editors. Improving food safety through a one health approach: workshop summary. Institute of Medicine (US). Washington (DC): The National Academy Press; 2012. p. 331–49. Available at http://www.ncbi.nlm.nih.gov/books/NBK114485/.
23. Dellit TH, Owens RC, McGowan JE Jr, et al. Infectious Diseases Society of America and the Society for Healthcare Epidemiology of America guidelines for developing an institutional program to enhance antimicrobial stewardship. Clin Infect Dis 2007;44:159–77.
24. Canadian Committee on Antibiotic Resistance. Infection prevention and control best practices for small animal veterinary clinics. 2008. Available at: www.wormsandgermsblog.com/uploads/file/CCAR%20Guidelines%20Final(2).pdf. Accessed August 10, 2014.
25. Keuleyan E, Gould M. Key issues in developing antibiotic policies: from an institutional level to Europe-wide. European Study Group on Antibiotic Policy (ESGAP), Subgroup III. Clin Microbiol Infect 2001;7(Suppl 6):16–21.
26. Hindler JF, Stelling J. Analysis and presentation of cumulative antibiograms: a new consensus guideline from the Clinical and Laboratory Standards Institute. Clin Infect Dis 2007;44:867–73.
27. Teale CJ, Moulin G. Prudent use guidelines: a review of existing guidelines. Rev Sci Tech 2012;31:343–54.
28. Guardabassi L, Jensen LB, Kruse H. Guide to antimicrobial use in animals. Oxford (England): Blackwell Publishing; 2008.
29. Giguère S, Prescott JF, Dowling PM. Antimicrobial therapy in veterinary medicine. 5th edition. Ames, Iowa: Wiley Blackwell; 2013.
30. Swedish Veterinary Association 2009. Guidelines for the clinical use of antibiotics in the treatment of dogs and cats. Available at: www.wormsandgermsblog.com/uploads/file/Policy%20ab%20english%2010b(2).pdf. Accessed August 10, 2014.
31. Danish Small Animal Veterinary Association 2013. Antibiotic use guidelines for companion animal practice. ISBN 978-87-870703-0-0. Available at: www.ddd.dk/organisatorisk/sektionsmaadyr/Documents/AntibioticGuidelines.pdf. Accessed August 10, 2014.
32. Sykes JE, Hartmann K, Lunn KF, et al. ACVIM small animal consensus statement on leptospirosis: diagnosis, epidemiology, treatment, and prevention. J Vet Intern Med 2011;25:1–13.

33. Greko C. Reductions of sales of antimicrobial for dogs—Swedish experiences. Eur J Comp Anim Pract 2013;23:55–60. Available at: http://www.fecava.org/ejcap.
34. Goff DA. iPhones, iPads, and medical applications for antimicrobial stewardship. Pharmacotherapy 2012;32:657–61.
35. Kaki R, Elligsen M, Walker S, et al. Impact of antimicrobial stewardship in critical care: a systematic review. J Antimicrob Chemother 2011;66:1223–30.
36. Prescott JF. The resistance *tsunami*, antimicrobial stewardship, and the golden age of microbiology. Vet Microbiol 2014;171:2013–8.
37. De Briyne N, Atkinson J, Pokludova L, et al. Factors influencing antibiotic prescribing habits and use of sensitivity testing among veterinarians in Europe. Vet Rec 2013. http://dx.doi.org/10.1136/vr.101454.
38. Van Belkum A, Dunne WM. Next-generation antimicrobial susceptibility testing. J Clin Microbiol 2013;51:2018–24.
39. Zankari E, Hasman H, Kaas RS, et al. Genotyping using whole-genome sequencing is a realistic alternative to surveillance based on phenotypic antimicrobial susceptibility testing. J Antimicrob Chemother 2013;68:771–7.
40. G8 Ministers Statement, London, June 12, 2013. Available at: www.gov.uk/government/publications/g8-science-ministers-statement-london-12-june-2013. Accessed August 10, 2014.

Zoonotic Disease Risks for Immunocompromised and Other High-risk Clients and Staff

Promoting Safe Pet Ownership and Contact

Jason W. Stull, VMD, MPVM, PhD[a,*], Kurt B. Stevenson, MD, MPH[b]

KEYWORDS

• Zoonoses • Pet • Immunocompromised • One health • Child • Pregnant • Elderly

KEY POINTS

- Pets are important members of many households, including those with people at increased risk for pet-associated infectious disease (ie, <5 or ≥65 years of age, pregnant, or immunocompromised).
- Additional attention to pet selection, contact, and husbandry, and to personal hygiene can reduce the likelihood of pet-associated disease, and is especially important for households with high-risk individuals.
- Veterinary staff are well positioned to educate clients on methods to reduce pet-associated disease.
- To be most effective, veterinary staff must be aware of high-risk clients (or their household members) so they can provide targeted education and recommendations.
- Veterinarians and physicians must work together to effectively reduce pet-associated infections.

INTRODUCTION: NATURE OF THE PROBLEM

Pet ownership is common. In North America, more than 50% of households own cats or dogs, with other species (eg, birds, reptiles/amphibians, exotic companion mammals such as hamsters) frequently reported.[1,2] Similar statistics have been reported for households in other countries.[3–7] These numbers likely severely underestimate the frequency of animal contact by individuals, as reported in one study in which 37% of non–pet-owning households had a member with frequent animal contact.[1]

The authors have nothing to disclose.

[a] Department of Veterinary Preventive Medicine, College of Veterinary Medicine, The Ohio State University, 1920 Coffey Road, Columbus, OH 43210, USA; [b] Department of Internal Medicine, Wexner Medical Center, Colleges of Medicine and Public Health, The Ohio State University, 410 West 10th Avenue, Columbus, OH 43210, USA
* Corresponding author.
E-mail address: jason.stull@cvm.osu.edu

Vet Clin Small Anim 45 (2015) 377–392
http://dx.doi.org/10.1016/j.cvsm.2014.11.007 vetsmall.theclinics.com

The mental and physical benefits of pet ownership and contact are documented in the literature.[8–11] Although findings vary between studies, numerous health benefits, including reduction in stress, anxiety, loneliness, and depression, have been associated with animal interaction.[8] These benefits extend to numerous populations, including children, the elderly, and the immunocompromised, and include individuals in institutions and the community. Children brought up with companion animals often have better social skills, self-esteem, and empathy than children without pets.[9] In adults and the elderly, studies have documented an association between pets and reduced risk of cardiovascular disease and improved psychological and physical well-being.[10] Health benefits are also well documented in individuals who are immunocompromised. Such individuals may spend considerable time alone, and thus are especially vulnerable to mental and physical illness. Among individuals infected with the human immunodeficiency virus (HIV), domestic animals have been shown to serve as sources of support and affection and protect against loneliness.[11] In all of these groups, the perceived importance of pets is clear, with patients and family members typically very attached to household pets, regardless of species.[12]

Despite these benefits, companion animals are a potential source of infectious agents to people (zoonoses). The exact number of pathogens that can be spread through direct or indirect pet contact is constantly changing as the available testing methodologies and appreciation for transmission dynamics evolve; however, there is evidence that at least 70 human pathogens are likely to be, at least in part, pet associated.[13] The severity of pet-associated illness is variable, ranging from unapparent colonization to permanent health sequelae or even death. Pet-associated zoonotic disease risks are present for anyone having contact with pets or their environments, including pet owners, nonowners, and those working in pet care and housing facilities (eg, veterinary clinics, pet shops, animal breeding facilities).[1,14–16] However, those at greatest risk for infection may be the same individuals with the most to gain from the benefits of pet contact.[17] This apparent conflict between pet-associated health benefits and risks has become an important health care issue and human health care providers may make overly cautious pet contact recommendations that the family veterinarian does not support or owners are unwilling to follow.[18] Veterinarians may be asked for advice from human health care providers in forming recommendations for a patient's pet or may be in a position to educate an owner or staff member on disease risk. For these reasons, veterinary staff have an obligation to inform themselves on this topic so that they can contribute their expertise. In addition, in some circumstances there are potential legal ramifications should clients or staff become ill from pet contact (see article by Marsh and Babcock in this issue).

APPROACH/GOALS

The risk for disease of these pet-associated pathogens in people follows the typical epidemiologic pattern of infectious diseases:

1. Specific human hosts are at increased disease risk.
2. Specific sources (species and ages of pets) and ownership behaviors are responsible for the greatest risk of disease.
3. Transmission is typically by direct/indirect contact with the pet and their body fluids or ingestion of animal fecal material, but may also be by respiratory or vector exposure.

Precautions directed toward the groups at greatest risk of disease and that are designed to alter the species of pets owned and the behaviors of owners that are most likely to cause disease should prevent illness. Understanding potential modes of transmission can also allow specific instructions to reduce risk. Given the importance of pet contact for human health and the strong bond between people and their pets, the approach is to promote safe pet ownership.

EPIDEMIOLOGY OF PET-ASSOCIATED INFECTIONS

Although pet-associated zoonoses can occur in any individual, people at the extremes of age (<5 years; ≥65 years), pregnant women, or people with immunocompromised conditions are at the greatest risk of disease (referred to as high-risk hereafter). The increased risk for these individuals is imparted through an immune system that is not functioning at the same capacity as that of an immunocompetent individual.[19] Children and some individuals with development disabilities often have suboptimal hygiene practices or higher-risk animal contacts that further increase risk. Numerous causes can result in an immunocompromised state, the degree of which varies between and within conditions. Examples of causes for an immunocompromised state include:

- Congenital immunodeficiencies (ie, those that result from genetic causes)
- Transplants (bone marrow and solid organ)
- Infectious diseases (eg, HIV infection)
- Metabolic diseases (eg, diabetes mellitus, chronic kidney failure)
- Splenectomy
- Cancers
- Treatment with immunosuppressive drugs or chemotherapeutics

It is estimated that up to 20% of the North American population has some degree of immunosuppression[20]; given the nature of exposure and recommendations, a more useful estimate may be the proportion of households with at least 1 individual at high risk (estimated as 59% of households in one study).[1]

People at high risk for pet-associated diseases often have more severe disease, experience symptoms for a longer duration, or experience more severe or unexpected complications than other people.[21,22] For example:

- Individuals infected with HIV are at 20 to 100 times greater risk of *Salmonella* bacteremia than those without HIV infection.[21]
- *Capnocytophaga canimorsus* is a member of the normal oral bacterial flora of dogs and cats. Alcoholics, asplenic individuals, and immunocompromised individuals are at risk for severe (often fatal) *C canimorsus* infection following dog/cat licks or bites.[23]
- Individuals with hematologic malignancies are twice as likely to be infected with *Campylobacter* than those without cancer and illness is more likely to be severe and prolonged in these individuals.[22]
- *Bordetella bronchiseptica* can cause severe illness in immunocompromised individuals,[24] whereas others rarely experience disease.
- Patients with advanced HIV infection and, primarily, cat exposure are at increased risk for infection with *Bartonella* spp with associated cutaneous bacillary angiomatosis and peliosis hepatitis.[25] *Bartonella* infection may be an underrecognized cause of fever in patients with acquired immunodeficiency syndrome (AIDS).[26]

Although numerous pathogens are suspected to be partly transmitted from pets, based on the severity of disease and relative frequency of identified disease in high-risk individuals, fewer are typically thought to be of particular concern (**Box 1**).[19,27–32]

Box 1
Pet-associated pathogens of particular concern for high-risk individuals

- *Bartonella* spp (including *Bartonella alsatica, Bartonella clarridgeiae, Bartonella henselae, Bartonella vinsonii* subspp)
- *Campylobacter jejuni*
- *C canimorsus*
- *Cryptosporidium* spp
- Dermatophytes (*Microsporum canis, Trichophyton mentagrophytes*)
- *Giardia duodenalis* (certain assemblages)
- *Salmonella* spp
- *Pasteurella multocida*
- *Toxoplasma gondii*

Despite the increased disease risk, few studies have determined precisely what proportion of human disease is attributable to pets, a figure that would be helpful in guiding risk-based decision making. For instance, it is estimated that 14% of all human illness caused by common enteric pathogen groups is attributable to direct or indirect animal contact,[33] with pets likely responsible for a low proportion of this. The true scope of pet-associated disease remains indefinable in part because of a shortage of locally or nationally reportable pet-associated pathogens and complicating factors such as multiple non–pet-exposure sources and frequent subclinical shedding by pets. Many experts project that pet-associated disease incidence is likely low,[1,17,27] although even this infrequent occurrence results in important and severe disease in people at high risk.

Numerous studies have helped to define specific exposures and behaviors that increase pet-associated zoonotic disease risk. These risks include species of pet, age of pet, and husbandry-related and hygiene-related aspects of pet ownership and contact.

Species

Through public health outbreak investigations, case reports for reportable zoonotic pathogens, and data on pathogen carriage, several pet species have been identified as posing an increased risk for associated disease. Reptiles, amphibians, rodents, exotic species (eg, hedgehogs), and young poultry (eg, chicks) have been implicated in several nationwide and international human salmonellosis outbreaks.[34] In these outbreaks, the increased risk for particular groups is highlighted because children accounted for a high proportion of cases (35%–70%), with high rates of hospitalization (26%–35%); occasionally cases resulted in the death of the child. The risks from reptiles and amphibians are particularly well documented. These species are estimated to be responsible for 11% of salmonellosis cases among persons less than 21 years of age.[35] In one study, 17% of state-reported reptile-associated salmonellosis cases were documented in children less than or equal to 1 year of age, emphasizing the potential for reptile-associated *Salmonella* to be readily transmitted without direct reptile contact.[36] Rodents and young poultry may also pose a risk for lymphocytic choriomeningitis virus and *Campylobacter*, respectively.

Age of Pet

Juvenile (<6 months of age) dogs and cats are more likely to shed zoonotic pathogens than older individuals. In particular, studies have documented an increased human disease risk for *Campylobacter* and *Bartonella henselae* with ownership of puppies[37,38] and kittens.[39]

Husbandry

Numerous studies have associated the feeding of raw meat, raw eggs, and raw animal product foods and treats with an increased risk for shedding *Salmonella* in dogs.[40] In one study, dogs fed raw animal product food or treats were 5 times as likely to shed *Salmonella* in their feces than dogs not fed these items.[41] *Salmonella* outbreaks in people have been associated with these practices, typically from direct exposure to contaminated items.[42] In addition, these risks are compounded by feeding pets in the kitchen, as documented in an outbreak of salmonellosis in infants involving *Salmonella*-contaminated pet food.[43] Other husbandry practices may also increase disease risk. For instance, unsupervised free access to outdoor environments (eg, unfenced roaming) allows hunting, eating garbage or feces, and access to nonpotable water, and these are risk factors for pets to acquire zoonotic organisms such as *Toxoplasma gondii* and *Leptospira interrogans*, and inadequate ectoparasite and endoparasite control (eg, ticks, worms) may increase the risk for zoonotic pathogens.[44,45]

Hygiene

Hand hygiene (washing with soap or use of alcohol-based hand sanitizers) is the cornerstone of prevention for contact-transmitted infectious diseases. This benefit similarly extends to the prevention of many animal-associated infections. Anderson and colleagues[46] found that veterinary personnel who reported washing their hands after handling horses thought to have infectious diseases had one-third the risk of colonization with methicillin-resistant *Staphylococcus aureus* (MRSA) than those that did not report this practice. Close contact with pets, specifically face licking by dogs and cats, is a source of transmission of several potentially zoonotic opportunistic pathogens.[47,48] In particular, bacteria such as *Pasteurella* spp and *C canimorsus* normally inhabit the oral cavity of most (if not all) dogs and cats, and the transmission of these organisms can result in life-threatening disease in high-risk individuals.[23,49]

High-risk Veterinary Clinic Staff

The veterinary clinic environment can also be a source of pet-associated disease. It is perhaps not surprising that individuals who work with animals are at increased risk from infectious diseases.[50] During their careers, approximately two-thirds of veterinarians report a major animal-related injury resulting in lost work or hospitalization.[14,51] In 2 US-based studies, 28% to 47% of veterinarians reported having contracted a zoonotic infection during the course of their veterinary work, of which ~45% were medically confirmed; the zoonoses most frequently reported included dermatophytosis, bartonellosis, and cat and dog bite infections.[52,53] In addition, several studies suggest an increased risk of infection for veterinarians (compared with control groups) for numerous zoonotic pathogens (eg, *Brucella canis*, *Bartonella* spp).[14,54–56] Within-clinic zoonotic transmission of pathogens such as MRSA and *Salmonella* has been reported, affecting pets, clinic staff, and clients of small-animal veterinary clinics.[57–59] When zoonotic pathogen exposure does not immediately result in disease, colonization may occur, with an increased chance for disease at a later date. Ishihara and colleagues[60] reported that veterinary staff and students who had contact with known MRSA-positive companion animals were more likely to be colonized with MRSA compared with those without this exposure. The disease risks for high-risk veterinary clinic staff have not been specifically evaluated, but are likely increased as documented in the general population.

CHALLENGES

Pet Ownership and Practices

As previously described, pets provide many health benefits and supportive functions for individuals and families. High-risk individuals, and households with these individuals, are perhaps in greatest need for these benefits because of social isolation, depression, or other benefits of the human-animal bond, but they are also at greatest risk for pet-associated infections.[8,11,19] Given these benefits, it is perhaps unsurprising that the frequency and type of pet ownership and contact in households with high-risk individuals is similar to those in the general population. Studies indicate that 50% to 60% of households with high-risk individuals in North America[1,17,18] and elsewhere[61] have pets, with the distribution of species mirroring that of the general population; dogs and/or cats are the most common pets, but other species (eg, reptiles, birds, exotics, rodents) are also reported.[17,61] The frequency with which pet species of higher concern for zoonotic transmission are reportedly owned by households with high-risk individuals is alarming (rodents/exotics, 46%; reptiles, 55%).[12] A study among households with children diagnosed with cancer noted that 20% of households acquired a new pet after their child was diagnosed, more than 70% of which acquired a high-risk pet, including young dogs/cats, rodents, reptiles, and amphibians.[17] Furthermore, of those that acquired a new pet, 13% did not have a pet at the time their child was diagnosed and 17% of current non–pet owners planned to acquire a pet in the next year. This fluidity in pet ownership can be a challenge, because human health care providers may not provide pet recommendations to current non–pet owners.

In addition to species owned, pet husbandry practices that increase zoonotic disease risk have frequently been documented among households with high-risk members. High-risk foods and treats (ie, raw eggs, raw meat, or raw animal product treats) were fed to dogs in more than 20% of households with children diagnosed with cancer (Jason W. Stull, 2014, unpublished) and immunocompromised children frequently cleaned up pet feces.[61] Furthermore, husbandry practices among households with high-risk members seem to be overall no more stringent than those practiced by households with lower-risk individuals, such as the feeding of raw animal product food/treats, uncontrolled outdoor access of dogs/cats, and parasite control.[12] Children less than the age of 5 years were 4 times as likely to be licked on the face by the household dog than were older children; an unsurprising finding given differences in size and mobility, but nonetheless concerning because of reports of lick-associated infections in young children.[49]

Zoonotic Disease Knowledge and Education

Despite an increased risk for pet-associated disease, the level of knowledge of pet-associated disease risks of high-risk individuals is limited. Similar to the general public, individuals who are high risk (or have a high-risk household member) are minimally aware of the potential for pets to transmit important pathogens to people.[1,17] This lack of awareness is perhaps expected because a minority (<36%) of high-risk pet owners recall having previously received education on pet-associated infections or ways to prevent these infections.[1,17,18] This finding is supported by a study by Hill and colleagues[62] who found that 94% of surveyed US physicians stated that they never or rarely initiated discussions about zoonoses with patients with HIV infection or AIDS. Furthermore, few veterinary (~58%) and physician (4%) practices have educational materials on zoonotic diseases available to clients/patients.[52,62] However, high-risk individuals seem to be open to such educational opportunities from veterinary staff.[1,17]

In order to provide targeted education and recommendations to clients with high-risk household members, veterinarians need to be aware of their clients' immune status and the presence of high-risk household members or others who frequently have contact with household pets (eg, friends/relatives), including those outside of the home (eg, pets involved in animal-assisted activities or therapy). However, it seems that veterinarians and their staff infrequently gather this information from clients. In one study, 66% of veterinarians (205 of 310) were not aware of their clients' immune status,[63] and in another only 25% of surveyed veterinarians stated that a client had ever disclosed their HIV infection or AIDS diagnosis, with the investigators attributing this to HIV-related stigma and failure to view veterinarians as a source of zoonotic disease information.[62] In a study of pet owners whose children had been recently diagnosed with cancer, most (55%) had taken a pet to a veterinarian since the child had been diagnosed; however, few (14%) recalled the veterinarian asking about the child's medical condition.[17] When veterinary staff did ask, all of the respondents informed the veterinarian about their child's medical condition and some (38%) disclosed the child's medical condition even when not asked by the veterinarian. Therefore, at least in this situation, if asked, clients are likely to provide information to assist in determining the high-risk status of household members, but without querying, many clients do not provide this information.

Perhaps one of the largest challenges of pet-associated zoonotic infections is that this topic is at the intersection of veterinary and human medicine. In order to effectively address this area, multiple disciplines (eg, physicians, veterinarians, public health workers) need to communicate. This communication not only needs to occur at the national/international level but also at the individual patient/client level to ensure that risks are effectively communicated and preventive measures addressed, drawing on the expertise of the entire health care team. However, multiple evaluations of this area document poor interdisciplinary communication.[62,63] Veterinarians' interaction with other health professions is typically low, particularly with physicians (reported on average as "no interaction" to "rare interaction" among practicing veterinarians in a US-based survey).[64] In a US-based study, 100% of physicians and 97% of veterinarians claimed to never or rarely contact individuals of the other profession when looking for advice on zoonotic disease risks or cases.[62] However, many practicing veterinarians seem to recognize the utility and importance of promoting interactions with physicians in order to enhance patient care and growth of the profession as well as provide expertise to physicians in zoonotic diseases.[64]

PREVENTION

People at high risk for pet-associated diseases often have more severe disease, and diagnosis in these individuals is often complicated by a delayed or limited serologic response or atypical presentation.[19,21,28] For these reasons, prevention of pet-associated disease is especially important in high-risk individuals. As indicated previously in this article, there are several challenges that make pet-associated risk reduction particularly difficult with high-risk individuals. These challenges include the frequent occurrence of high-risk pet ownership/contact practices, limited knowledge and education of pet-associated risks and prevention practices, limited communication between the health professions, and veterinarians' limited knowledge of clients' high-risk status. Steps to address these challenges and ultimately help veterinary staff reduce pet-associated disease risk are:

1. Identifying clients who are, or live in a household with, high-risk individuals.
2. Obtain up-to-date medical and husbandry histories for all pets owned by, and having contact with, high-risk individuals.
3. Educate high-risk owners on risks posed by the specific pets and husbandry practices.
4. Provide clear guidelines targeting the risks and pet contact situation.
5. Encourage clients to contact their physicians to discuss disease risks; consider suggesting that clients provide physicians with veterinarian's contact information to discuss, if interested.
6. Remain receptive to communication from physicians.
7. Encourage physicians caring for high-risk individuals (HIV-care providers, transplant medicine/surgeon practitioners, oncologists, and so forth) to add questioning about pet exposure as a routine part of their patient evaluation checklist. This questioning can provide a vehicle for increased communication by physicians with veterinarians.

Identifying and Educating High-risk Clients

Techniques that use passive (eg, pamphlets, signs) and active (intake questionnaire) formats may be effective in encouraging clients to disclose the immune status of individuals in their households. Likely a combination of both passive and active approaches may be needed. Zoonotic disease brochures and posters are available from several sources (listed later). Such resources help clients to self-identify their increased disease risk (potentially alerting them to the utility of disclosing this information) as well as providing them with basic education on the topic. In-clinic signs highlighting available support services, such as human-animal disease education, may also be useful.

Some investigators advocate using intake questionnaires to obtain information for the client's household.[65] Intake questionnaires may include questions about pet husbandry and whether there are any children less than 5 years of age; elderly people; people with immune problems; or women who may be, or are planning to become, pregnant.[65] However, veterinary clinic staff must recognize that any client personal health information may be considered confidential and protected under privacy laws. The greatest concerns focus on how this information is secured and provided to other individuals (eg, clinic staff, other veterinary clinics). As such, veterinary clinics need to decide how such information is recorded, if at all. If client personal health information is recorded, it is best to keep it general and ensure that clients are aware of (and provide written consent) why the information is requested; how the information will be used; and, if included in the patient's record, whether it may be transmitted to other veterinary clinics as part of the patient's record. This consent should be reviewed with the client on a regular basis, to ensure that it is up to date and that clients are comfortable in providing any sensitive information. This discussion can also include encouraging high-risk patients to consult with their physicians and specialty providers (eg, HIV-care providers, transplant medicine/surgeon practitioners, oncologists). Patients may also grant permission to their physicians to have them directly speak with the veterinarian. Consulting with a lawyer is warranted when considering instituting such polices (see article by Marsh and Babcock elsewhere in this issue).

Determining the high-risk status of household members is a key first step in reducing pet-associated infections. However, to be successful, veterinarians and their staff must be comfortable with providing recommendations to assist clients in reducing disease risks. Veterinarians and clinic staff are encouraged to become familiar with and stay up to date on pet-associated diseases.

Guidelines for Pet Ownership and Contact

Being at high risk or having such an individual in a household is not a contraindication to having a pet or pet contact. However, individuals who are high risk, and households with such individuals, should be more cautious than other pet owners in ensuring that their pets remain healthy and follow precautions to reduce transmission of pathogens from pets. These owners should also be aware of signs that suggest disease in their pets, encouraged to seek veterinary advice as soon as such signs are apparent, and have knowledge of preventive health measures that they can immediately use before receiving recommendations from their veterinarian or physician (eg, reduce contact between high-risk individuals and animals with diarrhea, use strict hand hygiene).

Multiple resources provide recommendations for reducing pathogen transmission from pets to high-risk individuals.[19,20,27,29–32,66–69] Pet contact guidelines can be categorized into providing additional attention to (1) personal hygiene, (2) types and ages of animals, and (3) pet health and husbandry practices (**Box 2**). These guidelines are general; several recently published resources should be consulted for targeted information for specific human and veterinary medical conditions[13,65] and additional sources are cited later in this article. Other guidelines are available for reducing pet-associated disease in health care facilities, such as for pets involved in animal-assisted interventions[70,71]; veterinarians are encouraged to become familiar with these guidelines in order to provide an additional resource in these situations. Clients who have specific questions about the health risk to household members should be encouraged to consult their physicians and specialty providers (HIV-care providers, transplant medicine/surgeon practitioners, oncologists, and so forth). In such situations, given their expertise in pet and husbandry-related aspects of disease risk, veterinarians are encouraged to offer their assistance to the physician and remain receptive to direct communication with the physician, keeping the subject focused on general zoonotic disease education and providing the specifics on animal-related aspects of disease (see article by Marsh and Babcock elsewhere in this issue).

In situations in which a specific zoonotic disease is diagnosed or highly suspected in a pet owned by a client with a high-risk household member, the veterinarian should provide the client with general recommendations to reduce disease risk and encourage the patient to consult with their physician and specialty providers (see **Box 2**). Information to provide to the owner includes:

- Mode of pathogen transmission
- Duration of pathogen shedding in pets
- General information regarding the risk of disease transmission to people (especially high-risk individuals) and prevention methods
- Encouragement for clients to inform their physicians of a potential exposure and seek their advice

Printed materials and suggested Web sites should be provided to clients to reinforce disease risks and recommended preventive measures (examples are listed later). All conversations and materials provided to clients on this topic (eg, general recommendations for pet ownership or contact, pet diagnostics, therapy, prevention) should be accurately summarized in the client's record and, if the client is at high risk for infection and consents, forwarded to the client's physician. These notes

Box 2
Pet contact guidelines for households with high-risk individuals

Personal hygiene

- Wash hands after handling animals or their environment; supervise hand washing for children less than 5 years old.
- Avoid contact with pets' feces and animal-derived pet treats by wearing gloves or using a plastic bag when having contact with these items.
- Promptly wash bites and scratches from animals; do not allow pets to lick open wounds, broken skin, mucous membranes (eg, discourage face licking), or medical devices such as intravascular catheters.
- Have someone who is not at high risk clean litter boxes/cages/aquariums (if that is not possible, wear gloves); do not dispose of aquarium water in sinks used for food preparation or in bathtubs.
- Ensure that playground sandboxes are kept covered when not in use.

Types and ages of animals

- Avoid contact with dogs and cats less than 6 months of age or strays.
- Avoid contact with animals with diarrhea.
- Avoid contact with young farm animals (eg, petting zoos).
- Avoid contact with reptiles, amphibians, rodents, and baby poultry (chicks and ducklings), and anything that has been in contact with these animals; preferably these animals should not be kept in the households of high-risk individuals. If these animals or their environment are touched, strict attention to hand hygiene is important.
- Reptiles, amphibians, rodents, and baby poultry should not be permitted to roam freely through a home or living area and should be kept out of kitchens and food-preparation areas.
- Exercise caution when playing with dogs and cats to limit scratches; keep pets' nails short (declawing is not recommended).
- When acquiring a new pet, seek mature animals with a known history from established vendors.
- Avoid contact with exotic pets and nonhuman primates.
- When visiting other households or locations with pets, take the same precautions with those pets.
- If the immunocompromised state may be transient or variable, consider waiting to acquire a new pet until immune suppression is stable; those who work with animals (veterinarians, laboratory workers, pet store employees, farmers, or slaughterhouse workers) should alter work practice during periods of maximal immunosuppression.

Pet health and husbandry

- Have any new pets examined by a veterinarian before being brought into the household.
- Spay/neuter pets to help decrease roaming tendencies and behavioral issues.
- Keep cats indoors; change litter boxes daily; keep litter boxes away from kitchens or other areas where food preparation and eating occur.
- Keep dogs confined when possible; walk on leash to prevent hunting and eating garbage or feces.
- Feed only canned or dry commercial food or well-cooked home-prepared food; any dairy or animal-based (egg, meat) products or treats should be cooked or (high-pressure) pasteurized.
- Feed pets in a designated nonkitchen area.

- Prohibit access to nonpotable water, such as surface water or toilet bowls.
- Follow routine preventive care, including steps to control and prevent ectoparasites and endoparasites (eg, ticks, fleas, gastrointestinal parasites) as indicated by the area.
- Clean bird cage linings daily; wear disposable gloves (with or without surgical mask) when handling; dampen cage litter with water (mist) to decrease generation of dust.
- Clean small rodent cages frequently.
- Regularly (eg, weekly) launder pet bedding.
- Seek veterinary care at first sign of illness in an animal.

provide continuity of care for other staff members attending to the pet and client and provide support for potential legal action should zoonotic illness occur in household contacts (see article by Marsh and Babcock in this issue). In addition, when zoonotic diseases are identified, all in-contact clinic staff and, if necessary, public health authorities should be notified.

High-risk Veterinary Clinic Staff

The prevention methods discussed earlier apply equally to clinic members who may be at increased risk for pet-associated infections. In addition, such individuals should discuss any necessary work restrictions and precautions with their physicians. In general, high-risk individuals who work in small-animal hospitals should avoid handling patients with suspected or known infectious diseases. Such individuals should strictly follow infection control principles, including hand hygiene and use of personal protective equipment. Based on the level of immunosuppression, routine glove use may be considered when handling all animals; however, strict hand hygiene (washing with soap and water or alcohol-based hand sanitizer) after every patient contact and immediately after removing gloves is critical. Gloves should always be worn when having contact with animal fluids or feces. Prevention of animal bites, scratches, or sharps injuries is important. Given their increased disease risk and limited hygiene, children less than 5 years of age should not be permitted in veterinary hospital patient care areas. Training for all staff on pet-associated zoonotic disease risks and prevention within and outside the veterinary clinic should be required and documented. Staff knowledge on this topic should be assessed periodically.

SUMMARY

Pets are important members of many households, including those with people at greater risk for pet-associated infectious disease (ie, <5 or ≥65 years of age, pregnant, or immunocompromised). Additional attention to pet selection, contact, husbandry, and hygiene can reduce the likelihood of pet-associated disease, and is especially important for households with high-risk individuals. Veterinary staff are well positioned to educate clients on methods to reduce pet-associated disease. To be most effective, veterinary staff must be aware of high-risk clients (or their household members) so they can provide targeted education and recommendations. Veterinarians and physicians must work together to effectively reduce pet-associated infections.

RESOURCES

Centers for Disease Control and Prevention. Gastrointestinal (enteric) diseases from animals. Available at: http://www.cdc.gov/zoonotic/gi/index.html.

Centers for Disease Control and Prevention. Healthy pets healthy people. Available at: http://www.cdc.gov/healthypets/index.html.

Grace SF. Assessing client risk for zoonotic disease transmission – questions to ask. North American Veterinary Committee. Clinician's brief 2008 Apr. Available at: http://www.cliniciansbrief.com/columns/39/assessing-client-risk-zoonotic-disease-questions-ask.

National Association of State Public Health Veterinarians Animal Contact Compendium Committee 2013. Compendium of measures to prevent disease associated with animals in public settings, 2013. J Am Vet Med Assoc 2013;243(9):1270–88. Available at: http://avmajournals.avma.org/doi/full/10.2460/javma.243.9.1270.

Pets are wonderful support. Safe pet guidelines: a comprehensive guide for immunocompromised animal guardians. Available at: http://www.pawssf.org.

Worms and germs blog. Resources – pets. Available at: http://www.wormsandgermsblog.com.

Writing Panel of Working Group, Lefebvre SL, Golab GC, et al. Guidelines for animal-assisted interventions in health care facilities. Am J Infect Control 2008;36(2):78–85. Available at: http://www.sciencedirect.com/science/article/pii/S019665530700781X.

Souza MJ. Zoonoses, public health and the exotic animal practitioner. Vet Clin North Am Exot Anim Pract 2011:14.

REFERENCES

1. Stull JW, Peregrine AS, Sargeant JM, et al. Household knowledge, attitudes and practices related to pet contact and associated zoonoses in Ontario, Canada. BMC Public Health 2012;12(1):553.
2. American Veterinary Medical Association. U.S. pet ownership & demographics sourcebook. Schaumburg, IL: American Veterinary Medical Association; 2007.
3. Butler JR, Bingham J. Demography and dog-human relationships of the dog population in Zimbabwean communal lands. Vet Rec 2000;147(16): 442–6.
4. Downes M, Canty MJ, More SJ. Demography of the pet dog and cat population on the island of Ireland and human factors influencing pet ownership. Prev Vet Med 2009;92(1–2):140–9.
5. Slater MR, Di Nardo A, Pediconi O, et al. Cat and dog ownership and management patterns in central Italy. Prev Vet Med 2008;85(3–4):267–94.
6. Murray JK, Browne WJ, Roberts MA, et al. Number and ownership profiles of cats and dogs in the UK. Vet Rec 2010;166(6):163–8.
7. Alves MC, Matos MR, Reichmann Mde L, et al. Estimation of the dog and cat population in the State of Sao Paulo. Rev Saude Publica 2005;39(6):891–7.
8. Friedmann E, Son H. The human–companion animal bond: how humans benefit. Vet Clin North Am Small Anim Pract 2009;39(2):293–326.
9. Melson GF, Schwarz RL, Beck AM. Importance of companion animals in children's lives–implications for veterinary practice. J Am Vet Med Assoc 1997; 211(12):1512–8.
10. Friedmann E, Thomas SA. Pet ownership, social support, and one-year survival after acute myocardial infarction in the Cardiac Arrhythmia Suppression Trial (CAST). Am J Cardiol 1995;76(17):1213–7.
11. Siegel JM, Angulo FJ, Detels R, et al. AIDS diagnosis and depression in the Multicenter AIDS Cohort Study: the ameliorating impact of pet ownership. AIDS Care 1999;11(2):157–70.

12. Stull JW, Peregrine AS, Sargeant JM, et al. Pet husbandry and infection control practices related to zoonotic disease risks in Ontario, Canada. BMC Public Health 2013;13(1):520.
13. Weese JS, Fulford MB. Companion animal zoonoses. Ames, Iowa: Wiley-Blackwell; 2011.
14. Baker WS, Gray GC. A review of published reports regarding zoonotic pathogen infection in veterinarians. J Am Vet Med Assoc 2009;234(10):1271–8.
15. Knust B, Ströher U, Edison L, et al. Lymphocytic choriomeningitis virus in employees and mice at multipremises feeder-rodent operation, United States, 2012. Emerg Infect Dis 2014;20(2):240–7.
16. Halsby KD, Walsh AL, Campbell C, et al. Healthy animals, healthy people: zoonosis risk from animal contact in pet shops, a systematic review of the literature. PLoS One 2014;9(2):e89309.
17. Stull JW, Brophy J, Sargeant JM, et al. Knowledge, attitudes, and practices related to pet contact by immunocompromised children with cancer and immunocompetent children with diabetes. J Pediatr 2014;165:348–55.e2.
18. Conti L, Lieb S, Liberti T, et al. Pet ownership among persons with AIDS in three Florida counties. Am J Public Health 1995;85(11):1559–61.
19. Mani I, Maguire JH. Small animal zoonoses and immunocompromised pet owners. Top Companion Anim Med 2009;24(4):164–74.
20. Trevejo RT, Barr MC, Robinson RA. Important emerging bacterial zoonotic infections affecting the immunocompromised. Vet Res 2005;36(3):493–506.
21. Hung CC, Hung MN, Hsueh PR, et al. Risk of recurrent nontyphoid *Salmonella* bacteremia in HIV-infected patients in the era of highly active antiretroviral therapy and an increasing trend of fluoroquinolone resistance. Clin Infect Dis 2007;45(5):e60–7.
22. Gradel KO, Norgaard M, Dethlefsen C, et al. Increased risk of zoonotic *Salmonella* and *Campylobacter* gastroenteritis in patients with haematological malignancies: a population-based study. Ann Hematol 2009;88(8):761–7.
23. Gaastra W, Lipman LJ. *Capnocytophaga canimorsus*. Vet Microbiol 2010; 140(3–4):339–46.
24. Ner Z, Ross LA, Horn MV, et al. *Bordetella bronchiseptica* infection in pediatric lung transplant recipients. Pediatr Transplant 2003;7(5):413–7.
25. Spach DH, Koehler JE. *Bartonella*-associated infections. Infect Dis Clin North Am 1998;12(1):137–55.
26. Koehler JE, Sanchez MA, Tye S, et al. Prevalence of *Bartonella* infection among human immunodeficiency virus-infected patients with fever. Clin Infect Dis 2003; 37(4):559–66.
27. Angulo FJ, Glaser CA, Juranek DD, et al. Caring for pets of immunocompromised persons. Can Vet J 1995;36(4):217–22.
28. Kotton CN. Zoonoses in solid-organ and hematopoietic stem cell transplant recipients. Clin Infect Dis 2007;44(6):857–66.
29. Pickering LK, Marano N, Bocchini JA, et al. Exposure to nontraditional pets at home and to animals in public settings: risks to children. Pediatrics 2008;122(4): 876–86.
30. Yokoe D, Casper C, Dubberke E, et al. Safe living after hematopoietic cell transplantation. Bone Marrow Transplant 2009;44(8):509–19.
31. Kaplan JE, Benson C, Holmes KH, et al. Guidelines for prevention and treatment of opportunistic infections in HIV-infected adults and adolescents: recommendations from CDC, the National Institutes of Health, and the HIV Medicine Association of the Infectious Diseases Society of America. MMWR Recomm Rep 2009; 58(RR-4):1–207.

32. Lappin MR. Pet ownership by immunocompromised people. Compend Contin Educ Vet 2002;24(5A):16–25.
33. Hale CR, Scallan E, Cronquist AB, et al. Estimates of enteric illness attributable to contact with animals and their environments in the United States. Clin Infect Dis 2012;54(Suppl 5):S472–9.
34. Centers for Disease Control and Prevention. Gastrointestinal (enteric) diseases: selected multistate outbreak investigations linked to animals and animal products. 2014. Available at: http://www.cdc.gov/zoonotic/gi/outbreaks.html. Assessed December 7, 2014.
35. Mermin J, Hutwagner L, Vugia D, et al. Reptiles, amphibians, and human *Salmonella* infection: a population-based, case-control study. Clin Infect Dis 2004; 38(Suppl 3):S253–61.
36. Whitten T, Bender JB, Smith K, et al. Reptile-associated salmonellosis in Minnesota, 1996–2011. Zoonoses Public Health 2014. [Epub ahead of print]. http://dx.doi.org/10.1111/zph.12140.
37. Mughini Gras L, Smid JH, Wagenaar JA, et al. Increased risk for *Campylobacter jejuni* and *C. coli* infection of pet origin in dog owners and evidence for genetic association between strains causing infection in humans and their pets. Epidemiol Infect 2013;141(12):2526–35.
38. Tenkate TD, Stafford RJ. Risk factors for *Campylobacter* infection in infants and young children: a matched case-control study. Epidemiol Infect 2001;127(3):399–404.
39. Breitschwerdt EB. Bartonellosis: one health perspectives for an emerging infectious disease. ILAR J 2014;55(1):46–58.
40. Freeman LM, Chandler ML, Hamper BA, et al. Current knowledge about the risks and benefits of raw meat-based diets for dogs and cats. J Am Vet Med Assoc 2013;243(11):1549–58.
41. Leonard EK, Pearl DL, Finley RL, et al. Evaluation of pet-related management factors and the risk of *Salmonella* spp. carriage in pet dogs from volunteer households in Ontario (2005–2006). Zoonoses Public Health 2011;58(2):140–9.
42. Centers for Disease Control and Prevention (CDC). Human salmonellosis associated with animal-derived pet treats–United States and Canada, 2005. MMWR Recomm Rep 2006;55(25):702–5.
43. Behravesh CB, Ferraro A, Deasy M 3rd, et al. Human *Salmonella* infections linked to contaminated dry dog and cat food, 2006-2008. Pediatrics 2010;126(3): 477–83.
44. Chomel B. Emerging and re-emerging zoonoses of dogs and cats. Animals 2014; 4(3):434–45.
45. Nicholson WL, Paddock CD, Demma L, et al. Rocky Mountain spotted fever in Arizona: documentation of heavy environmental infestations of *Rhipicephalus sanguineus* at an endemic site. Ann N Y Acad Sci 2006;1078:338–41.
46. Anderson ME, Lefebvre SL, Weese JS. Evaluation of prevalence and risk factors for methicillin-resistant *Staphylococcus aureus* colonization in veterinary personnel attending an international equine veterinary conference. Vet Microbiol 2008; 129(3–4):410–7.
47. Forsblom B, Sarkiala-Kessel E, Kanervo A, et al. Characterisation of aerobic gram-negative bacteria from subgingival sites of dogs–potential bite wound pathogens. J Med Microbiol 2002;51(3):207–20.
48. Stull JW, Sturgeon A, Costa M, et al. Metagenomic investigation of the oral microbiome of healthy dogs. Vet Microbiol 2013;162(2–4):891–8.
49. Kobayaa H, Souki RR, Trust S, et al. *Pasteurella multocida* meningitis in newborns after incidental animal exposure. Pediatr Infect Dis J 2009;28(10):928–9.

50. Haagsma JA, Tariq L, Heederik DJ, et al. Infectious disease risks associated with occupational exposure: a systematic review of the literature. Occup Environ Med 2012;69(2):140–6.
51. Scheftel JM, Elchos BL, Cherry B, et al. Compendium of veterinary standard precautions for zoonotic disease prevention in veterinary personnel: National Association of State Public Health Veterinarians Veterinary Infection Control Committee 2010. J Am Vet Med Assoc 2010;237(12):1403–22.
52. Lipton BA, Hopkins SG, Koehler JE, et al. A survey of veterinarian involvement in zoonotic disease prevention practices. J Am Vet Med Assoc 2008;233(8):1242–9.
53. Jackson J, Villarroel A. A survey of the risk of zoonoses for veterinarians. Zoonoses Public Health 2012;59(3):193–201.
54. Monroe PW, Silberg SL, Morgan PM, et al. Seroepidemiological investigation of *Brucella canis* antibodies in different human population groups. J Clin Microbiol 1975;2(5):382–6.
55. Kumasaka K, Arashima Y, Yanai M, et al. Survey of veterinary professionals for antibodies to *Bartonella henselae* in Japan. Rinsho Byori 2001;49(9):906–10.
56. Lantos PM, Maggi RG, Ferguson B, et al. Detection of *Bartonella* species in the blood of veterinarians and veterinary technicians: a newly recognized occupational hazard? Vector Borne Zoonotic Dis 2014;14(8):563–70.
57. Wright JG, Tengelsen LA, Smith KE, et al. Multidrug-resistant *Salmonella* Typhimurium in four animal facilities. Emerg Infect Dis 2005;11(8):1235–41.
58. Cherry B, Burns A, Johnson GS, et al. *Salmonella* Typhimurium outbreak associated with veterinary clinic. Emerg Infect Dis 2004;10(12):2249–51.
59. Weese JS, Dick H, Willey BM, et al. Suspected transmission of methicillin-resistant *Staphylococcus aureus* between domestic pets and humans in veterinary clinics and in the household. Vet Microbiol 2006;115(1–3):148–55.
60. Ishihara K, Shimokubo N, Sakagami A, et al. Occurrence and molecular characteristics of methicillin-resistant *Staphylococcus aureus* and methicillin-resistant *Staphylococcus pseudintermedius* in an academic veterinary hospital. Appl Environ Microbiol 2010;76(15):5165–74.
61. Abarca VK, Lopez Del PJ, Pena DA, et al. Pet ownership and health status of pets from immunocompromised children, with emphasis in zoonotic diseases. Rev Chilena Infectol 2011;28(3):205–10.
62. Hill WA, Petty GC, Erwin PC, et al. A survey of Tennessee veterinarian and physician attitudes, knowledge, and practices regarding zoonoses prevention among animal owners with HIV infection or AIDS. J Am Vet Med Assoc 2012;240(12):1432–40.
63. Grant S, Olsen CW. Preventing zoonotic diseases in immunocompromised persons: the role of physicians and veterinarians. Emerg Infect Dis 1999;5(1):159–63.
64. Root Kustritz MV, Molgaard LK, Tegzes JH. Frequency of interactions between veterinarians and other professionals to guide interprofessional education. J Vet Med Educ 2013;40(4):370–7.
65. Rabinowitz P, Conti L. Human-animal medicine. Clinical approaches to zoonoses, toxicants, and other shared health risks. Maryland Heights, MO: Saunders; 2010.
66. Glaser CA, Angulo FJ, Rooney JA. Animal-associated opportunistic infections among persons infected with the human immunodeficiency virus. Clin Infect Dis 1994;18(1):14–24.
67. Hemsworth S, Pizer B. Pet ownership in immunocompromised children–a review of the literature and survey of existing guidelines. Eur J Oncol Nurs 2006;10(2):117–27.

68. National Association of State Public Health Veterinarians Animal Contact Compendium. Compendium of measures to prevent disease associated with animals in public settings, 2013. J Am Vet Med Assoc 2013;243(9):1270–88.
69. Avery RK, Michaels MG. Strategies for safe living after solid organ transplantation. Am J Transplant 2013;13(s4):304–10.
70. Writing Panel of Working Group, Lefebvre SL, Golab GC, et al. Guidelines for animal-assisted interventions in health care facilities. Am J Infect Control 2008; 36(2):78–85.
71. Lefebvre SL, Peregrine AS, Golab GC, et al. A veterinary perspective on the recently published guidelines for animal-assisted interventions in health-care facilities. J Am Vet Med Assoc 2008;233(3):394–402.

Legal Implications of Zoonotic Disease Transmission for Veterinary Practices

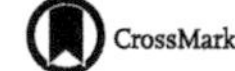

Antoinette E. Marsh, MS, PhD, JD[a,*], Sarah Babcock, DVM, JD[b]

KEYWORDS

• Liability • Zoonoses • Negligence • Malpractice • Standard of care

KEY POINTS

- Owners should be educated when a zoonotic agent is suspected or diagnosed relative to the animal's health and its human contacts and their potential need for physician referral.
- Advisories should be recorded in the animal's medical record. If required by law, report the occurrence of zoonotic disease to the appropriate regulatory agency and keep copies of reports.
- Actions and documents serve as legal evidence in opposition to a claim of malpractice, professional negligence, or complaints to the state veterinary practice licensing boards.
- Veterinarians should develop and engage in opportunities to build relationships with other health professionals to facilitate the communication needed to minimize zoonotic disease transmission.

INTRODUCTION: NATURE OF THE PROBLEM

Veterinarians' service to promote public health and zoonotic disease control traces back to when the profession primarily provided professional services for food production and horses used in transportation. Now, small animal practitioners are a vital link in public health as it relates to pets and other domestic animals intentionally brought into close proximity to people and their homes. Animals may be subclinical carriers of one or more zoonotic agents. Many immunocompromised clients do not seem outwardly different than the general pet-owning public. Thus, some risk of zoonotic disease infection is ever-present. However, if someone is injured by a zoonotic

The authors have nothing to disclose.

[a] Veterinary Preventive Medicine, College of Veterinary Medicine, The Ohio State University, 1900 Coffey Road, Columbus, OH 43210, USA; [b] Animal & Veterinary Legal Services, PLLC, 32750 South River Road, Harrison Township, MI 48045, USA

* Corresponding author.

E-mail address: Marsh.2061@osu.edu

Vet Clin Small Anim 45 (2015) 393–408

http://dx.doi.org/10.1016/j.cvsm.2014.11.008 vetsmall.theclinics.com

0195-5616/15/$ – see front matter

pathogen and it is attributed to a veterinarian's negligence, the individual or members of the victim's family could file a claim and may recover a monetary amount through litigation or settlement (Karen Wernette, AVMA-PLIT, 2014, personal communication).[1] There are no absolute guarantees to legal-proof veterinary practice standards as it relates to zoonotic diseases and human injury. One cannot assume a veterinarian is automatically negligent when a zoonotic pathogen is diagnosed in an owner when the likely animal reservoir is the household pet. It solely depends on the facts of the case.

To minimize the risk of liability, what is required of the veterinarian who examines a pet? Does it matter if the pet is healthy or is diagnosed with a zoonotic pathogen? Is it merely to state to the animal's owner that the animal is healthy, dispense the necessary preventative care vaccines/dewormers/ectoparasite control or the necessary prescription/treatment, and assume all is well when the client and the animal leave the facilities? Unfortunately, there are many potential variables that may complicate this scenario. What could go wrong with this picture? Outwardly appearing healthy animals do transmit zoonotic agents. What are the legal obligations of the veterinarian to the client, to the disease-monitoring governmental agency, and to the clinic employees? How does a veterinarian minimize the risk of adverse legal consequences associated with professional malpractice or a complaint to their veterinary medical board (VMB)? Are the consequences elevated if it involves a zoonotic agent?

The authors explore these questions, providing some general guidelines to avoid or at least generate the means to refute a claim should a complaint be alleged against the veterinarian.

APPROACH/GOALS

The veterinarian is well suited to address the risks posed by zoonotic diseases caused by pathogens that are shared between people and animals. This paper analyzes the legal role and responsibilities private practice veterinarians have in public health regarding zoonotic agents carried or transmitted by their patients.

Defining the Legal Duties of the Veterinarian

The practice of veterinary medicine is defined and regulated by different mechanisms, depending on the country. Some countries have a national board (college or association), such as Panama and Costa Rica, whereas Argentina and the United States maintain provincial or state veterinary medical boards (VMBs) (Ramiro Toribio, College of Veterinary Medicine, The Ohio State University, 2014, personal communication). These boards generally oversee the practice of veterinary medicine and determine whether and what sanctions are imposed for failure to comply with the laws, regulations, and standards established (Ramiro Toribio, College of Veterinary Medicine, The Ohio State University, 2014, personal communication).[2] Increasingly, within the United States, individual state VMBs are referring to the American Veterinary Medical Association (AVMA) Principles of Veterinary Medical Ethics in their review of deviations from accepted conduct.[3] Additionally, there are legal duties under general tort law (damage, injury, wrongful acts done willfully, negligently, or in circumstances involving strict liability) applicable to veterinarians, including their duty as employers to provide safe work environments.

A duty, in the context of the law, is established when a veterinarian enters into a veterinary-client-patient relationship. It is uncertain how far that duty extends beyond the immediate health needs of the pet and the information given to the owner. Does it extend to others in close proximity to the pet and, if so, how far? This question forecasts an evolving area, based on potential changes to animal law. As is far too common with legal challenges, there are no absolutes as the facts of the case and changes in law rapidly evolve. Thus, veterinarians could face civil courts (owner driven), state licensing boards (public protection), state occupational health safety agency/commission (protection of the workforce), or criminal adjudication (punishment for intentional serious crime) when their work involves a zoonotic agent and an adverse event occurs.

Defining the Veterinarian's Role in Public Health

Veterinary medical ethics and the veterinarian's oath of the AVMA outline the ethical duties of veterinarians related to public health. The AVMA Principles of Veterinary Medical Ethics states "the responsibilities of the veterinary profession extend beyond individual patients and clients to society in general."[4] It elaborates on this principle to state that veterinarians are encouraged to provide their services for activities that protect public health. The veterinarian's oath states "I solemnly swear to use my scientific knowledge and skills for the benefit of society, ...the promotion of public health, and advancement of medical knowledge."[5] Thus, the rudiments of the ethical duty begin with the oath for veterinarians to promote public health, including the mitigation or prevention of the transmission of zoonotic pathogens.

One Health is the integrative effort of multiple disciplines working locally, nationally, and globally to attain optimal health for people, animals, and the environment. When considering the veterinarian's traditional role in food safety and newer roles in environmental health, one might call the veterinarian the Super One Health Professional. Globally, veterinarians play a critical role in the detection and prevention of diseases. For example, the Global Early Warning System coordinates the alert and response mechanisms of international human and animal health organizations to assist in prediction, prevention, and control of animal disease threats, including zoonoses.[6] Multidisciplinary risk assessment to include veterinarians provides added value to global early warning of zoonotic disease. This worldwide strategy of One Health for expanding interdisciplinary collaborations and communications in all aspects of health care for humans, animal, and the environment is embraced by the veterinary profession.[7] How does the individual community-practicing veterinarian fit into the One Health strategy? Has the professional or legal duty of a veterinarian changed or been expanded by the acceptance of the role of veterinarians in public health and the One Health effort, and is there a professional or legal duty to this concept of One Health? These questions are important as the threshold for a breach of legal duty depends on if the standard of care is less than what a reasonable veterinarian would have done under similar circumstances based on expert testimony.[3] Defining the standard of care in companion animal medicine as it relates to public health and the role of the veterinarian in One Health is challenging. The accepted standard of care may vary in the future as the profession further establishes the veterinarian's role and leadership in One Health.

CHALLENGES

Liability

Negligence is a tort action whereby one injured individual assigns fault of the injury to another. The violation of duty can be the result of a failure to act, failure to act appropriately, or failure to exercise the degree of care that an ordinary, reasonable, and prudent person would have taken under similar circumstances. If a reasonable person could foresee injury or harm to another, one may be held responsible for the resulting harm through their actions or inactions when a duty exists and harm happens. Essentially, a duty or obligation requires one to conform to certain standards of conduct to protect others against unreasonable risks.

Professional liability arises under malpractice and is an extension of the law of negligence. Malpractice occurs if a veterinarian performs professional services that are less than the standard expected of a prudent veterinarian exercising due care and diligence under similar circumstances. Veterinarians may face a claim of ordinary negligence (as an ordinary person) or malpractice (as a professional), depending on the injured party and how it happened. The authors' focus is on veterinary malpractice in the context of a zoonotic disease and the rendering of professional services to a client-owned animal.

Veterinary Malpractice: A Duty, Breach, Causation, and Damages

The increasing interdependence between humans and animals raises the potential for zoonotic pathogen transmission and, with it, an expansion in the number and variety of related legal claims. To date, most claims related to zoonotic diseases have arisen in conjunction with animal attacks and exposure or potential exposure to rabies.[3]

The following 4 elements (A, B, C, and D) must be present to sustain a claim of malpractice:

A duty
*B*reach of the applicable professional standard of care (duty)
*C*ausation and *D*amages

A duty

The authors briefly discussed this earlier, but the presence of the veterinarian-client-patient relationship creates a duty for the veterinarian to adhere to certain standards of care for patients. If there is no relationship, the veterinarian owes no duty to the patients or the owners. Acceptance of a case creates this duty, which is viewed in the law as an implied contract, making the practitioner responsible to use the skills and care of the ordinary, reasonable, and prudent practitioner.[8] For example, the AVMA Principles of Veterinary Medical Ethics are clear that the veterinarian and client have the right to establish or decline a veterinarian-client-patient relationship.[9] It is also clear that the veterinarian should first consider the needs of patients, but that does not alleviate the idea that there may be a duty to the client as well.[10] One may argue that the veterinarian's role includes protecting the health of the animal and educating the owner about risks posed by the presence of a known zoonotic agent.

Breach of a duty

For an owner to prevail in a malpractice claim based on a violation of the duty of care, the animal's owner must prove that "the veterinarian failed to use such reasonable skill, diligence, and attention as may ordinarily be expected of careful, skillful and trustworthy persons in the profession."[3,11] Testimony from an expert who can attest to what persons of similar training and expertise would do under similar circumstances is required to establish what is reasonable under a certain set of circumstances.[12] A veterinarian who holds himself or herself out as an expert (eg, board-certified specialist) will be expected to adhere to a higher level of care.

Generally, a veterinarian will not ordinarily be held liable because of some unforeseeable or unfavorable result. Regarding the element of a zoonotic disease, it is not clear how the responsibility of a veterinarian to the patients and the owners based on this duty may be inferred under a specific set of facts. If the veterinarian's conduct, diagnosis, or advised treatment is less than the acceptable standard of care regarding a suspected or diagnosed zoonotic pathogen, the owner may have a claim against the veterinarian.

Standard of care is established by the expert opinion provided by another veterinarian who will review the facts of the case. Substandard care is the failure to "use such reasonable skill, diligence, and attention as might ordinarily have been expected of a careful, skillful, and trustworthy person in the profession."[11] If most veterinarians make deworming recommendations to feline or canine owners and provide the owners with educational materials on the risks of ocular and visceral larval migrans in children associated with environmental contamination by *Toxocara* ova, then the standard of care is to provide such information and education. If very few to no veterinarians provide specific zoonotic information on methicillin-resistant *Staphylococcus pseudintermedius* (MRSP) because of the rare occurrence of human infection, then a lack of detailed recommendations would not be a breach, under a normal situation, particularly when the veterinarian has no knowledge of immunocompromised household members in close proximity with the infected pet. A recommendation of hand washing after handling the MRSP colonized dog as with any pet may be sufficient to meet the standard of care.[13] In contrast, documented methicillin-resistant *Staphylococcus aureus* (MRSA) in a dog with an owner in a known immunocompromised group would require a more thorough and thoughtful conversation to educate the client, followed by record notation of the professional advisement.

The law does not require the veterinarian to be infallible.[14] In contrast, expert opinion is not needed in a prima facie case whereby a claim is evident from the facts and the "very nature of the acts complained of bespeak improper treatment and malpractice."[50] There is a distinction between an error of judgment and negligence.[8] If a veterinarian makes an error in judgment after applying the appropriate standard of care, then liability may not be imposed. In contrast, if the error in judgment is a result of applying substandard care as determined by the ordinary, reasonable, and prudent veterinarian, then it is malpractice.

Burden of proof

There are distinctions in the burden of proof regarding a professional malpractice claim filed in a civil court as compared with a criminal proceeding or a licensing board disciplinary action. In a civil case, the plaintiff must establish their claim by a preponderance of the evidence, a lower threshold when compared with beyond a reasonable doubt for most criminal evidence. A licensing board does not always publish or provide the burden of proof used to evaluate a filed complaint in a disciplinary matter (Theresa Stir, Ohio State Veterinary Medical Licensing Board, 2014, personal communication).[2]

Causation

The causation element involves (1) whether the alleged substandard conduct is the actual cause of the injuries and (2) if the conduct is the proximate cause (also referred to as the *legal cause*). Proximate cause is a policy determination whereby the court may deem it unfair to hold an individual liable for all consequences resulting from an initial breach of duty. Generally, foreseeable injury is an important part of the proximate cause analysis. The questions to ask are the following: Given the situation's criteria, could one predict (foresee) the potential injuries? Did the specific outcome in the case result directly from the errors, actions, or inactions on the part of the veterinarian, performing at less than the acceptable standard of care? For example, in a case whereby a dog died of a severe infection originating from a urinary tract infection, the court concluded that the veterinarian's actions were not the proximate cause of death.[15] The plaintiff alleged professional negligence for failing to perform a urinalysis, and this breach of the standard of care proximately caused the dog's death. Expert witness testimony indicated that a urinalysis would have only identified the presence of bacteria and would not have identified the specific bacteria strain and its antibiotic susceptibility. The urine culture and antibiotics used by this veterinarian were appropriate for the situation. Therefore, the lack of a urinalysis (alleged proximate cause) would not have affected the initial treatment and rapid adverse outcome of the case (severe bacterial infection following a laminectomy and postoperatively inserted urine catheter).

Damages

The monetary award for a successful negligence claim consists almost exclusively of compensatory money paid to the injured party.[3] Under some statutes, attorney fees can be awarded.[3] The purpose of awarding compensatory damages in negligence cases is to restore the injured plaintiff and not punish the negligent defendant, although punitive damages are sometimes allowed if the actions were intentional or reckless. Insurance may only cover negligent and not intentional actions; coverage will be governed by the terms in the insurance policy. Compensatory damages for actions that result in an injury to humans could include general damages for pain and suffering and special (economic) damages relating to past and future medical bills, lost wages, and loss of future earning capacity.[3] Some professionals in the veterinary-legal field report seeing an increase in considering the awarding of noneconomic damages and an increase in the scrutiny over which standards of care are evaluated as well as the number of lawsuits filed against veterinarians.[16] Nonetheless, direct and indirect losses resulting from the alleged malpractice must be quantified and justified.[17]

PREVENTION

Pitfalls to Avoid with Client-Patient Activities

Although there are many hurdles to a successful malpractice claim, here are a few examples in the context of zoonotic diseases that may highlight where a veterinarian's conduct may less than the acceptable standard of care.

Bad records = poor defense

First and foremost, maintenance of complete and accurate records to demonstrate the standard of care followed, provided, and recommended for patients are useful and invaluable evidence. A 2014 special report in the *Journal of the American Veterinary Medical Association* found that, from 2005 to 2011, the second greatest number of disciplinary actions taken by state VMBs were in response to improper record keeping.[2]

If a client declines a recommended course of action and a problem is likely anticipated (foreseeable), this is an example of when documentation is advisable. Any legal liability release form should be reviewed by an attorney who is licensed to practice where it is to be used. Consent forms should be tailored to patients, with additional information provided to the client in a printed pamphlet and referenced in the executed consent form. Documenting details should be standard practice whenever clients refuse a recommended courses of treatment whether of a zoonotic risk or a general procedure. Documentation is even more important when there is a health risk to clients or human household members. It would be difficult to defend a claim if no such notation is made in the patient record.[16]

Failure to recommend preventive measures

Many veterinarians fail to recommend preventive measures for common zoonotic diseases because of a belief that such pathogens carry minimal risk or that owners may refuse the recommended preventive measures.[18–20] The risk of zoonotic diseases may seem negligible because of a very low incidence. In a legal context, though, the risk is calculated by considering both the frequency and the severity of the harm. Thus, even for uncommon (yet known) zoonotic diseases, the risk may be considered great if the potential damage associated with the disease is high.[3] Courts may use a cost-benefit analysis to determine whether a veterinarian is liable for the injury to a pet or owner. Thus, when minimal expenditure of resources by the veterinarian or staff could have prevented severe harm, the court may be more inclined to find the veterinarian at fault and liable for resulting damages.[3]

This argument proved successful in bringing a product liability suit against a pet store for selling a parasitized puppy.[21,22] Product liability and veterinary malpractice are different legal claims. Nevertheless, a veterinarian may find it difficult to persuade a court that he or she should not be held liable for blindness in a child resulting from ocular larval migrans caused by *Toxocara canis* when the circumstances suggest the infection was acquired from the family puppy and nothing but routine vaccinations were noted in the record. However, providing information and educating a client about ways to avoid zoonotic risks and advocating a recommended deworming schedule could potentially have prevented the child's condition. In contrast, a zoonotic claim that involved children infected with *Escherichia coli* at a fair petting zoo was determined in favor of the defendant as the defendant took affirmative actions to protect the fair patrons. These actions included using several veterinarians who worked to protect the health and safety of the fair visitors. The veterinarians put up additional signage and hand sanitizers after a prefair risk assessment revealed the need for these educational and preventive measures after touching the animals.[23]

The veterinarian may negate a malpractice claim by documenting that there was no breach of professional duty or omission of required professional action to prevent unreasonable risk of harm.[23] By removing the *B* from the 4 elements (A, B, C, and D), a claim will fail. By way of example, after a thoughtful discussion with the client who still declines preventive measures, it is essential that this refusal be documented. Ultimately, it is the client who provides treatment consent after receiving adequate warnings and information about the risk both to the pet and the household members. One needs to consider how a situation would seem retrospectively if harm did occur and what an ordinary, reasonable, and prudent veterinarian would have done with a foreseeable harm.

Failure to take appropriate samples or quarantine an animal

In a case against a veterinarian treating a dairy cow with neurologic disease, the veterinarian failed to include the cow's cerebellum and brain stem for rabies testing, and the laboratory results came back inconclusive. Nine people received rabies prophylaxis. The veterinarian failed to meet the standard of care, and his insurance company paid more than $95,000 to cover the medical expenses for the 9 people exposed.[24]

In *Placko v Fawver*, the plaintiff alleged the veterinarian was negligent in taking proper measures to confine a rabies-suspected cat that had bitten a child.[25] The cat died while in a third-party's care, and the carcass was lost. The crucial disputed issues of the case centered on communications between the individual responsible for quarantining the cat and the veterinarian who made the confinement request.

The court stated that the veterinarian was under a duty to provide information that the cat was a possible rabies carrier and was being confined for this reason. Furthermore, under the facts of the 1977 case, it was the veterinarian's duty to provide information as to what to do if the cat died during confinement. In present day, rabies reporting statutes explicitly define the responsibilities when a veterinarian suspects rabies.

Failure to avoid client exposures while in the examination room

When to have a client in an examination room is a difficult question to answer as clinics have different physical layouts, procedures for acquiring pet history, and availability of technical staff. Most would agree that when a veterinarian is aware or is warned that an animal may become aggressive, biting and scratching and subsequent wound infection is a risk. Owners not involved in restraint can get injured through a bite or scratch while in a room with a distressed animal. In a fractious cat case, the owner was not requested to help restrain the cat, yet the cat bit the owner. The veterinarian's insurance carrier paid out $17,199 for the client's lost wages and $8,281 for out-of-pocket medical expenses related to the infected cat bite.[26] When a risk of injury to the client is likely present, request that the client leaves the examination room or take the animal to another room for the procedure. Restraining an animal on the owner's property can result in liability to the veterinarian, as is what occurred with a bull undergoing fertility testing. A chute gate flew open and hit the owner, who subsequently required extensive treatment. The owner alleged that the veterinarian was negligent for not properly latching the gate, and the case settled with the injured owner receiving $33,000.[27] This latter case may be atypical in that it was the animal owner's facilities. Nonetheless, veterinarians in their own practice facility are ultimately responsible for the safety of those around them, including the safety of clients who bring animals into the clinic.

Failure to advise clients on the dangers of exotic pets, atypical pets, or high-risk pets

The increase in popularity of exotic rodents and other pocket pets has resulted in importation of live foreign wildlife into other locations.[28] Because these species are commonly unregulated and caught in the wild, these pets may pose various health threats to their owners.[29] Wild animals distributed through the commercial pet trade are associated with outbreaks of human infections, and these nontraditional pet animal species may serve as a reservoir or a vector for the introduction of new pathogens.[30] A lack of familiarity with a given species may limit a veterinarian's ability to detect health threats or make appropriate health recommendations. Clients who own any species that is outside the veterinarian's professional expertise may require the veterinarian to refer the client to a colleague with the necessary expertise.[3] Failure to provide this information or referral may be considered a breach of duty, creating liability.

Failure to advise clients on risky pet husbandry and care

One might argue that the ultimate decision for the care of the pet belongs to the owner. Nonetheless, if the veterinarian inquires as to the food type, exercise, day boarding, and other animal contact in a wellness check, it may be advisable to provide the client with educational materials on zoonotic risks or situations whereby the animal is at risk for acquiring an infection that then may be passed along to the owner. Owners cite veterinarians as the most common source of information about pet health, care, and nutrition.[31] For example, an owner does not allow their Labrador retriever to swim in a local drainage pond; nonetheless, this same dog attends a dog day care with kiddy pools where various dogs are in and out of standing water. The owner may understand the risk of *Giardia* or other water-borne pathogens contaminating the local drainage pond but may not appreciate the potential risk of *Giardia* or *Leptospira* at the dog day care facility or misunderstand *Giardia* assemblages or species-specific genotypes. Raw-food diets or prey hunting are other areas where the veterinarian may be held responsible for failing to advise the client of the risks if the veterinarian knew this risk. A 2008 study states, "Veterinarians have the responsibility (duty) of ensuring that clients understand the risks when they feed this type of food (raw meat)."[31] The results of a 2002 Canadian study demonstrated 30% of the dogs shed *Salmonella* after consuming a bone and raw-food diet; the investigators warned of a public health concern, especially for those with young children, the aged, or other people who may have compromised immune systems.[32]

If the veterinarian sends the client home with medication, requiring pill or administration of an injection to a fractious animal, then the veterinarian should advise the client about the potential of bites, scratches, and needle sticks. If a veterinary practice dispenses or prescribes injectable treatments, education regarding safe handling practices, including safe administration, needle handling, and disposal should be provided and documented. This is also discussed elsewhere in this issue, by Gibbons and colleagues.[33] Should the veterinarian know the client is immune compromised, the veterinarian should be especially thoughtful when giving advice along with the subsequent documentation in the patient record. Additional steps regarding needle safety are provided in Gibbons and MacMahon, Workplace Safety and Health for the Veterinary Health care Team. Some practices allow clients to return used needles and syringes to the clinic in a rigid, plastic, small lid-opening container if injections are part of the pet's ongoing care. Some pharmacies will dispense Sharps containers with a return disposal fee included. Whatever mechanism is used, clients need to be told about syringe and needle handling and disposal, and the information should be included in the discharge instructions and clinic record.

Stull and colleagues[34] reported on pet husbandry and infection-control practices, whereby 14% of reptile-owning households allowed the pet to roam through the kitchen or washed it in the kitchen sink. Does the veterinarian have the duty to warn the owner of the human-disease risks associated with kitchen sink reptile husbandry practices? Retrospectively during litigation, one could argue that the veterinarian, serving in a professional capacity, failed to counsel the owner of the substantial likelihood of *Salmonella* shedding by an otherwise outwardly appearing healthy reptile. Would a veterinarian, serving as an expert witness, testify that the standard of care is to give a warning or not to warn about *Salmonella*? From a legal standpoint, communicating and documenting this communication about risky husbandry practices may not always lead to owner compliance, yet the veterinarian's duty is better satisfied.

Failure to advise clients to seek care from a physician

It is important for veterinarians to provide clients with information regarding a suspected zoonotic disease and advise them to seek medical attention. Failing to recommend a client seek care from his or her physician may legally be viewed as a breach of the standard of care when a reasonable veterinary professional would make this recommendation.[3] Nonetheless, veterinarians are not permitted to give medical advice to clients or practice human medicine in any form (physical examination, suggesting a diagnosis, or taking a medical history *of the owner*).[16] Dr Mani, veterinarian, and Dr Maguire,[35] human physician, advocate that the veterinarian "strongly advise owners about the threats of animal-to-human transmission of a variety of infectious agents," and "[p]hysicians must also recognize the disease in humans."[35] These investigators suggest the veterinarian "closely question owners about human household members exhibiting similar clinical signs to the veterinary patient."[35] Here is an example when there is no bright-line legal rule to follow on questioning the human client relative to the human side of the zoonotic infection. If in doubt before crossing the line, educate the client and recommend the owner visit with their human physician, then document the pathogen, zoonotic potential, and your recommendations to the owner to seek physician evaluation relative to the contact with the suspect or infected animal.

This challenging area is where national veterinary associations may need to take the lead. Without a bright line, it will be on an individual judgment basis that a veterinarian must decide what to ask, what to record, and how confidentiality, if required, will be maintained if it involves the human and not the animal. Admittedly, this area is ripe for a legal challenge. For example, if an MRSA infection occurs within the household members, including the pet and a person, how does the veterinarian handle the information and provide satisfactory treatment options? This question is open for debate. Without disclosure of the owner or pet identity, consultation with colleagues and academic resources may provide some protective shell should a claim of malpractice arise, as one's peer and academic resources would be the expert witnesses.

More than a decade ago, survey results demonstrated a disconnection between the veterinary and human medical professions, evidencing a lack of communication between the two professionals on zoonotic diseases.[36,37] Veterinary programs have made advancements. Today, veterinary education programs include a complete course or a series of lectures regarding zoonotic agents; it is no longer a meat-hygiene course. A reasonable prudent veterinarian would advise a client of zoonotic risks associated with a suspected infectious companion animal.

Client communication strategies

How to discuss with a client the potential for zoonotic disease transmission may be a difficult conversation, considering the strong message that pets are now family members. The challenge is how not to frighten the owner, yet provide useful information. One recommendation is to "ask clients whether they are interested in discussing the risks of pet ownership among individuals who might be at higher risk of being infected with diseases transmitted from pets to humans."[38] Data suggest the public still requires education in this area.[34]

Liability Potential in the Workplace

Without adequate controls, zoonotic agents pose a risk to the veterinarian, other staff members, and any human or animal visitor to the clinic.

Bad employee = more than a nuisance

Under the doctrine of respondeat superior, the clinic owner or supervising veterinarian can be responsible for the negligence of an associate veterinarian or others working under their supervision. Veterinarians must use reasonable care in selecting new employees.[39] To establish the employer's liability in a negligent hiring case, the complainant must prove that (1) the employee causing the injury was unfit for the tasks assigned; (2) the employer's hiring or keeping the unqualified employee was the proximate cause of the injury; and (3) the employer knew, or should have known, of the employee's unfitness.[39]

Work-related zoonotic infections

Veterinarians may be held liable for harm to employees who contract zoonotic diseases in the course of their employment. Several studies report veterinarians having been infected with a zoonotic disease in practice, such as 102 out of 216 veterinarians in Oregon and 105 out of 371 veterinarians in Washington.[38,40,41] Under the US Occupational Safety and Health Act, employers are required to provide a safe workplace for employees. This is also discussed elsewhere in this issue, by Gibbons and Colleagues. This protection should also extend to other personnel in the workplace, such as volunteers, and should cover a variety of occupational hazards, including exposure to potentially infectious materials. For example, leptospirosis can be transmitted to people from animals through direct contact with infectious urine. In a 1986 New Jersey case, a kennel employee died after contracting leptospirosis at a veterinary facility.[42] A suit was initiated claiming the veterinarian failed to provide a safe workplace, although the case subsequently settled outside of the court with the parties reaching a confidential settlement for an unknown financial amount. The risk for transmission of a zoonotic disease in the workplace may be even greater if the practice has a patient that poses a higher risk and/or comes in contact with multiple clinic staff. For example, during the 2003 US outbreak of monkeypox infection, veterinarians and their staff represented more than 25% of affected humans. To avoid liability, veterinary practices should consider what preventive measures need to be taken to provide safe work conditions.[43] Finally, care must be taken to avoid discrimination of employees who must restrict their work so as to avoid exposure to a zoonotic agent and to determine whether limited to no exposure will impact their ability to perform essential job tasks.[44] Veterinary clinics should implement appropriate infection-control practices, document training to all staff members, including volunteers, and enforce the use of personal protection equipment and responsible practices that promote a safe workplace. A 2008 study demonstrated that most veterinarians (69.0%–88.1%) did not have a written infection-control policy.[45] One resource that may be used to draft a written infection-control policy for a practice is the Compendium of Veterinary Standard Precautions for Zoonotic Disease Prevention in Veterinary Personnel. This document (updated in 2010) provides guidelines for infection-control practices and includes a model infection control plan for veterinary practices to adapt to use in their facility.[46,47] A private practice may insert additional sections directly relevant to their setting or deleting sections, such as dental procedures, that it may not provide.

Training and personal protective equipment are used to mitigate a work-related risk of injury. A record of each employee and volunteer's training should be maintained, and record retention time will vary by state. A variety of infection-control training resources are available through the Internet.[48,49] Access and use of personal protective equipment should be encouraged. Risk management consists of anticipating, recognizing, and eliminating problems.[39,50] Documenting this can serve as supportive evidence should a claim arise.

When employers disregard workers' safety, placing themselves and others at risk, the practice owner should immediately deal with this problem and document the measures to mitigate the problem. A chemistry professor at the University of California, Los Angeles had faced up to 4.5 years in prison if convicted in a 2008 laboratory fire that killed a research assistant who was handling a chemical and not wearing a protective coat, and her sweater melted onto her skin.[51] The professor was the direct supervisor and was ultimately responsible for the safety of personnel. The California Division of Occupational Safety and Health fined the University $32,000 after determining the worker was not properly trained and should have been wearing a laboratory coat.[52]

Weese and Prescott[53] assessed laboratory and biosafety practices and determined a substantial number of veterinary clinics used unsafe laboratory practices when working with microbial cultures. They noted deficiencies in the location, general biosafety practices, culture practices, and supervision. If the practice owner knowingly ignores these deficiencies, from a risk management position, the liability for that clinic just increased significantly.

When an accident does occur, whether with a zoonotic agent exposure or a slip and fall, there are steps that can be taken to avoid future accidents and assist should the injured employee make a claim.[54] Although there may be an assumption that this is part of the job, there are several actions an employer can take to protect their employees and minimize their potential risk of acquiring a zoonotic pathogen.

Workers' Compensation and Employee Injuries

An employee may be barred from suing his or her veterinary employer for injuries associated with a workplace-acquired disease or injury if a worker's compensation claim is made and the parties are subject to workers' compensation laws. In *Oliver v Scamps Pet Center*, the court found that there was evidence to support a claim that psittacosis was an occupational disease under workers' compensation law.[55] In *Frey v Gunston Animal Hospital*, the veterinary technician won her appeal from an earlier decision by her state Workers' Compensation Commission when they denied her claim for reimbursement for the cost of rabies prophylaxis treatment after the veterinary hospital where she was employed erroneously disposed of a euthanized feral cat displaying neurologic disease.[56] Early in the course of the cat's treatment, Frey pilled the cat without gloves; there was a good chance that saliva came into contact with her scratched hands. The Court of Appeals reviewed the Workers' Compensation Commission decision and the procedures the veterinarian pursued following the staff member's exposure and how the case was then handled by the insurer and the commissioner:

> *When the veterinarian-owner learned of Frey's exposure to the cat, she contacted several experts in rabies epidemiology because of her concern for Frey, who was unvaccinated. After those experts recommended rabies treatment for Frey, Frey received injections to prevent rabies infection. The hospital's workers' compensation insurer concluded, however, that Frey's condition did not result from an accidental injury or occupational disease and declined to pay for the treatment.*[56]

The deputy commissioner denied the cost of reimbursement for Frey's $ 1,765 treatment.

> *The deputy commissioner ruled that Frey did not have an occupational disease because she was never diagnosed with rabies. In addition, the deputy commissioner ruled that Frey did not sustain an injury by accident and that Frey was seeking benefits for prophylactic treatments.*

The appellate decision recognized that the provisions of the Workers' Compensation Act is to carry out its humane and remedial purposes of affording compensation to employees who suffer accidental injuries resulting from hazards in the work environment. The court found the evidence proved a compensable injury by accident for which she was entitled to recover the expenses incurred for the rabies treatment. *Frey* is in contrast to the cases presented in the earlier section, "Failure to take appropriate samples or quarantine an animal." Frey did not file a claim against her employer, as it seems the employer took reasonable measures to mitigate Frey's risk of rabies after the incident. Frey, as an employee, was seeking recovery through a workers' compensation claim.

Workers' compensation laws vary (A comprehensive discussion of the worker's compensation topic is beyond the scope of this review).[1] Although not strictly employees, volunteers serve important roles in veterinary clinics. Under workplace safety and risk of liability, consideration should be given to volunteers. Some basic questions include the following: Are volunteers considered employees under your workers compensation laws? Does your insurance carrier cover volunteers? Veterinary practice owners should consult their insurance carriers and perhaps an experienced employment law attorney before accepting volunteer workers.[57]

Requirements to Report Zoonotic Diseases

In most jurisdictions, there are legal requirements to report certain zoonotic diseases to the appropriate authority. These requirements vary greatly among jurisdictions. Not only do these requirements vary but also the agency to which they are reported varies, as does interagency reporting, such as between a department of health and department of agriculture.

Thus, the burden is on veterinarians to be familiar with the requirements in location where they practice. It is advised that the practice check periodically for updates in requirements and changes in statutes and make the information about reporting easily located in the clinic with the necessary agency contacts. There are potential penalties if a veterinarian fails to report as prescribed. Under law, a veterinarian's license may be revoked or suspended. Fines or criminal penalties could also be imposed.[58]

SUMMARY

Zoonotic diseases are important both from a public health point of view and because of the effects they may have on veterinary licensure discipline and litigation. Staying current on zoonotic pathogens is an important continuing education component. The increased concerns about zoonotic diseases will have legal implications for veterinarians who fail to do the following: (1) diagnose, prevent, or treat zoonotic diseases in animals; (2) advise their clients who potentially have been exposed to consult their physician; (3) provide a safe work environment; and (4) report diseases as required by law. Veterinarians should err on the side of caution, documenting communications with clients, training of clinic staff, and keeping copies of reports submitted to governmental agencies. Essentially, effective communications go a long way toward avoiding liabilities associated with zoonotic agents.

REFERENCES

1. Tannenbaum J. Medical-legal aspects of veterinary public health in private practice. Semin Vet Med Surg (Small Anim) 1991;6(3):175–85.
2. Babcock SL, Doehne JR, Carlin ER. Trends in veterinary medical board state disciplinary actions, 2005-2011. J Am Vet Med Assoc 2014;244(12):1397–402.
3. Babcock S, Marsh A, Lin J, et al. Legal implications of zoonoses for clinical veterinarians. J Am Vet Med Assoc 2008;233:1556–62.
4. Principles of veterinary medical ethics of the AVMA, principle II. Professional behavior K. Available at: https://www.avma.org/KB/Policies/Pages/Principles-of-Veterinary-Medical-Ethics-of-the-AVMA.aspx. Accessed August 13, 2014.
5. Veterinarian's oath. Available at: https://www.avma.org/KB/Policies/Pages/veterinarians-oath.aspx. Accessed August 13, 2014.
6. The global health security agenda. Available at: http://www.globalhealth.gov/global-health-topics/global-health-security/ghsagenda.html. Accessed August 13, 2014.
7. One health initiative. Available at: http://www.onehealthinitiative.com. Accessed August 13, 2014.

8. Geyer L. Malpractice and liability. Vet Clin North Am Small Anim Pract 1993;23(5): 1027–52.
9. Principles of veterinary medical ethics of the AVMA, principle II. Professional behavior E. Available at: https://www.avma.org/KB/Policies/Pages/Principles-of-Veterinary-Medical-Ethics-of-the-AVMA.aspx. Accessed August 13, 2014.
10. Principles of veterinary medical ethics of the AVMA, principle II. Professional behavior A. Available at: https://www.avma.org/KB/Policies/Pages/Principles-of-Veterinary-Medical-Ethics-of-the-AVMA.aspx. Accessed August 13, 2014.
11. Bailey C. Annotation, veterinarian's liability for malpractice. 71 ALR 4th 811, 1989.
12. Carter v. Louisiana State University. 520 So.2d 383 (La. 1988).
13. Dogs for pet owners. Available at: http://www.wormsandgermsblog.com/uploads/file/M3%20Dogs%20-%20Owner.pdf. Accessed September 5, 2014.
14. Turner v. Benhart. 527 So.2d 717 (Ala. 1988).
15. Lauderbaugh v. Gellasch, 2008 Ohio 6500 (Oh. 2008).
16. Lacroix C, Clark M. Everyday zoonosis can lead to everyday lawsuits for veterinarians. Suppl Veterinary Forum (Suppl) 2008;25(3A):24–30.
17. Shane S. Jurisprudence for ratite practitioners. Vet Clin North Am Food Anim Pract 1998;14(3):525–31.
18. Kornblatt A, Schantz P. Veterinary and public health considerations in canine roundworm control: a survey of practicing veterinarians. J Am Vet Med Assoc 1980;177:1212–5.
19. Harvey J, Roberts J, Schantz P. Survey of veterinarians' recommendations for treatment and control of intestinal parasites in dogs: public health implications. J Am Vet Med Assoc 1991;199(6):702–7.
20. Stull J, Carr A, Chommel B. Small animal deworming protocols, client education, and veterinarian perception of zoonotic parasites in western Canada. Can Vet J 2007;48:269–76.
21. Worrell v. Animal Kingdom, 563 A.2d 1387 (Conn. 1989).
22. Worrell v. Animal Kingdom, Case No. 0272077. The MA, CT, RI Verdict Reporter 1993;2:474.
23. Rolan v. N.C. Dep't of Agric. & Consumer Servs, 756 S.E.2d 788 (N.C. 2014).
24. AVMA PLIT. Inadequate tissue provided for rabies testing. Production Medicine 2013.
25. Placko v. Fawver. 371 N.E.2d 187 (Ill. 1977).
26. AVMA PLIT. Cat bite infects owner's hand. Professional liability: 2011:4.
27. AVMA PLIT. Rancher Injuried and Unconscious after Fractious Bull Bangs Open Gate. Winter 2012.
28. Chomel B. Zoonoses of pocket pets and other unusual veterinary species. In: Proc 144th Annu Conv Am Vet Med Assoc. Washington, DC, July 14–18, 2007.
29. Johnson-Delaney C. Safety issues in the exotic pet practice. Vet Clin North Am Exot Anim Pract 2005;8(3):515–24.
30. Smolinski M, Hamburg M, Lederberg J. Microbial threats to health: emergence, detection, and response. Washington, DC: National Academies Press; 2003.
31. Laflamme D, Abood S, Fascetti A, et al. Pet feeding practices of dog and cat owners in the United States and Australia. J Am Vet Med Assoc 2008;232(5): 687–94.
32. Schlesinger D, Joffe D. Raw food diets in companion animals: a critical review. Can Vet J 2011;52(1):50–4.
33. Weese J, Jack D. Needlestick injuries in veterinary medicine. Can Vet J 2008; 49(8):780–4.

34. Stull J, Peregrine A, Sargeant J, et al. Pet husbandry and infection control practices related to zoonotic disease risks in Ontario, Canada. BMC Public Health 2013;13:520. Available at: http://wwww.biomedcentral.com/1471-2458/13/520. Accessed August 13, 2014.
35. Mani I, Maguire JH. Small animal zoonoses and immunocompromised pet owners. Top Companion Anim Med 2009;24(4):164–74.
36. Gauthier JL, Richardson DJ. Knowledge and attitudes about Zoonotic helminths: a survey of Connecticut pediatricians and veterinarians. Compend Contin Educ Pract Vet 2002;24(Suppl):4–9.
37. Grant S, Olsen C. Preventing zoonotic disease in immunocompromised persons: the role of physicians and veterinarians. Emerg Infect Dis 1999;5:159–63.
38. Lipton B, Hopkins S, Koehler J, et al. A survey of veterinarian involvement in zoonotic disease prevention practices. J Am Vet Med Assoc 2008;233: 1242–9.
39. Copeland J. Employer-employee relations. Vet Clin North Am Small Anim Pract 1993;23(5):957–74.
40. Croft D, Sotir M, Williams C, et al. Occupational risks during a monkeypox outbreak, Wisconsin, 2003. Emerg Infect Dis 2007;13(8):1150–7.
41. Jackson J, Villarroel A. A survey of the risk of zoonoses for veterinarians. Zoonoses Public Health 2012;59:193–201.
42. Fiala J. CDC study: DVM fail lepto safety practices. DVM News-Magazine 2006.
43. Nienhaus A, Skudlik C, Seidler A. Work-related accidents and occupational diseases in veterinarians and their staff. Int Arch Occup Environ Health 2005;78: 230–8.
44. Burnett v. Univ of Tenn-Knoxville, No. 3:09-CV-017, 2010 U.S. Dist. LEXIS 40666 (E.D. Tenn. April 26, 2010).
45. Wright J, Jung S, Holman R, et al. Infection control practices and zoonotic disease risks among veterinarians in the United States. J Am Vet Med Assoc 2008;232(12):1863–72.
46. Elchos B, Scheftel J. Discussion of the compendium of veterinary standard precautions: preventing zoonotic disease transmission in veterinary personnel. Zoonoses Public Health 2008;55(8–10):526–8.
47. Scheftel J, Elchos B, Cherry B, et al. Compendium of veterinary standard precautions for zoonotic disease prevention in veterinary personnel: National Association of State Public Health Veterinarians Veterinary Infection Control Committee 2010. J Am Vet Med Assoc 2010;237(12):1403–22.
48. Zoonotic diseases. Available at: http://www.cfsph.iastate.edu/. Accessed August 12, 2014.
49. Available at: http://www.wormsandgermsblog.com/. Accessed August 12, 2014.
50. AVMA PLIT. Behavioral safety-six observation techniques to prevent incidents at your practice. Safety Bulletin 2013;21.
51. Bronstad A. Campus, professor lawyer up to fight criminal negligence charges following lab death. Natl Law J January 23, 2012.
52. Bronstad A. UCLA professor avoids prison in fatal lab fire. Natl Law J 2014.
53. Weese J, Prescott J. Assessment of laboratory and biosafety practices associated with bacterial culture in veterinary clinics. J Am Vet Med Assoc 2009; 234(3):352–8.
54. AVMA PLIT. Incident reporting and investigating when employees are injured. Safety Bulletin 2014;22.
55. Oliver v. Scamps Pet Center, 126 Ore. App. 541, 868 P.2d 794 (Ore. 1994)

56. Frey v. Gunston Animal Hospital, 39 Va. App. 414, 573 SE2d 307 (Va. 2002).
57. Flemming D. Dog bites veterinarian: the legal issues. J Am Vet Med Assoc 2004; 225(5):695–7.
58. Hannah H. Communicable disease–the veterinarian's duty to report, to confine, to disclose. J Am Vet Med Assoc 1992;201(1):40–1.

Workplace Safety and Health for the Veterinary Health Care Team

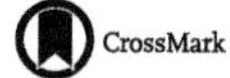

John D. Gibbins, DVM, MPH[a,*], Kathleen MacMahon, DVM, MS[b]

KEYWORDS

- Occupational safety • Occupational health • Regulations • Needlestick injuries
- Hazardous drugs • Animal bites

KEY POINTS

- Employers should develop and implement a comprehensive safety and health program, including written standard operating procedures, that address occupational safety and health risks that are specific to their clinic. This program should be consistent with national, regional, state, and other applicable standards and regulations.
- A written infection control plan is an important component of a comprehensive veterinary clinic safety and health program.
- Management commitment, employee involvement, and initial and refresher training for staff on all aspects of the program are keys to success.
- Many resources are available to help employers develop clinic guidelines to prevent occupational injuries and illnesses from bites and scratches, sharps, and hazardous drugs, as well as other hazards commonly encountered in veterinary medicine. Some of these resources are provided at the end of this article.

INTRODUCTION

Veterinary practice is associated with a large number of potential chemical, biological, physical, and psychological hazards that vary with the workplace setting and the type of tasks performed. Veterinary employers are responsible for ensuring that workplace hazards are identified and evaluated, from animal-related hazards to chemical

---

The authors have nothing to disclose.
The findings and conclusions in this report are those of the authors and do not necessarily represent the views of the National Institute for Occupational Safety and Health.
[a] Division of Surveillance, Hazard Evaluations, and Field Studies, National Institute for Occupational Safety and Health, Centers for Disease Control and Prevention, 1090 Tusculum Avenue, MS R-10, Cincinnati, OH 45226, USA; [b] Education and Information Division, National Institute for Occupational Safety and Health, Centers for Disease Control and Prevention, 1090 Tusculum Avenue, MS C-14, Cincinnati, OH 45226, USA
* Corresponding author.
E-mail address: jgibbins@cdc.gov

Vet Clin Small Anim 45 (2015) 409–426
http://dx.doi.org/10.1016/j.cvsm.2014.11.006
0195-5616/15/$ – see front matter Published by Elsevier Inc.

exposures. Employers should develop and implement a comprehensive, customized, written safety and health program to address and prevent those hazards. A program that identifies and addresses recognized workplace hazards is an important step toward preventing workplace illnesses and injuries. Training employees about the hazards they are exposed to and encouraging them to report work-related illnesses and injuries are important aspects of an effective safety and health program. A written infection control plan is an important component of a comprehensive safety and health program.

The principles of occupational safety and health are universal and many of the recognized hazards are found worldwide in veterinary clinics. This article focuses on workplace standards in the United States but other countries have similar workplace standards and guidance.

The elements and principles of workplace standards relevant to veterinary clinics are reviewed, including the US Occupational Safety and Health Administration (OSHA) Recordkeeping, Hazard Communication, Personal Protective Equipment, Respiratory Protection, and Bloodborne Pathogens Standards. Information about selected veterinary safety and health hazards is presented, including sharps injuries, animal bites and scratches, and hazardous drug exposures. Strategies to reduce the potential for adverse safety and health effects of workplace hazards and resources for training and education are provided. Information about the cost of work-related injuries and illnesses and the economic incentives of an effective safety and health program that prevents these costly incidents is presented. Additional information about each of these topics is provided in the Resources section.

GENERAL CLINIC PREVENTION

Developing an Occupational Safety and Health Program

Developing and implementing a comprehensive workplace safety and health program that identifies and addresses the serious hazards of each workplace is an important foundation for preventing illnesses and injuries. Management commitment and employee involvement in the development, communication, and implementation of the program are critical to its success (**Box 1**). A worksite evaluation that assesses all workplace activities and processes is needed to identify workplace hazards. It is helpful to consider the typical hazards that are found in many veterinary workplaces; however, it is also important to identify any additional or different potential hazards in each specific workplace. Employers should develop written standard operating procedures that address the hazards in their workplace. International and national resources with information about common hazards found in veterinary clinics are provided in the Resources section.

Box 1
Safety and health program critical elements

1. Management commitment and employee involvement
2. Worksite analysis to identify hazards
3. Hazard prevention and control
4. Training for employees, supervisors, and managers

From OSHA. OSHA fact sheet: effective workplace safety and health management systems. 2014. Available at: https://www.osha.gov/Publications/safety-health-management-systems.pdf. Accessed July 5, 2014.

Assistance with a workplace hazard evaluation can be obtained from a professional consultant trained in industrial hygiene or other occupational safety and health professional (see Resources). Before hiring a consultant, individuals should consider evaluating the consultant's experience in veterinary clinic settings and asking for references from colleagues in the veterinary profession. In the United States, OSHA has a consultation program that provides assistance with workplace compliance. The US National Institute for Occupational Safety and Health (NIOSH) may help evaluate workplace health hazards if requested by employees, employee representatives, or employers through its Health Hazard Evaluation program. NIOSH may provide assistance and information by phone and in writing, or may visit the workplace to assess exposure and employee health. Based on their findings, NIOSH recommends ways to reduce hazards and prevent work-related illness (see Resources).

Having an illness and injury reporting system in place and encouraging employees to report work-related incidents is a key component of an occupational safety and health program. Evaluating and analyzing these incidents can help refine and tailor the safety and health program to the workplace-specific hazards of concern. A reevaluation of workplace hazards should be conducted periodically and after any change in a process, material, or equipment to ensure the program is current and effective.

A written infection control plan is a critical component of a comprehensive safety and health program because it protects employees from potential biological hazards in veterinary practice. Important elements of an infection control program include

- Identifying and recognizing potential biological hazards
- Applying the hierarchy of controls, including elimination, substitution, engineering controls, administrative controls, and personal protective equipment (PPE), to prevent and reduce risks (**Box 2**)
- Training employees about their risks and how to prevent or minimize them
- Reporting and recording of workplace-related injuries and illnesses.

Occupational Safety and Health Standards

Overview

Workplace standards that apply to veterinary clinics depend on the potential hazards in the clinic. Even for those employers who may not be required to comply with some standards, voluntarily following the provisions of the relevant standards is important to prevent or minimize work-related injuries and illnesses. The standards presented here include Recordkeeping, Hazard Communication, Personal Protective Equipment, Respiratory Protection, and Bloodborne Pathogens. Adhering to these standards reinforces an infection control plan and contributes to a comprehensive safety and health program. Additional workplace standards may apply to veterinary clinics depending on the potential hazards in the facility such as noise, radiation, and waste anesthetic gases (see Resources).

Employers should be aware of local, state, regional, and federal workplace regulations that apply to their practice. In the United States, in addition to federal OSHA, 25 states, Puerto Rico, and the Virgin Islands have OSHA-approved state plans. State plans set workplace safety and health standards that are at least as effective as comparable federal standards. They can also promulgate standards covering hazards not addressed by federal standards. For example, California has an Aerosol Transmissible Diseases Standard, the first US standard to protect workers from occupational exposure to infectious diseases that can be transmitted by inhaling air that contains viruses, bacteria, or other infectious agents. It was designed to make recommended infection control practices legally enforceable. There is no similar federal standard.

Box 2
Examples of the hierarchy of controls for infection control

The hierarchy of controls should be followed to most effectively protect workers from hazards. These controls are listed in decreasing order of effectiveness; elimination is the most effective control. An example of each type of control is provided.

Elimination

- Remove the hazard from the workplace
  - Do not admit animals with potential high-risk zoonotic diseases if the facility is not properly equipped.

Substitution

- Switch to the use of a less risky hazard.
  - Switch to the use of needleless devices.

Engineering controls

- Prevent exposure to a hazard or place a barrier between the hazard and the worker.
  - Install a dedicated ventilation system for isolation rooms.

Administrative controls

- Implement changes in work practices and management policies.
  - Require rabies preexposure vaccination for high-risk workers.

PPE

- Use gloves, safety eyewear, masks, hearing protection, respirators, or other protective equipment when other controls cannot effectively reduce exposures.
  - Wear nonlatex gloves when handling animals with skin lesions.

Adapted from NIOSH. NIOSH veterinary safety and health hazard prevention and infection control. 2014. Available at: http://www.cdc.gov/niosh/topics/veterinary/hazard.html. Accessed August 7, 2014.

Summarized below is information about workplace occupational safety and health regulations with a focus on US standards. The principles of occupational safety and health are universal but regulations and requirements may vary by country, region, or state. Each employer should be informed about the occupational safety and health regulations that apply to their clinic. Additional information about each of the workplace standards summarized below is provided in the Resources section.

Employer responsibility for workplace safety and health

Employers are responsible for identifying and assessing the serious, recognized hazards in their workplace, and preventing and minimizing the risks to workers exposed to these hazards. Various groups can be exposed to hazards in veterinary clinics, including full-time workers, temporary workers, interns, volunteers, and observers. The legal obligations to protect these individuals vary with the country, region, or state. For example, some US OSHA state plans may extend coverage to certain volunteers and other workers exempt from federal OSHA authority. Employers should know and follow the regulations that apply to their facility. Workers' compensation and other insurance provisions vary. Regardless, employers are encouraged to include all personnel, whatever their employment status, in their occupational safety and health programs. Individuals should not be allowed to participate in clinic activities that they have not been trained and equipped for. This may lead to excluding some individuals, such as one-time or occasional observers, from certain activities because of the burden of training and providing protection.

Some workers, such as immunocompromised or pregnant workers, may require additional considerations and protections. See elsewhere in this issue for information about zoonotic disease risk in these populations by Stull and Stevenson and discussion about the legal implications of zoonotic disease transmission in veterinary practices by Marsh and Babcock.

In the United States, the Occupational Safety and Health (OSH) Act of 1970 mandates that US employers provide employees with a safe and healthy workplace. The General Duty Clause of the OSH Act Section 5(a)(1) requires that every employer provide employment and a place of employment that is free from recognized hazards that cause or are likely to cause death or serious physical harm to employees (**Box 3**). It is intended to protect employees against those hazards that an employer's industry is aware of but for which there are no established standards. Examples of hazards for which OSHA has applied the General Duty Clause include occupational exposure to infectious diseases such as tuberculosis. When a hazard-specific OSHA standard is available, such as those described below, it would apply and be enforced rather than the General Duty Clause.

Recordkeeping

Maintaining records of workplace injuries and illnesses is an important component of a workplace safety and health program. In the United States, the OSHA Recordkeeping Regulation (29 CFR Part 1904) requires employers to prepare and maintain records of serious workplace injuries and illnesses (**Box 4**). Injuries and illnesses that should be recorded include those that result in time away from work, restricted work, transfer to another job, loss of consciousness, or medical treatment beyond first aid. OSHA provides specific forms (Forms 300, 300A, and 301) to record work-related incidents (see Resources). An incident is considered work-related if an event or exposure in the employee's work environment caused or contributed to the condition, or if a preexisting injury or illness is significantly aggravated by the employee's work environment. All employers covered by the OSH Act must report the death of any employee from a work-related incident or the in-patient hospitalization of 3 or more employees as a result of a work-related incident to OSHA within 8 hours. Employers cannot retaliate or discriminate against a worker for reporting an injury or illness.

All small businesses with up to 10 employees are exempt from compliance with the Recordkeeping regulation. However, reporting and recording workplace injuries and illnesses is an important component of a comprehensive safety and health program.

Box 3
Employer responsibility for workplace hazards, US OSHA General Duty Clause

1. A workplace hazard is present to which employees were exposed
2. The hazard is recognized by the employer or employer's industry
3. The hazard causes or is likely to cause serious harm or death
4. Feasible methods exist to substantially reduce the hazard

From OSHA. Letter of interpretation: elements necessary for a violation of the General Duty Clause. 2003. Available at: https://www.osha.gov/pls/oshaweb/owadisp.show_document?p_table=interpretations&p_id=24784. Accessed June 30, 2014.

Box 4
Recordkeeping for work-related injuries and illnesses

1. Collect relevant information about the incident
   - US OSHA Form 301: Injury and Illness Incident Report
2. Maintain a log of work-related injuries and illnesses to document information about incidents
   - US OSHA Form 300: Log of Work-related Injuries and Illnesses
3. Summarize the year's incidents at the end of the calendar year
   - US OSHA Form 300A: Summary of Work-related Injuries and Illnesses
   - Post in the workplace between February 1 and April 30
4. Review and analyze incidents to inform prevention and control of future incidents

Recording this information provides employees with information about hazards and incidents in the workplace and allows targeting of hazards that may need additional emphasis to prevent future incidents. A working group made up of employer and employee representatives can be established to discuss work-related incidents in a constructive and nonpunitive manner to help prevent future incidents. Employee privacy should be maintained to the greatest extent possible.

Hazard Communication Standard

Training workers about the chemicals they are exposed to is a critical component of a workplace safety and health program. In the United States, the OSHA Hazard Communication Standard (29 CFR 1910.1200) requires that employers of workers who handle, store, or use potentially dangerous chemicals develop a written hazard communication program (**Box 5**). A hazardous chemical is any chemical classified as a physical hazard (eg, flammable gas or gas under pressure), health hazard (eg, eye irritant or carcinogen), simple asphyxiant, combustible dust, pyrophoric gas, or hazard not otherwise classified (see Resources). The standard applies to all hazardous chemicals on the premises, whether they are currently in use or stored. This standard is known as the right-to-know law. It ensures that employees exposed to chemicals are informed of the hazards associated with the chemicals and the precautions that should be used when handling them. The Hazard Communication Standard does

Box 5
US OSHA hazard communication program steps

1. Learn the standard and identify responsible staff.
2. Prepare and implement a written hazard communication program.
3. Ensure containers, including secondary containers, are labeled.
4. Maintain safety data sheets for all hazardous workplace chemicals.
5. Inform and train employees; document the training.
6. Evaluate and reassess the program.

From OSHA. OSHA fact sheet: steps to an effective hazard communication program for employers who use hazardous chemicals. 2014. Available at: https://www.osha.gov/Publications/OSHA3696.pdf. Accessed June 30, 2014.

not apply to household consumer products when they are used in the workplace similar to consumer use. That is, the workplace exposure has a similar duration and frequency as consumer exposure. For example, if window cleaner is used in a similar quantity and a similar frequency as used by a consumer it would be exempt.[1] Other products, such as hydrogen peroxide, if used in greater quantities and more frequently than consumer use would not be exempt.

The US OSHA Hazard Communication Standard was updated in 2012 to align with the United Nations' Globally Harmonized System of Classification and Labeling of Chemicals (GHS), an international standardized approach to hazard communication (see **Box 6**). The GHS provides a common approach to classifying chemicals and communicating hazard information on labels and safety data sheets (previously called material safety data sheets). It provides a basis for harmonization of chemical rules and regulations at the national and international levels. Different countries are at various stages of considering and implementing GHS. The revised US standard, known as the right-to-understand law, provides employees with consistent and understandable information on the appropriate handling and safe use of hazardous chemicals. By June 2015, US employers will be required to comply with all modified provisions of the revised standard. US employers were required to have trained employees on the new label elements and safety data sheet format by December 2013 (see Resources).

Personal protective equipment

PPE is an important control for protecting workers when engineering, work practice, and administrative controls are not feasible or do not provide sufficient protection against workplace hazards. In the United States, the OSHA Personal Protective Equipment Standard (29 CFR 1910.132) requires that PPE be provided at no cost to the employee. Employers should clean, repair, and replace PPE as needed.

Worker training about PPE should include the following information:

- When it is needed
- What type is needed
- How to put it on, adjust, wear, and take it off
- Its limitations
- Its proper care, maintenance, useful life, and disposal.

Box 6
Major changes to the US OSHA Hazard Communication Standard, 2012

- Hazard classification: Chemical manufacturers and importers are required to determine the hazards of the chemicals they produce or import.
- Labels: Chemical manufacturers and importers must provide a label that includes a signal word, pictogram, hazard statement, and precautionary statement for each hazard class and category.
- Safety Data Sheets: The new format requires 16 specific sections, ensuring consistency in presentation of important protection information.
- Information and training: Employees should have been trained by December 2013 on the new label elements and safety data sheet format, in addition to the current training requirements.

From OSHA. OSHA fact sheet: hazard communication standard final rule. 2014. Available at: https://www.osha.gov/dsg/hazcom/HCSFactsheet.html. Accessed August 7, 2014.

If PPE is used, a PPE program should be implemented, including the following elements:

- The hazards present
- The selection, maintenance, and use of PPE
- The training of employees
- Monitoring of the program to ensure its ongoing effectiveness.

Respiratory protection

A respirator is a specific type of PPE that protects employees from inhaling dangerous substances, such as chemicals and infectious particles. Unlike surgical masks, respirators are specifically designed to provide respiratory protection by forming a tight seal against the wearer's skin and filtering out airborne particles, including pathogens.[2] Surgical masks are not respirators; they do not form a tight seal against the skin or filter very small airborne pathogens.[2] An example of when a respirator may be needed is when a clinic employee is exposed to a zoonotic respiratory pathogen such as avian influenza.

Respirators should only be used when all other controls, including engineering controls, are not feasible. Engineering control systems, such as adequate general ventilation or using local ventilation to remove contaminants from the air, are the preferred control methods for reducing worker inhalation exposures. Selecting the right respirator requires an assessment of the workplace operations, processes, or environments creating the respiratory hazard. Selection of an appropriate respirator and its proper wear and use are critical to its effectiveness. The specific respiratory hazard and its airborne concentrations should be assessed by an industrial hygienist or experienced safety professional before choosing a respirator (see Resources).

In the United States, respirators should only be used in the context of a complete written respiratory protection program as required by the OSHA Respiratory Protection Standard. Fit-testing, medical evaluation, and the other OSHA-required procedures are essential to assure that the respirator will achieve the required protection. The OSHA standard sets requirements for the fit-testing of respirators to ensure a proper seal is maintained between the respirator's sealing surface and the wearer's face. The OSHA standard also contains requirements for determining that workers can use respirators safely, for training and educating employees in the proper use of respirators, and for maintaining respirators properly.

Employees may choose to wear a respirator even if it is not required by the employer or the OSHA standard. Employers who allow voluntary respirator use must make sure the worker is medically able to use the respirator, the respirator does not create a hazard, and the respirators are properly cleaned, stored, and maintained. Employers must provide the respirator users with the information contained in the OSHA Respiratory Protection Standard 1910.134, Appendix D (revise to Appendix D). Veterinary clinics located outside of the United States should follow standards established by their regulatory organizations (see Resources).

Bloodborne pathogens standard

Protecting workers from bloodborne pathogens is another important component of a comprehensive workplace safety and health program. In the United States, the OSHA Bloodborne Pathogens Standard (29 CFR 1910.1030) protects employees from potentially infectious organisms that may be present in blood. Although this standard applies primarily to occupational exposures to human blood, occupational exposures to animal blood used for research and known to be infected with the human immunodeficiency virus (HIV), hepatitis B virus, or hepatitis C virus are also covered.[3,4] The standard does not protect workers from exposure to blood from companion animals, other domestic animals, animals in zoos, or research animals not known to be infected with these pathogens.

The US National Association of State Public Health Veterinarians (NASPHV) recommends voluntary compliance with the OSHA Bloodborne Pathogens Standard to protect employees working in veterinary or other animal settings.[5] Standard precautions, good work practices, engineering controls, and the proper use of PPE should be considered to prevent or minimize occupational exposures to animal blood because of the potential risk of transmission of zoonotic pathogens (see later discussion).

SELECTED HAZARDS AND PREVENTION

Information about sharps, needlestick injuries, and animal bites and scratches, and strategies for prevention are provided below. For information about other common hazards see the Resources section.

Sharps

Developing, implementing, and consistently following safe sharps handling procedures is a key component of a clinic's infection control and occupational health program. Needlestick and sharps injury (NSI) prevention receives a great deal of attention and research in human medicine, primarily due to the risk posed from HIV and viral hepatitis infections. However, NSIs are also a common occurrence in veterinary medicine: 64% to 93% of veterinary personnel report at least 1 NSI in their career.[6] An Australian survey of 664 veterinarians found that approximately 75% reported at least 1 NSI in the previous 12 months.[7] Syringe and suture needles were the most common cause of NSIs in this study. Reported risk factors for exposure to an NSI that was previously used (contaminated) were female gender, working in small or mixed animal practice, less experience, and working more hours and/or seeing more patients per week.[8]

In human and veterinary medicine, many NSIs go unreported and are often only reported if complications occur.[6,8]

Potential complications from NSI in veterinary medicine include:

- Direct physical trauma with potential for nerve damage, especially to the fingers and hands
- Secondary wound infection due to contamination with infectious agents from the animal's skin
- Injection of syringe contents that may contain killed or modified live vaccines; antibiotics; hazardous drugs, such as chemotherapeutic agents and hormones; sedatives; and anesthetics, such as ketamine and narcotics. Effects can range from local irritation to severe systemic and fatal effects[9]
- Transmission of zoonotic pathogens.

Much less is known about the potential for zoonotic infections from NSI in veterinary medicine than bloodborne pathogen infections widely recognized as occupational hazards in human medicine. However, there are case reports of infection with *Bartonella* species in veterinarians associated with NSI.[10,11] The potential for zoonotic transmission through NSIs for organisms such as arboviruses or *Blastomyces* or for newly emerging infectious diseases is also a concern.[12]

The OSHA bloodborne pathogens standard does not apply to animal blood except in certain cases where animals are used for research on human bloodborne pathogens. However, the use of sharps (as well as animal bites) in veterinary practice poses the potential for staff and clients to be exposed to human blood. If an NSI involves a needle or other sharp contaminated with human blood, the bloodborne pathogens standard does apply. For this reason, clinics should have an exposure control plan for human blood as part of their overall infection control plan and should voluntarily comply with the OSHA bloodborne pathogens.[5] OSHA provides a fact sheet with guidelines about developing an exposure control plan at: https://www.osha.gov/OshDoc/data_BloodborneFacts/bbfact01.pdf.

Preventing Needlestick and Other Sharps Injuries

Practical steps can be taken to reduce and prevent NSI in veterinary clinics (**Boxes 7** and **8**). In addition to these steps, employers and individuals who serve as the clinic infection control coordinator should evaluate the availability and feasibility of implementing safety devices such as retractable needles or needleless devices when appropriate.

Animal Bites and Scratches

According to the American Veterinary Medical Association Professional Liability Insurance Trust (AVMA PLIT) injury from animal contact accounted for 82% of workers' compensation claims filed between January 1, 2007 and June 30, 2011. Workers'[13] in 2012, 48% of all claims were due to injuries from dogs, with an average cost of $3192, and 46% were due to cat injuries, with an average cost of $1580 (Andrew Starrenburg, HUB International Limited, 2014, personal communication). In 2008, the average cost of a dog bite–related hospital stay was $18,200.[14] In approximately 75% of dog and cat bites in the veterinary clinic setting in 2012, wounds were to the fingers or thumbs, hands, lower arms, or wrists (HUB International Limited, 2014, personal communication). Bite wounds to fingers, hands, and wrists are higher-risk due to the greater potential of bone, joint, tendon, or nerve involvement. These wounds can result in infections or nerve damage and lead to long-term disability

Box 7
Steps for reducing needlestick and sharps injuries

- Educate all employees and volunteers about safe sharps handling and potential adverse health effects from needlestick injuries; periodic refresher training is also necessary.
- Educate clients about safe handling and disposal if sharps are to be used for home treatment (such as subcutaneous fluid administration).
- Use trained personnel, not clients, to restrain animals; this protects staff and clients.
- Do not recap needles unless necessary as part of a medical procedure such as a fine needle aspirate. If necessary, use a one-hand scoop method or use forceps to recap the needle (see **Box 8**).
- Place approved sharps containers in easily accessible and visible areas where sharps are used.
- Promptly dispose of used sharps in approved containers.
- Never try to remove anything from a sharps container; do not overfill containers.
- Ensure employees and volunteers report all injuries. Record information about the incident. Analyze and discuss how the injury occurred to help prevent future incidents.
- Dispose of sharps containers and materials and/or medical waste in accordance with laws and ordinances specific to the locale (ie, country, region, state).

Adapted from Weese JS, Jack DC. Needlestick injuries in veterinary medicine. Can Vet J 2008;49:780–4.

Box 8
Procedure for recapping needle when medically indicated (one-handed scoop technique)

- Place needle cap on horizontal surface such as a table top
- Hold syringe with attached needle in one hand
- Use the needle to scoop up the cap without using the other hand
- Secure cap by pushing against a hard surface or by using forceps

Adapted from Scheftel JM, Elchos BL, Cherry B, et al. Compendium of veterinary standard precautions for zoonotic disease prevention in veterinary personnel: National Association of State Public Health Veterinarians Veterinary Infection Control Committee 2010. J Am Vet Med Assoc 2010;237(12):1403–22.

and inability to perform intricate tasks such as surgery. Bite wounds may result in more severe secondary infections in immunocompromised people.

A survey of certified veterinary technicians (CVTs) in Minnesota evaluated work-related injuries to include animal bites.[15] Among CVTs who reported bite-related injuries, the bite injury rate was significantly higher for respondents less than 26 years of age.[15] The rate of bite injury was also higher in this study for those who reported they believed work-related injuries could not be prevented. This suggests that education about injury prevention in general, and bite prevention in particular, may be beneficial for veterinary technicians.

A wide variety of aerobic and anaerobic bacteria have been cultured from dog and cat bite wounds, with polymicrobial infections commonly seen.[16] Such mixed infections can present challenges for antimicrobial therapy and patient management.

The most common pathogen implicated in animal bites is *Pasteurella multocida*; numerous evaluations have found the bacteria in the oral cavity of most healthy cats. Cats are the main reservoir for *Bartonella henselae*, the agent most commonly associated with cat-scratch disease. *B clarridgeiae* has also been associated with clinical cat-scratch disease, and should be considered in patients who demonstrate negative serology for *B henselae* when cat scratch-disease is suspected.[17] Although rare, serious infections and deaths have been seen from the zoonotic transmission of the agents responsible for tularemia (*Francisella tularensis*) and plague (*Yersinia pestis*).[17–19] Human cases of sporotrichosis have been associated with cat bites and scratches as well as exposure to infected cats in which no wound was reported, such as administering medications.[20] Blastomycosis has been reported in a veterinary assistant following a dog bite.[21]

Rabies in dogs and cats is rare in the United States. In 2012, approximately 92% of the 6162 rabid animals reported to the Centers for Disease Control and Prevention were in wildlife.[22] Rabid cats (257) outnumbered rabid dogs (84); 1 human case was reported and was attributed to bat exposure in the United States and symptom development, treatment, and diagnosis abroad.[22] However, rabies risk to animals and humans varies considerably by country and region; it is important to know the regional epidemiology of rabies to appropriately manage disease risk in workers. Preexposure vaccination should be offered to veterinary staff, especially high-risk workers, such as those in frequent contact with potentially rabid bats, raccoons, skunks, cats, dogs, or other high-risk species.[23] Vaccination of employees who handle high-risk animals in addition to bite prevention is a cornerstone of an infection control program given the high human case fatality ratio and the high cost if postexposure prophylaxis is not given in a timely manner. Animal rabies vaccination programs are also crucial given the availability of an inexpensive and highly effective vaccine for dogs and cats.

Due to the potential for atypical and mixed infections following bite wounds, individuals who are bitten or who develop nonspecific health symptoms when working with animals should inform their health care provider about their occupational history.

As discussed previously regarding sharps, animal bite wounds and scratches have the potential to expose clinic staff and clients to human blood. Clinics should have an exposure control plan for human blood and body fluids, and instruct employees about potential hazards and safe first aid techniques for responding to situations in which they may be exposed to human blood. Numerous organizations, such as the American Red Cross, offer courses in bloodborne pathogen training, first aid, and cardiopulmonary resuscitation that can assist in staff education.

Prevention of Animal Bites and Scratches

Appropriate animal restraint during all procedures is key for the safety of the animal and for clinic personnel who are doing the restraining and/or performing medical procedures. All staff should be trained on the proper methods of animal restraint for all species they will work with. Although some studies have shown that veterinary staff still commonly rely on clients to assist in animal restraint,[24] this practice is discouraged. Although clients often want to help and feel their involvement may cause less stress for their pet, allowing clients to restrain animals puts both clinic staff and the client at risk and exposes the clinic owner to liability should a bite, scratch, NSI, or other type of injury occur. Physical restraints, such as muzzles, bite-resistant gloves, restraint bags, sedation, and anesthesia, should be used when appropriate. Aggressive tendencies should be noted in the patient's medical records and posted on cages. The use of color-coded collars also allows clinic staff to readily recognize potentially aggressive animals. Situational awareness and remaining alert to changes in animal behavior is key because animals may react in unexpected ways when in a new environment or if ill or in pain. As with other types of occupational injuries, bites and scratches should be reported to supervisors and appropriate first aid and medical treatment provided. An investigation into the circumstances that led to the bite or scratch should occur with the goal of preventing future occurrences. Human and veterinary health care providers should follow the appropriate reporting requirements to animal control, public health, or other officials for investigation of animal bites. Information about injury prevention training resources and development of a formal, written animal bite response policy are provided at the end of this article.

Hazardous Drug Exposures

Drugs are classified as hazardous if studies in animals or humans indicate that exposures to them have a potential for causing cancer, developmental or reproductive toxicity, or harm to organs. Hazardous drugs, as defined by NIOSH, include drugs that are known or suspected to cause adverse health effects from exposures in the workplace.[25] Most hazardous drugs used in small animal clinical practice are antineoplastic agents; however, some antiviral agents, hormones, and bioengineered drugs are also considered hazardous. NIOSH, in coordination with other organizations, maintains and periodically updates the NIOSH List of Antineoplastic and Other Hazardous Drugs in Healthcare Settings.[26] This list may not be all-inclusive because, first, drugs used by a facility may receive Food and Drug Administration approval and enter the market place after this list was released, and, second, this list of hazardous drugs was developed for human health care settings.

There is a great deal of overlap in hazardous drugs used in human and veterinary medicine, especially in the area of antineoplastic agents. However, some drugs that should be considered hazardous may be used exclusively in veterinary medicine, such as xylazine and tilmicosin. Tilmicosin is an antibiotic used to treat bovine respiratory disease that has been associated with serious adverse effects and fatalities from accidental injection or suicide.[27] Additionally, some drugs may be listed under a drug name that may not be commonly recognized in veterinary medicine; for example, prostaglandin F_2 alpha (Lutalyse) is listed as dinoprostone.

Prevention of Hazardous Drug Exposures

For these reasons, and to ensure compliance with the OSHA Hazard Communications Standard, employers must develop and maintain a list of all pharmaceuticals and chemicals to include hazardous drugs that is specific to their facility. Sources of information that can be used to develop a hazardous drug inventory include the NIOSH list (see previous discussion), safety data sheets (formerly known as material safety data sheets), package inserts, drug manufacturers, professional organizations, and the medical literature.

In addition to developing a drug inventory list, employers are responsible for providing initial and refresher training on the safe handling and potential health effects of hazardous drugs to their employees. This training should be documented by the employer and delivered in a format that enhances comprehension and ensures that employees consistently follow safe practices. The use of written standard operating procedures and checklists are tools to help ensure safe drug administration for both the animal and employees. Safe work practices are important for all employees. Precautions are especially important for women who may be or become pregnant, and employees who may be immunocompromised. Resources for training are listed at the end of this section.

The safe handling of hazardous drugs requires a cradle-to-grave approach. Applying the hierarchy of controls (elimination, substitution, engineering, administrative, and PPE) to the following steps in hazardous drug administration, where appropriate, is recommended (**Box 9**).

Chemotherapy spill kits should be located wherever drugs are handled or stored in the facility. Cages should be labeled to alert staff that an animal has been treated with chemotherapeutic agents so precautions can be followed. In larger hospitals with more staff who may work in other departments of the hospital such as radiology, consider using a color-coded collar that identifies the animal as having recently received chemotherapy to alert staff and remind owners that precautions with waste should be followed for at least 48 to 72 hours following treatment with most drugs.[28] With proper planning, training of staff, and written standard operating procedures, veterinarians can ensure that employees are protected from hazardous drug exposures while providing excellent care for their clients and their pets.

Box 9
Steps in hazardous drug administration in which controls are needed

- Hazardous drug delivery to the clinic
- Drug preparation for administration (intravenous and oral)
- Drug transport in the clinic
- Drug administration to the animal
- Cleaning of tables, counters, floors, cages, and runs
- Disposal of animal waste, body fluids, and drug administration supplies such as intravenous bags
- Laundering of bedding, scrubs, smocks, and lab coats

SUMMARY

1. Veterinary employers should develop and implement a comprehensive workplace safety and health program, including written standard operating procedures that address occupational safety and health risks that are specific to their clinic. This program should be consistent with national, regional, state, and other applicable standards and regulations.
2. A written infection control plan is an important component of a comprehensive clinic safety and health program. Management commitment, employee involvement, and initial and refresher training for staff on all aspects of the program are keys to success.
3. Many resources are available to help employers develop clinic guidelines to prevent occupational injuries and illnesses from bites and scratches, sharps, and hazardous drugs, as well as other hazards commonly encountered in veterinary medicine. Some of these resources are provided at the end of this article.

RECOMMENDED RESOURCES

Veterinary Occupational Hazards

- International Labour Organization Occupational Safety and Health: http://www.ilo.org/safework/lang–en/index.htm
- World Health Organization Occupational Health: http://www.who.int/occupational_health/en/
- European Agency for Safety and Health at Work: https://osha.europa.eu/en
- Canadian Centre for Occupational Health and Safety: http://www.ccohs.ca/
- Canada Labour Program Health and Safety: http://www.labour.gc.ca/eng/health_safety/
- United Kingdom Health and Safety Executive: http://www.hse.gov.uk/index.htm
- OSHA International: https://www.osha.gov/international/
- NIOSH Veterinary Safety and Health topic page: http://www.cdc.gov/niosh/topics/veterinary/
- NORA Healthcare Sector Veterinary Goals: http://www.cdc.gov/niosh/nora/comment/agendas/hlthcaresocassist/
- NASPHV Veterinary Standard Precautions Compendium: http://www.nasphv.org/Documents/VeterinaryPrecautions.pdf
- Human-Animal Medicine textbook, Occupational Health of Animal Workers (chapter): http://www.sciencedirect.com/science/book/9781416068372

Safety and Health Programs

- OSHA Safety and Health Program Management Guidelines: https://www.osha.gov/pls/oshaweb/owadisp.show_document?p_table=FEDERAL_REGISTER&p_id=12909
- OSHA Fact Sheet: Voluntary Safety and Health Program Management Guidelines: https://www.osha.gov/OshDoc/data_General_Facts/vol_safetyhealth_mngt_.pdf
- OSHA Sample Safety and Health Program for Small Business: https://www.osha.gov/SLTC/etools/safetyhealth/mod2_sample_sh_program.html
- NASPHV Model Infection Control Plan for Veterinary Practices: http://www.nasphv.org/Documents/ModelInfectionControlPlan.doc
- AVMA Guidelines for Veterinary Practice Facilities: https://www.avma.org/KB/Policies/Pages/Guidelines-for-Veterinary-Practice-Facilities.aspx
- OSHA On-site Consultation: https://www.osha.gov/dcsp/smallbusiness/consult.html
- NIOSH Health Hazard Evaluation Program: http://www.cdc.gov/niosh/hhe/

OSHA Business Case for Safety and Health: https://www.osha.gov/dcsp/products/topics/businesscase/index.html

US OSHA Standards

OSHA Law and Regulations: https://www.osha.gov/law-regs.html

State OSHA Programs: https://www.osha.gov/dcsp/osp/

OSHA Small Business Handbook: https://www.osha.gov/Publications/smallbusiness/small-business.html

OSHA Safety and Health Training Resources: https://www.osha.gov/dte/library/index.html

General Duty Clause

Occupational Safety and Health Act of 1970—General Duty Clause: https://www.osha.gov/pls/oshaweb/owadisp.show_document?p_id=3359&p_table=oshact

Recordkeeping

OSHA Recordkeeping Standard: https://www.osha.gov/recordkeeping/index.html

OSHA Recordkeeping Training Presentations: https://www.osha.gov/recordkeeping/RKpresentations.html

OSHA Injury and Illness Recordkeeping Forms: https://www.osha.gov/recordkeeping/RKforms.html

Hazard Communication

OSHA Hazard Communication: https://www.osha.gov/dsg/hazcom/index.html

OSHA Small Entity Compliance Guide for Employers that Use Hazardous Chemicals: https://www.osha.gov/Publications/OSHA3695.pdf

OSHA Fact Sheet: Training Requirements for the Revised Hazard Communication Standard: https://www.osha.gov/Publications/OSHA3642.pdf

OSHA Model Plans and Programs for the OSHA Bloodborne Pathogens and Hazard Communications Standards: https://www.osha.gov/Publications/osha3186.html

OSHA Interpretation: Hazard Communication Standard in veterinary practice: http://www.osha.gov/pls/oshaweb/owadisp.show_document?p_table=INTERPRETATIONS&p_id=21120

OSHA Interpretation: Hazard Communication Standard and veterinary drugs: https://www.osha.gov/pls/oshaweb/owadisp.show_document?p_table=INTERPRETATIONS&p_id=21343

Personal Protective Equipment

OSHA Personal Protective Equipment: https://www.osha.gov/SLTC/personalprotectiveequipment/index.html

Respiratory Protection

OSHA Small Entity Compliance Guide for the Respiratory Protection Standard: https://www.osha.gov/Publications/3384small-entity-for-respiratory-protection-standard-rev.pdf

OSHA Sample Respiratory Protection Program: https://www.osha.gov/Publications/3384small-entity-for-respiratory-protection-standard-rev.pdf

OSHA Respiratory Protection Training Videos: https://www.osha.gov/SLTC/respiratoryprotection/training_videos.html

NIOSH Respirators: http://www.cdc.gov/niosh/topics/respirators/

NIOSH Respirators For Respirator Users: http://www.cdc.gov/niosh/npptl/respusers.html

NIOSH Podcast: General Instructions for Disposable Respirators: http://www2c.cdc.gov/podcasts/player.asp?f=11298

NIOSH Poster: How to Properly Put On and Take Off a Disposable Respirator: http://www.cdc.gov/niosh/docs/2010-131/

Bloodborne Pathogens and Needlestick and Sharps Injuries

CDC Sharps Safety for Healthcare Settings: http://www.cdc.gov/sharpssafety/

OSHA Bloodborne Pathogens and Needlestick Prevention: https://www.osha.gov/SLTC/bloodbornepathogens/index.html

OSHA Model Plans and Programs for the OSHA Bloodborne Pathogens and Hazard Communications Standards: https://www.osha.gov/Publications/osha3186.html

OSHA Standards Interpretation: Application of the Bloodborne Pathogens Standard to Veterinary Clinics: http://www.osha.gov/pls/oshaweb/owadisp.show_document?p_table=INTERPRETATIONS&p_id=24608

Resources for pet owners, veterinary staff, and public health personnel can be found at Worms and Germs blog: www.wormsandgermsblog.com.

Bites and Scratches

The American Red Cross offers online and classroom training on first aid, bloodborne pathogens, and cardiopulmonary resuscitation: http://www.redcross.org/

The American VeterinaryMedical Association dog bite prevention materials for staff and clients: https://www.avma.org/public/pages/Dog-Bite-Prevention.aspx

Employee training modules and tools on a variety of topics to include animal restraint and bite prevention: http://avmaplit.com/Default.aspx?id51609

Hazardous Drugs

Documents and Web sites

NIOSH Occupational Exposure to Antineoplastic Agents: http://www.cdc.gov/niosh/topics/antineoplastic/

National Veterinary Cancer Registry: http://nationalveterinarycancerregistry.org/

Veterinary Cancer Society: http://www.vetcancersociety.org/members/

NIOSH Workplace Solutions: Medical Surveillance for Healthcare Workers Exposed to Hazardous Drugs: http://www.cdc.gov/niosh/docs/wp-solutions/2013-103/pdfs/2013-103.pdf

NIOSH Workplace Solutions: Safe Handling of Hazardous Drugs for Veterinary Healthcare Workers: http://www.cdc.gov/niosh/docs/wp-solutions/2010-150/pdfs/2010-150.pdf

AVMA Disposal of Hazardous Pharmaceutical Wastes: https://www.avma.org/Advocacy/National/Federal/Pages/Disposal-of-Hazardous-Pharmaceutical-Wastes.aspx

Books

Crump K, Thamm, D. Cancer chemotherapy for the veterinary health team. Wiley-Blackwell. ISBN 978-0-8138-2116-0.

REFERENCES

1. OSHA. OSHA frequently asked questions: hazard communication. 2014. Available at: https://www.osha.gov/html/faq-hazcom.html. Accessed August 7, 2014.

2. OSHA. OSHA standards interpretation: application of the bloodborne pathogens standard to veterinary clinics. 2002. Available at: https://www.osha.gov/pls/oshaweb/owadisp.show_document?p_table=INTERPRETATIONS&p_id=24608. Accessed July 5, 2014.
3. NIOSH. Respirator awareness: your health may depend on it, personal protective equipment for healthcare workers. Cincinnati (OH): U.S. Department of Health and Human Services, Centers for Disease Control and Prevention, National Institute for Occupational Safety and Health, DHHS (NIOSH); 2013. Publication No. 2013-138.
4. OSHA. OSHA fact sheet: OSHA's bloodborne pathogens standard. 2011. Available at: https://www.osha.gov/OshDoc/data_BloodborneFacts/bbfact01.pdf. Accessed July11, 2014.
5. NASPHV. Compendium of veterinary standard precautions. J Am Vet Med Assoc 2010;237(12):1403–22.
6. Weese JS, Faires M. A survey of needle handling practices and needlestick injuries in veterinary technicians. Can Vet J 2009;50(12):1278–82 [PubMed: 20190978].
7. Leggat PA, Smith DR, Speare R. Exposure rate of needlestick and sharps injuries among Australian veterinarians. J Occup Med Toxicol 2009;4(25) [PubMed: 19712488].
8. Haiduven DJ, Simpkins SM, Phillips ES, et al. A survey of percutaneous/mucocutaneous injury reporting in a public teaching hospital. J Hosp Infect 1999;41(2): 151–4 [PubMed: 10063478].
9. Thompson RN, McNicholl BP. Needlestick and infection with a horse vaccine. BMJ Case Rep 2010;2010:1–2 [PubMed: 22767480].
10. Lin JW, Chen CM, Chang CC. Unknown fever and back pain caused by *Bartonella henselae* in a veterinarian after a needle puncture: a case report and literature review. Vector Borne Zoonotic Dis 2011;11(5):589–91 [PubMed: 20569013].
11. Oliveira AM, Maggi RG, Woods CW, et al. Suspected needlestick transmission of *Bartonella vinsonii* subspecies *berkhoffii* to a veterinarian. J Vet Intern Med 2010; 24(5):1229–32 [PubMed: 20695992].
12. Weese JS, Jack DC. Needlestick injuries in veterinary medicine. Can Vet J 2008; 49:780–4 [PubMed: 18978971].
13. JAVMA News. AVMA PLIT lists top claims for business insurance. October 15, 2012. Available at: https://www.avma.org/News/JAVMANews/Pages/121015m.aspx. Accessed December 8, 2014.
14. Holmquist L, Elixhauser A. Emergency department visits and inpatient stays involving dog bites, 2008. Rockville (MD): Agency for Healthcare Research and Quality; 2010. Available at: http://www.hcup-us.ahrq.gov/reports/statbriefs/sb101.pdf. Accessed June 23, 2014.
15. Nordgren LD, Gerberich SG, Alexander BH, et al. Evaluation of factors associated with work-related injuries to veterinary technicians certified in Minnesota. J Am Vet Med Assoc 2014;245(4):425–33 [PubMed: 25075827].
16. Abrahamian FM, Goldstein EJ. Microbiology of animal bite wound infections. Clin Microbiol Rev 2011;24(2):231–46 [PubMed: 21482724].
17. Kordick DL, Hilyard EJ, Hadfield TL, et al. *Bartonella clarridgeiae*, a newly recognized zoonotic pathogen causing inoculation papules, fever, and lymphadenopathy (cat scratch disease). J Clin Microbiol 1997;35(7):1813–8 [PubMed: 9196200].
18. Weinberg AN, Branda JA. Case 31–2010: a 29-year-old woman with fever after a cat bite. N Engl J Med 2010;363(16):1560–8 [PubMed: 20942673].

19. Gage KL, Dennis DT, Orloski KA, et al. Cases of cat-associated human plague in the Western US, 1977–1998. Clin Infect Dis 2000;30:893–900 [PubMed: 10852811].
20. Dunstan RW, Langham RF, Reimann KA, et al. Feline sporotrichosis: a report of five cases with transmission to humans. J Am Acad Dermatol 1986;15(1):37–45 [PubMed: 3722508].
21. Gnann JW, Bressler GS, Bodet CA, et al. Human blastomycosis after a dog bite. Ann Intern Med 1983;98(1):48–9 [PubMed: 6848043].
22. Dyer JL, Wallace R, Orciari L, et al. Rabies surveillance in the United States during 2012. J Am Vet Med Assoc 2013;243(6):805–15 [PubMed: 24004227].
23. CDC. Human rabies prevention—United States, 2008: recommendations of the Advisory Committee on Immunization Practices. MMWR Recomm Rep 2008; 57(RR-3):1–28 [PubMed: 18496505].
24. Anderson M. Video observation of infection control practices in veterinary clinics and apetting zoo, with emphasis on hand hygiene and interventions to improve hand hygiene compliance [Ph.D Thesis]. Ontario (Canada): University of Guelph; 2013.
25. NIOSH. NIOSH Alert: preventing occupational exposures to antineoplastic and other hazardous drugs in health care settings. Cincinnati (OH): U.S. Department of Health and Human Services, Centers for Disease Control and Prevention, National Institute for Occupational Safety and Health, DHHS (NIOSH); 2004. Publication No. 2004–165.
26. NIOSH. NIOSH List of antineoplastic and other hazardous drugs in healthcare settings 2012. Cincinnati (OH): U.S. Department of Health and Human Services, Centers for Disease Control and Prevention, National Institute for Occupational Safety and Health, DHHS (NIOSH); 2012. Publication No. 2012-150 (June 2012).
27. Veenhuizen MF, Wright TJ, McManus RF, et al. Analysis of reports of human exposure to Micotil 300 (tilmicosin injection). J Am Vet Med Assoc 2006;229(11): 1737–42 [PubMed: 17144818].
28. NIOSH, Couch J, Gibbins J, et al. Health hazard evaluation report: CHEMOTHERAPY drug evaluation at a veterinary teaching hospital–Michigan. Cincinnati (OH): U.S. Department of Health and Human Services, Centers for Disease Control and Prevention, National Institute for Occupational Safety and Health, NIOSH; 2012. HETA No. 2010-0068-3156.

Index

Note: Page numbers of article titles are in **boldface** type.

Vet Clin Small Anim 45 (2015) 427–435
http://dx.doi.org/10.1016/S0195-5616(15)00012-1 vetsmall.theclinics.com
0195-5616/15/$ – see front matter

G

H

I

L

M

N

O

P

Q

R

S

Printed and bound by CPI Group (UK) Ltd, Croydon, CR0 4YY
07/10/2024
01040499-0003